D0235593

WENNER-GREN
INTERNATIONAL SYMPOSIUM SERIES

VOLUME 54

BRAIN AND READING

BRAIN AND READING

**Structural and Functional Anomalies in
Developmental Dyslexia with Special Reference to
Hemispheric Interactions, Memory Functions,
Linguistic Processes and Visual Analysis in Reading**

Proceedings of the Seventh International Rodin Remediation Conference
at the Wenner-Gren Center, Stockholm, and Uppsala University,
June 19–22, 1988

Edited by

Curt von Euler
*Nobel Institute for Neurophysiology
Karolinska Institute, Stockholm, Sweden*

Ingvar Lundberg
*Department of Psychology
University of Umeå, Umeå, Sweden*

and

Gunnar Lennerstrand
*Department of Ophthalmology
Karolinska Institute, Stockholm, Sweden*

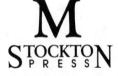

STOCKTON PRESS

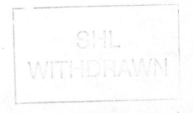

First published 1989

Published by
THE MACMILLAN PRESS LTD
Houndmills, Basingstoke, Hampshire RG21 2XS
and London
Companies and representatives
throughout the world

Printed in Great Britain by
Camelot Press, Southampton

British Library Cataloguing in Publication Data
International Rodin Remediation Conference.
(7th : 1988 : Wenner-Gren Center and
Uppsala University)
Brain and reading
1. Man. Dyslexia
I. Title   II. Euler, Curt von   III.
Lundberg, Ingvar   IV. Lennerstrand, Gunnar
616.85′53
ISSN 0083–7989
ISBN 0–333–48892–X

Published in the United States and Canada by
Stockton Press, 15 East 26th Street, New York, NY 10010
Library of Congress Cataloging-in-Publication Data available
ISBN 0–935859–69–1

Contents

I. Introductory Chapters

II. Hemispheric Specializations and Interactions

Contributors and Invited Participants

John Annett
Dept of Psychology
University of Leicester
Leicester LE1 7RH
UK

Marian Annett
Dept of Psychology
University of Leicester
Leicester LE1 7RH
UK

Dorothy M. Aram
Dept of Pediatrics
Rainbow Childrens Hospital
2101 Adelbert Road
Cleveland, OH 44106
USA

William Baker
340 Linden street
Wellesley Hills, MA 02181
USA

Eric Bateson
The Forman School
Litchfield, CT 06759
USA

Giovanni Berlucchi
Università di Verona
Istituto di Fisiologia Umana
Strada Le Grazie
I-37132 Verona
Italy

Marianne Bernadotte
Villagatan 10
S-114 32 Stockholm
Sweden

Elizabeth Browning
31 Elthiron Road
London SW6 4BW
UK

Alfonso Caramazza
Cognitive Neuropsychology Lab
Cognitive Science Center
The Johns Hopkins Univ
Baltimore, MD 21218
USA

Lars Cernerud
School Health Service Bureau
Box 22007
S-104 22 Stockholm
Sweden

Gunilla Cernerud
Dept of Ophtalmology
Maria Clinics
Wolmar Yxkullsgatan 25
S-116 50 Stockholm
Sweden

Otto-Detlev Creutzfeldt
Dept of Neurobiology
Max-Planck-Institute for
  Biophysical Chemistry
D-3400 Göttingen-Nikolaus,
Berg
West Germany

Thord Dahlbom
Dept of Pedagogy
Box 2109
S-750 02 Uppsala
Sweden

Casey Dorman
Massachusetts Hospital School
3, Randolph Street
Canton, MA 02021
USA

Stephan Ehlers
Dept of Child and Youth
  Psychiatry
Univ of Gothenburg
S-402 35 Gothenburg
Sweden

Mildred El Azazi
Dept of Ophtalmology
Huddinge Hospital
S-141 86 Huddinge
Sweden

Carsten Elbro
Center for Audiologopedi
Univ of Copenhagen
Njalsgade 86
DK-2300 Copenhagen 5
Denmark

Olle Engstrand
Dept of Linguistics
Univ of Stockholm
S-106 91 Stockholm
Sweden

Berit Engström
Dept of Audiology
Karolinska Hospital
S-104 01 Stockholm
Sweden

Curt von Euler
Nobel Institute for
  Neurophysiology
Karolinska Institute
S-104 01 Stockholm
Sweden

Laurel Fais
The Forman School
Litchfield, CT 06759
USA

Gunnar Fant
Dept of Speech Transmission
The Royal Institute of
  Technology
S-100 44 Stockholm
Sweden

Hans Forssberg
Dept of Paediatrics
Karolinska Hospital
S-104 01 Stockholm
Sweden

Susan Fowler
Berkshire Dyslexia Association
2, Causman's Way
Tilehurst
Reading RG3 6PG
UK

Ove Franzén
Dept of Psychology
Univ of Uppsala
Box 227
S-752 20 Uppsala
Sweden

Douglas Frost
Section of Neuroanatomy
Yale Medical School
333, Cedar Street
New Haven, CT 06510
USA

Susan Gathercole
MRC Applied Psychology Unit
15, Chaucer Road
Cambridge, CB2 2EF
UK

Gad Geiger
International School for
  Advanced Studies, SISSA
Strada Cordera 11
I-34014 Trieste
Italy

Jürgen Gerling
Bernhard Landwehrmeyer
  Neurologische Universitäts-
  klinik mit Ab Neurophysiologie
Hansastr. 9
D-788 Freiburg
West Germany

Mirdza Germanis
Huddinge Hospital
Dept of Ophthalmology
S-141 86 Huddinge
Sweden

Kerstin Graffman
Dept of Medical Education
Karolinska Institute
S-104 01 Stockholm
Sweden

Ragnar Granit
Eriksbergsgatan 14
S-114 30 Stockholm
Sweden

Sten Grillner
Nobel Institute for
  Neurophysiology
Karolinska Institute
S-104 01 Stockholm
Sweden

Rudolf Groner
Univ of Bern
Institute of Psychology
Laupenstrasse 4
CH-3008 Bern
Switzerland

Anne-Lise Grung
Tokenesveien 25
3143 Kjöpmannskiaer
Norway

Tomas Hedqvist
Stockholms Skolförvaltning
Box 22007
S-104 22 Stockholm
Sweden

Torsten Husén
Armfeltsgatan 10, I
S-115 34 Stockholm
Sweden

Torleiv Høien
Nordisk Institutt for Lese-
  forskning
Eivindsholvg. 7
4340 Bryne
Norway

David H. Ingvar
Dept of Clinical Neurophysiology
University Hospital
S-221 85 Lund
Sweden

Christer Jacobson
Office of School Psychology
Alvesta
Box 501
S-342 01 Alvesta
Sweden

Allan Jansson
Dept of Applied Pedagogics
Box 5053
S-350 05 Växjö
Sweden

Lise Randrup Jensen
Center for Damages of the Brain
Univ of Copenhagen
Njalsgade 88
DK-2300 Copenhagen
Denmark

Barbro Johansson
Dept of Neurology
University Hospital
S-221 85 Lund
Sweden

Eva Johansson
Dept of Applied Pedagogics
Univ of Växjö
Box 5053
S-350 05 Växjö
Sweden

Birgitta Johnsen
Dept of Phoniatrics
Akademiska Hospital
S-751 05 Uppsala
Sweden

William Katz
Dept of Psychology
UCSD School of Medicine
La Jolla, CA 92093
USA

Mary-Louise Kean
Center for the Neurobiology
   of Learning and Memory
Univ of California
Irvine, CA 92717
USA

Doris Kelly
Berkshire Dyslexia Association
2, Causman's Way
Tilehurst
Reading RG3 6PG
UK

Sally Kemp
1802 South Cheynne
Tulsa, OK 7411
USA

Ursula Kirk
222, East 93rd Street
New York, N.Y. 10128
USA

Francisco Lacerda
Dept of Linguistics
Univ of Stockholm
S-106 91 Stockholm
Sweden

Hugo Lagercrantz
Nobel Institute for
   Neurophysiology
Karolinska Institute
S-104 01 Stockholm
Sweden

Theodor Landis
Neurologische Klinik
Universitätshospital
CH-8091, Zürich
Switzerland

Jan Petter Larsen
Dept of Neurology
Central Hospital in Rogeland
4011 Stavanger
Norway

Rolf Leanderson
Dept of Phoniatrics
Karolinska Hospital
S-104 01 Stockholm
Sweden

Gunnar Lennerstrand
Dept of Ophthalmology
Huddinge Hospital
S-141 86 Huddinge
Sweden

Jerome Y. Lettvin
Research Laboratory of
   Electronics, MIT
Cambridge, MA 02139
USA

Deborah L. Levy
Developmental Resource Center
2751 van Buren Street
Hollywood, FL 33020
USA

Caroline Liberg
Dept of Linguistics
Univ of Uppsala
S-751 20 Uppsala
Sweden

Alvin M. Liberman
Haskins Laboratories
New Haven, CT 06511
USA

Isabelle Y. Liberman
Haskins Laboratories
New Haven, CT 06511
USA

Björn Lindblom
Dept of Linguistics
Univ of Stockholm
S-106 91 Stockholm
Sweden

Rolf Lindgren
Dept of Linguistics
Univ of Stockholm
S-106 91 Stockholm
Sweden

Ingvar Lundberg
Dept of Psychology
Univ of Umeå
Rådhusesplanaden 2
S-901 87 Umeå
Sweden

Mary Manning-Thomas
Roosewood Cottage
47, North Perrott
Nr. Crewkerne
Somerset   TA18 7SG
UK

George McConkie
Center for the Study of Reading
51, Gerty Drive
Champaign, IL 61820
USA

Littleton M. Meeks
Meeks Associates, Inc.
P.O. Box 643   ·
Lincoln, MA 01773
USA

Gabriele Miceli
Dept of Neurology
University Catholica
Roma
Italy

Britt Mogård
Almgården, Sjövik
S-148 00 Ösmo
Sweden

Vernon B. Mountcastle
Dept of Neuroscience
The Johns Hopkins Univ
School of Medicine
725 North Wolfe Street
Baltimore, MD 21205
USA

Egon Nordman
Länsskolnämnden i Kronobergs Län
Klostergatan 13
S-352 31 Växjö
Sweden

Ulf Norrsell
Univ of Gothenburg
Dept of Physiology
S-400 33 Gothenburg
Sweden

Kerstin Norrsell
Dept of Ophtalmology
Sahlgrenska Hospital
S-413 45 Gothenburg
Sweden

Göte Nyman
Dept of Psychology
Univ of Helsinki
Ritarikatu 5
SF-00170 Helsinki 17
Finland

Jan Ober
Laboratory of Rehabilitation,
   Engineering and Biomechanics
ul Szeherezady 130/132
60-195 Poznan
Poland

George A. Ojeman
Dept of Neurological Surgery
Univ of Washington
Seattle, WA 98195
USA

Åke Olofsson
Dept of Psychology
Univ of Umeå
Rådhusesplanaden 2
S-901 87 Umeå
Sweden

Richard K. Olson
Dept of Psychology
Univ of Colorado
Boulder, CO 80309
USA

David Ottoson
Wenner-Gren Center Foundation
Sveavägen 166, 23 tr
S-113 46 Stockholm
Sweden

S.H.C. Peel
Guildford College of Technology
Dept of Hum & Soc Sciences
Stoke Park
Guildford, Surrey GU1 1EZ
UK

Charles G. Phillips
Aubrey House
Horton-cum-Studely
Oxford, OX9 1BU
UK

Keith Rayner
Univ of Massachusetts
Amherst, MA 01003
USA

Alix Richardson
University Laboratory of
  Physiology
Parks Road
Oxford OX1 3PT
UK

Patricia Riddle
University Laboratory of
  Physiology
Parks Road
Oxford OX1 3PT
UK

Arne Risberg
Dept of Speech Transmission
The Royal Institute of
  Technology
S-100 44 Stockholm
Sweden

John C. Rothwell
Dept of Neurology
Inst of Psychiatry
De Crespigny Park
Denmark Hill
London SE5 8AF
UK

Agneta Rydberg
Dept of Ophtalmology
Huddinge Hospital
S-141 86 Huddinge
Sweden

J.J.M. Sauter
Taveernelaan 1B
3735 KA Bosch en Duin
The Netherlands

Daisy Schalling
Dept of Psychiatry and
  Psychology
Karolinska Hospital
S-104 01 Stockholm
Sweden

William Schofield
Dept of Experimental Psychology
Univ of Cambridge
Downing Street
Cambridge, CB2 3EJ
UK

Jean Seabrook
Nat. SPELD Center
15 Rastrick Street
Christchurch
New Zealand

Gordon Sherman
Dept of Neurology
Beth Israel Hospital
330, Brookline Avenue
Boston, MA 02215
USA

Nancy Sonnabend
790, Baylston Street S.3H
Boston, MA 02199
USA

Lawrence Stark
Depts of Physiological
  Optics and Engineering Science
226, Minor Hall
Univ of California
Berkely, CA 94720
USA

Jarle Stedje
Elevvårdsbyrån
Skolförvaltningen
Box 22007
S-104 22 Stockholm
Sweden

John Stein
University Laboratory of
  Physiology
Parks Road
Oxford OX1 3PT
UK

Johan Sundberg
Dept of Music Acoustics
The Royal Institute of
  Technology
S-100 44 Stockholm
Sweden

Ulf Söderberg
Dept of Neurophysiology
Ulleråkers Hospital
S-750 15 Uppsala
Sweden

Paula Tallal
Center for Molecular and
  Behavioral Neuroscience
Newark, NJ 07102
USA

Per Uddén
Rodin Remediation Foundation
Hofstrasse 1
CH-6064 Kerns
Switzerland

Ingrid Uhler
Astreavägen 6
S-181 31 Lidingö
Sweden

Richard Wanderman
The Forman School
Litchfield, CT 06759
USA

Beryl Wattles
47, Barrow Road
Cambridge CB2 2AR
UK

Olof Wennhall
Central Hospital
Dept of Ophthalmology
S-721 89 Västerås
Sweden

Monica Westerlund
Dept of Paediatrics
Akademiska Hospital
S-751 85 Uppsala
Sweden

Barry Whitsel
Dept of Physiology
Univ of North Carolina
Chapel Hill, NC 27514
USA

Jan Ygge
Dept of Ophtalmology
Karolinska Hospital
S-104 01 Stockholm
Sweden

Eran Zaidel
Dept of Psychology
Univ of California
Los Angeles, Calif 90024
USA

Yehoshua Zeevi
Israel Inst of Technology
El Engineering Dept
Technicon City
Haifa
Israel

Robert Zenhausern
St. John's University
Psy.Lab. SB-15 Mariallac
Grand Central & Utopia P.Ways
Jamaica, NY 11439
USA

Sven Öhman
Dept of Linguistics
Univ of Uppsala
S-751 20 Uppsala
Sweden

Preface

The increasing awareness of the very severe problem that developmental dyslexia imposes both on the afflicted individuals and on the whole society has led to an intensified research interest. Until a decade or two ago most research efforts were directed at finding remedial and pedagogical solutions to the most apparent problems and diagnostic classifications based on the differences in symptomatic manifestations. Recently, however, the main focus of interest has been shifted into the midst of the fields of modern neurobiology, neuropsychology, and linguistics.

This book, like the topics of the cross-disciplinary conference on which it is based, reflects major advances in several different research areas elucidating the neurological anomalies and functional deficits underlying developmental dyslexia. Several of the chapters provide new basic knowledge about language development, phonetics and phonology, brain mechanisms involved in information processing, and strategies of visual analysis in reading. They provide important background for the chapters dealing more specifically with recent advances concerning the cognitive characteristics, deficits in linguistic capability and visuo-motor problems in individuals with specific developmental dyslexia. Thus, a special feature of this volume is the combination of different neurological, neuropsychological and psycholinguistic perspectives.

Several aspects on fetal brain development seem to be of immediate relevance for the understanding of the cause of developmental dyslexia. Of special interest in this regard are the early developmental anomalies that may affect, with some prevalence, the brain structures in the left hemisphere subserving language functions, including such linguistic processing as phonetic discrimination, phonemic categorization, "working memory" and other factors of importance for reading and writing.

Recent research on hemispheric specialization has shown that the right hemisphere possesses a surprising degree of linguistic capacity, but also that a functioning left hemisphere suppresses right-hemisphere involvement in language. The degree and distribution of this suppression depends on interhemispheric interactions. Developmental anomalies in dyslexics causing deficits in left hemispheric linguistic capacities may be associated with anomalies in interhemispheric dynamics and also with right hemisphere aberration in some visuomotor control functions. This would seem an important area of future research on dyslexia.

Although developmental dyslexia is often defined on the basis of the absence of other, non-verbal dysfunctions it now appears that some subtle associated deficits in various combinations can be detected in many dyslexics, especially with respect to attentional processes, discrete timing in perceptual, memory, motor functions, and the rapid processing and storing of both verbal and non-verbal perceptual information.

In the field of modern psycholinguistics there seems to be general agreement that linguistic capability depends on the proper operation of several different processing functions at different, hierarchially organized, cognitive levels such as the phonetic, phonemic, and grammar levels, each probably related to a particular brain mechanism. Memory functions seem to be of crucial importance in several of these functions. In most cases of developmental dyslexia the specific difficulties can be related to more or less subtle deficits in one or several of these linguistic subfunctions. In particular, many dyslexics have a reduced ability to get conscious access to the phonemic level. The very complex nature of the acoustic signal in spoken language, with little or no physical criterion for a phonetic segmentation, makes it difficult for certain children to become aware of the phonological structure and segmentation in speech.

The last section is devoted to problems related to strategies in visual analysis, eye movements and visuo-motor integration during reading in normal readers and dyslexics. Although there is little evidence that abnormal eye movements per se can be the cause of reading difficulties in developmental dyslexia, studies of the control of eye movements and saccadic strategies have provided new data on the information processing during different stages of the development of reading competence. (Dysfunction in right hemispheric mechanisms for retinal/oculomotor associations and visuospatial control is extensively dealt with also in a section on hemispheric specialization and interactions). Examination of the dynamics of eye movements and the co-ordination of the two eyes during reading might prove an important diagnostic tool, provided high precision binocular recording techniques are employed.

PREFACE

The book reflects our conviction that only multidisciplinary approaches to the problems of developmental dyslexia and trans-disciplinary interactions between scientists representing several different fields will open up avenues to new knowledge of this specific learning disability and find new effective methods for diagnosis and remediation.

The Editors

Acknowledgements

The 7th International Rodin Remediation Conference on which this volume is based was sponsored by the Wenner-Gren Foundation for Scientific Research, the Swedish Medical Research Council, the Swedish Research Council for Humanistic and Social Sciences, The Ministry for Education and The Academia Rodinensis Pro Remedia-tione. Their support is hereby gratefully acknowledged.

We are greately indebted to Ms Vanja Landin for her skilful and devoted work on preparing and organizing the conference. Our thanks are due also to Ms Gun Lennerstrand, Ms Björg Jakobs, and Ms Ulla Lindgren for their much appreciated organizational assistance.

"If, therefore, someone seriously wishes to investigate the truth of things, he ought not to select one science in particular; for they are all interconnected and interdependent; he should rather consider simply how to increase the natural light of his reason, not with a view to solving this or that scolastic problem, but in order that his intellect should show his will what decision it ought to make in each of life's contingences. He will soon be surprised to find that he has made far greater progress than those who devote themselves to particular studies and that he has achieved not only everything that the specialists aim at but also goals far beyond any they can hope to reach."

Rene Descartes
"Regulae ad directionen ingenii",
1628. (Transl. in "The phylosophical writings of Descartes",
1985. Eds: J.Cottingham, R.Stotthoff & D.Murdoch. Cambridge Univ.
Press, Cambridge, page 10)

I
Introductory Chapters

1
Neuroanatomical Findings in Developmental Dyslexia

Gordon F. Sherman, Glenn D. Rosen
and Albert M. Galaburda

INTRODUCTION

Developmental dyslexia is an operationally defined
condition (or group of conditions) characterized mainly
by difficulty with learning to read and the inability to
achieve expected reading levels.   In the restricted
definition of the disorder, the reading difficulty may
not be part of a more generalized disturbance of
sensorimotor function, intellectual capacity, thought and
affective processes, or cultural opportunity (Eisenberg,
1978).   Both dyslexic children and adults exhibit
abnormalities in spoken language as well as written
language, consisting predominantly of problems with oral
comprehension of syntactically complex sentences,
awareness of the phonological structure of words, and
working memory for linguistic objects (Kean, 1984). Most
experts in the field agree that dyslexia represents a
true behavioral anomaly, rather than simply an extreme
example of normal variation in reading competence (Hynd
and Cohen, 1983).

EPIDEMIOLOGY

The diagnosis of dyslexia, which is estimated to
apply to 5% of the schoolage population, can only be made
in children of at least 8 or 9 years, in the second or
third year of school, who demonstrate a reading age of
equal or greater than two years below expected level.
These figures, however, cannot address the frequency in
the population of anomalous cognitive structures involved
in reading acquisition and achievement, but rather
represents only those individuals that fail to
compensate. Earlier behavioral markers of the disorder,
capable of being detected in preschool years, are not

3

available currently, although they are a focus of active
research. Diagnosis in older individuals falls off
because of diminished screening and the arrival of
compensatory strategies that hide, but do not correct,
the underlying abnormalities.

   Dyslexia tends to run in families (De Fries et al.,
1978) and is diagnosed more commonly in boys (Finucci and
Childs, 1981), and an increased frequency is sometimes
seen among left-handed and ambidextrous individuals, and
likewise lefthandedness and ambidexterity is increased
among dyslexics (Geschwind and Behan, 1982). Other
disorders of learning are more commonly diagnosed in
dyslexics, e.g. stuttering and attention deficit
disorders, and ailments that implicate dysfunction of the
immune system, such as allergies and autoimmunity, are
reported to be more common in dyslexics and their
families (Geschwind and Behan, 1982) although others have
disputed some aspects of this claim (Pennington et al.,
1987).

NEUROANATOMICAL FINDINGS

   Anatomical studies of the dyslexic brain have been
made in living subjects and in autopsy cases. Computer-
assisted tomograms of the head (CT-scans) have shown
deviations from the expected pattern of brain asymmetry
ordinarily disclosed by these techniques. Prominence of
the left occipito-temporal region (occipital petalia) is
more commonly demonstrated in CT-scans of normal
subjects, however, this bias is not as strong among
dyslexics (Hier et al., 1978).

   Autopsy studies have been made on six male dyslexic
brains, and two types of deviation from expected norms
are seen: (1) absence of the usual pattern of cerebral
asymmetry of the language-related planum temporale; and
(2) focal developmental abnormalities of cortical
architecture, particularly in the left hemisphere's
perisylvian regions (Galaburda et al., 1985).

Cerebral Asymmetry:

   Gross and Architectonic Characteristics. Only about
fifteen percent of control brains at postmortem
examination show symmetry (10% difference between the
sides) of the planum temporale, a region on the
supratemporal plane containing auditory architectonic
areas. The remaining eighty-five percent show greater
than 10% asymmetry, with most (70%) in favor of the left

side (Galaburda et al, 1987a).   In all dyslexics coming to postmortem examination, the planum temporale was symmetrical (Galaburda et al., 1985).

Symmetry of the planum temporale may signify a distinct organization of the neural substrates underlying linguistic capacity.   Symmetry, rather than asymmetry, reflects a greater amount of language cortex, rather than simply the allocation of some of the left sided language cortex to the right hemisphere.   In a group of 100 brains, the total amount of planum (left plus right) was inversely correlated with the degree of planum asymmetry— the greater the asymmetry, the lesser the total area of the planum (Galaburda et al., 1987a).   This relationship also holds for brain asymmetry in the primary visual cortex of the rat (Galaburda et al., 1986), which shows the same relationship between total amount of right and left cortex and degree of asymmetry of this structure (see Figure 1).

Besides the measured differences in volume, general architectonic appearance does not differ between two asymmetric areas, and measures of cell packing density, proportions of different types of neurons, and laminar characteristics do not distinguish the two sides.   The studies of Scheibel (1984) on the golgi characteristics of neurons on the two asymmetric sides have disclosed subtle differences that cannot by themselves explain the often striking difference in volume (up to 300% in some human architectonic areas).   Therefore, it appears that asymmetry in the volume of homologous cortical architectonic areas can best be explained by side differences in the numbers of neurons (Galaburda et al., 1986a).

In addition, based on architectonic appearance alone, it is not possible to predict whether an area in a given brain will be symmetrical or asymmetrical. Instead, in Nissl stained preparations, what best differentiates between brains with symmetrical and asymmetrical areas is the presence in the asymmetrical case of a relatively small area containing fewer neurons on one side.   Conversely, a brain with symmetrical areas contains more neurons in total.

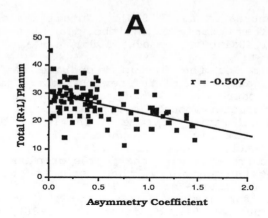

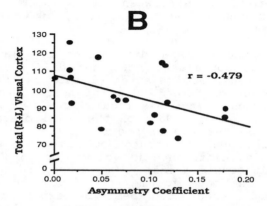

Figure 1 -   **A.**   Scatterplot indicating a negative
    correlation between asymmetry coefficient and volume of
    planum temporale in the human. As asymmetry increases,
    the total volume of the planum temporale decreases. N =
    100, p < 0.001, asymmetry coefficient = (R-
    L)/{(0.5)(R+L)}. **B.** Scatterplot indicating negative
    correlation between asymmetry coefficient and total volume
    of area 17 (primary visual cortex) of the rat. As is the
    case in the human, symmetric brain areas are larger than
    those that are asymmetric. N = 19, p < 0.05, asymmetry
    coefficient = (R-L)/{(0.5)(R+L)}.

        It has not been directly determined whether cell
number differences reflect a side difference in
production or in ontogenetic survival of neurons. If
asymmetric cell loss takes place, it is not clear whether
there is a random loss of neurons on one side as compared

with the other, producing essentially cortices of different surface extent and depth, or whether the loss is of columns of cells at the boundaries with adjacent architectonic areas; in the latter situation the loss may occur either by cell death or by assignment of columns of cells to the neighboring area through the shifting of the boundary line, similar to the observation in experimental deafferentiation of the visual cortex in the fetal monkey (Rakic and Williams, 1986).

Based on the above characteristics of brains with symmetric and asymmetric areas, it is possible that the brains of dyslexic individuals fail to pare down the number of neurons in the language areas of the normally minor hemisphere and are left with a neuronal overpopulation. These ·redundant neurons may not be functionally useful for language, as suggested by behavioral studies in dyslexics showing that brain lateralization for language is almost uniformly biased to the left in these subjects (Prior et al., 1983).

Connectional Characteristics. Brains of lefthanders are more often symmetrical than those of righthanders and also tend to have bigger corpora callosa (LeMay, 1977). Therefore, we investigated symmetric and asymmetric rat brains for possible differences in callosal connectivity. We found that the pattern of callosal terminations differs in the two types of brains. First, the density of callosal connections is greater in certain areas in the symmetric brains. In other words, the increase in the numbers of neurons in the minor side is accompanied by a disproportionate rise in the number of callosal terminations. Second, the patterns of terminations differ in the two cases; in the symmetrical brains the projections are organized more diffusely, whereas in the asymmetrical cases they tend to congregate in more discrete columns (Rosen et al., 1987). We suggest that in the dyslexic brain the language areas contain additional neurons in the minor hemisphere and that these additional neurons may contribute to patterns of interhemispheric connectivity that is both quantitatively and qualitatively different from that seen in asymmetric brains.

Cerebrocortical Microdysgenesis.

Examination of the cerebral cortex of six male dyslexic individuals has disclosed focal anomalies (microdysgenesis) in cortical architecture. These are attributed to causative agents acting in midgestation during early corticogenesis (McBride and Kemper, 1982).

The abnormality consists of focal accumulations of cells (neurons and glia) in layer I of the cerebral cortex (ectopias) often accompanied by subjacent distortion of the laminar and columnar cortical architecture (dysplasia). Moreover, the pial outline is often distorted into excrescences of ectopic cells (brain warts) or into abnormal, poorly laminated small gyri and sulci (microgyria). Abnormal collections of fibers commonly accompany the abnormal cell collections, and dilated small blood vessels (microangiomata) are also frequent. Distinct small areas of abnormality occur in large numbers in these brains (ranging from 30 to 100 per brain), and tend to cluster around the sylvian fissures. The left hemisphere is more severely affected, and within it, the frontal and temporal opercular regions contain the largest number of dysgenetic foci. Several congenital brain disorders have been reported to exhibit these types of anomaly, and autopsy studies in normal brains (free from obvious neurological disease) have demonstrated small numbers of anomalies in an occasional brain. Our own studies in normative brains (processed as the dyslexic brains) have demonstrated only a rare occurrence of focal dysgenesis and never more than two foci per affected brain (Kaufmann and Galaburda, 1987).

ANIMAL MODELS OF CEREBROCORTICAL MICRODYSGENESIS

We and others have examined the brains of immune defective strains of mice for the presence of congenital brain anomalies. The rationale for these studies is that dyslexia and immunological disorders (both allergic and autoimmune) are associated with lefthandedness . Thus, individuals who are either left-handed or not strongly right-handed have higher incidences of immune disorders, and non-righthandedness has been reported to be more common among dyslexics (Geschwind and Behan, 1982).

The prototype animal model for autoimmune disorders is the New Zealand Black (NZB) mouse. This animal develops an illness similar to the human systemic lupus erythematosus (SLE) and dies of its complications prematurely. Immunological abnormalities include the presence of autoantibodies and abnormalities of stem cells, macrophages, and T and B lymphocytes. In addition, these mice exhibit a variety of behavioral difficulties in learning active and passive avoidance responses (Nandy et al., 1983; Spencer et al., 1986).

The brains of a significant proportion of NZB mice show microdysgenesis that, under light microscopy, appears to be indistinguishable from the anomalies witnessed in the brains of dyslexics (Sherman et al.,

1985). Thus, these brains show nests of neurons and glia in layer I of the cerebral cortex, usually affecting only one hemisphere. Other strains of immune defective mice, e.g., the BXSB and hybrids among these strains also show abnormalities affecting different areas of the forebrain (Sherman et al., 1987a). In addition, problems with neuronal migration have been noted in the hippocampus of these mice (Nowakowski, 1986), and the morphology of these neurons is abnormal (Nowakowski and Sekiguichi, 1987).

We have argued that the dysgenesis present in the brains of dyslexics reflects widespread cortical disorganization. The first question regarding this claim is whether the nests of neurons in layer I are simply the result of abnormal migration and malposition of neurons. The organization of neuropeptides within the cortex of NZB mice suggests that the neurons comprising the layer I ectopias have not simply migrated inappropriately, but that their numbers have been regulated abnormally during corticogenesis (Sherman et al., 1987b). Thus, it appears that either too many VIP containing neurons are generated in association with the cortical anomaly, or that too many of these neurons are preserved after ontogenetic neuronal death. Evidence regarding the origin of the ectopias points to the late period of neuronal migration or shortly thereafter as the most likely time during which these abnormalities are produced (McBride and Kemper, 1982). This would suggest that the excessive number of VIP neurons is more likely to reflect abnormalities in developmental neuronal pruning than generation of excessive numbers of cells. Thus, neuronal ectopias may not only represent a disorder of neuronal malposition, but also represent a problem with regulation of neuronal numbers.

A corollary of the statement that neuronal ectopias reflect abnormal regulation of neuronal numbers during ontogenesis is that there is also abnormal regulation of numbers and types of neuronal connections. The presence in Nissl- and neurofilament-stained material of bundles of anomalous fibers supports this hypothesis. In addition, there is evidence that neuronal ectopias of the type seen in dyslexic brains and in the immune defective mice can be produced by injury during cortical development (for a discussion see Sherman et al., 1987a), at a time when connections are particularly vulnerable to the reorganizing effects of damage (Goldman and Galkin, 1978). Moreover, we have observed anomalous connections associated with spontaneously occurring microdysgenesis in a rat. Specifically, a rat that had received a callosal section in adult life showed an area of microgyria and layer I ectopia that contained abnormal callosal terminations. The normal callosal pattern in the part of the cortex that was affected in this animal is well layered and adopts a columnar pattern. However, in the affected cortex the terminations did not constitute a layered and columnar appearance, suggesting a failure of the normal pruning of connections during development, a failure to correct targeting errors, and/or sprouting of aberrant connections (Galaburda et al, 1987b).

ORIGIN OF CEREBROCORTICAL MICRODYSGENESIS

Instances of layer I ectopias, brain warts, microgyria and other related forms of cortical dysplasia have been described in a wide variety of congenital brain malformations having different etiologies, e.g., viral infections, x-irradiation, chromosomal disorders, physical and toxic injury, and, as mentioned above, a markedly restricted expression of the abnormality can be seen in allegedly normal brains, i.e., brains without documented neurological insult. Of all the known causes of this type of microdysgenesis, the only existing epidemiologic clue as to its origin in the brains of dyslexics (and in the immune-defective strains of mice) comes from the observation that affected families or cohorts have a higher than expected incidence of immune disorders. One such report states that the incidence of dyslexia among the offspring of women with the clinical diagnosis of SLE may reach as high as fifty percent (Lahita, personal communication). The mechanisms by which immune disorders and congenital abnormalities of cortical anatomy may come to be causally related are unclear. We have postulated that toxic antibodies may cross the placenta and damage the developing fetal brain to cause cortical microdysgenesis and trigger the process of cellular and connectional deregulation outlined above.

EPIGENETIC ROLE OF SEX HORMONES IN THE PATHOGENESIS OF THE BRAIN ANOMALIES

It has been argued that sex steroids play a pathogenetic role in dyslexia. This conclusion is tempting since the disorder is more commonly diagnosed in boys, and its significant occurrence in girls makes a Y-chromosome linkage impossible and an X-linked disorder unlikely. The only published studies linking the behavioral phenotype to the human genome implicates the autosomal fifteenth chromosome (Smith et al., 1983).

Studies on functional cerebral lateralization have demonstrated a different bias between the genders, with boys demonstrating a relatively right hemisphere and girls a relatively left hemisphere superiority. The male hormone testosterone has been attributed a role in this differential organization, and the alleged left hemisphere deficiencies in dyslexics have been interpreted as an extreme example of this bias. Moreover, there is ample support to the claim that male hormones modify immune activity, which led Geschwind and colleagues to propose a common role for the hormone in the production of anomalies in lateral organization of the brain and immune system abnormalities (Geschwind and Behan, 1982). However, to date, there is no evidence that sex steroids can produce cortical dysgenesis, and it is still difficult to reconcile the observation that immune disorders are more common in females with the more frequent expression of dyslexia in males.

The answer may turn out to be more complex than previously suspected. Testosterone may be involved in the regulation of cell and axonal pruning during ontogenesis through its actions as a trophic factor (Toran-Allerand, 1978), and thus may explain some of the anatomic abnormalities seen in the symmetrical and dysgenetic dyslexic brains. On the other hand, testosterone's ameliorating effects on autoimmunity, which would be expected to protect the male fetus, may lead to more severe involvement of female fetuses. In the latter case females would express either a more widespread learning deficiency not diagnosed as dyslexia, or may be wasted in the fetal stage. Preliminary data may support this contention (Galaburda et al., 1986b), but additional epidemiologic studies addressing issues of sex ratios in dyslexic families and histories of miscarriage will be needed to test these hypotheses.

IMPLICATIONS OF THE BEHAVIORAL DISORDER IN DYSLEXIA

The brains of dyslexics illustrate two anatomical findings that could separately alter language acquisition and linguistic performance as well as other cognitive capacities. There is an unexpectedly high prevalence of brain symmetry, with its attendant influence over cerebral lateralization for language, and there is dysgenesis of the left perisylvian cortices involved in language function. The absence of asymmetry is in it of itself a curiosity, since there is no strong evidence that this anatomical characteristic is detrimental to linguistic competence. The findings by Bever (1987), that the presence of lefthandedness in the families of

righthanders biases linguistic strategies away from a
strong reliance on syntactic operations, suggest that
symmetric brains may be so disposed. In normal discourse
this alone may not amount to language disability, but it
is easy to conceive that under some strongly constrained
situations the lack of ready access to syntactic
operations may constitute a risk for producing errors in
language performance similar to those exhibited by
dyslexics. The effect of brain symmetry on linguistic
capacity needs to be clarified, and currently available
neuroimaging techniques offer new opportunities for this
type of research.

     It is more intuitive to conclude that the
microdysgenesis that affects the perisylvian language-
related cortices plays the crucial role in the functional
disorder. This is particularly enticing in view of the
evidence that implicates abnormal cellular and
connectional organization of language related neuronal
assemblies, including interhemispheric relationships.
The abnormal assemblies are characterized by anomaly of
exuberance rather than of hypoplasia, and this
observation may shed light on questions about the
neurobiological substrates of language and their
development. Thus, it is possible that the kind of
phonological and syntactic ambiguity experienced by
dyslexics reflects noise generated by redundant and
otherwise exuberant pathways. However, this question
represents a special case of a more basic problem facing
modern neuroscience and cognitive science, which is that
of level at which complex cognitive capacities such as
language are represented in the nervous system, and how
can they be altered by physiological variation and
pathological influences.

     Yet the presence together of brain symmetry and
dysgenesis in the brains of dyslexics, conditions that
even singly are uncommon in the normal population,
suggests that their pathogenetic role in dyslexia may be
conjoint. Thus, it is possible that symmetry introduces
a risk for abnormal competency in some linguistic
operations, and that dysgenesis obliterates important
possibilities for compensation. In that case, it would
be expected that cases of dyslexia will appear that have
symmetry but left hemisphere early injury of a type
different from that illustrated by microdysgenesis. We
have analyzed one brain, that of a woman dyslexic, who
showed the combination of symmetry of the planum
temporale and multiple focal myelinated gliotic scars
involving the left perisylvian cortex, and attributed to
injury before the age of three years (Galaburda et al.,
1986b). Additional observations in autopsy material will
help to confirm this two-strike hypothesis.

REFERENCES

Bever, T. (1987). Paper presented at the 19th Conference of the Cognitive Sciences Society.

DeFries, J.C., Singer, S.M., Goch, T.T., and Lewitter, F.I. (1978). Familial nature of reading disability. Brit. J. Psychiatry, 132, 361-367.

Dvorak, K., Feit, J., and Jurankova, Z. (1978). Experimentally induced focal microgyria and status verrucosus deformis in rats--pathogenesis and interrelation histological and autoradographical study. Acta Neuropath., 44, 121-129.

Eisenberg, L. (1978). Definitions of dyslexia: Their consequences for research and policy. In Dyslexia — An Appraisal of Current Knowledge (eds. A.L. Benton and D. Pearl). Oxford University Press, New York.

Finucci, J.M. and Childs, B. (1981). Are there really more dyslexic boys than girls. In Sex Differences in Dyslexia (eds. I. Ansara, N. Geschwind, A. M. Galaburda, and N. Gartrell). Orton Dyslexia Society, Baltimore.

Galaburda, A.M., Aboitiz, F., Rosen, G.D., and Sherman, G.F. (1986a). Histological asymmetry in the primary visual cortex of the rat: Implications for mechanisms of cerebral asymmetry.Cortex, 22, 151-160.

Galaburda, A.M., Corsiglia, J., Rosen, G.D., and Sherman, G.F. (1987a). Planum temporale asymmetry, reappraisal since Geschwind and Levitsky. Neuropsychologia, 25, 853-868.

Galaburda, A.M., Rosen, G.D., Sherman, G.F., and Assal, F. (1986b). Neuropathological findings in a woman with developmental dyslexia. Ann. Neurol., 20, 170.

Galaburda, A.M., Rosen, G.D., and Sherman, G.F. (1987b). Connectional anomaly in association with cerebral microgyria in the rat. Soc. Neurosci. Abs., 13, 1601.

Galaburda, A.M., Sherman, G.F., Rosen, G.D., Aboitiz, F., and Geschwind, N. (1985). Developmental dyslexia: Four consecutive cases with cortical anomalies.Ann. Neurol., 18, 222-233.

Geschwind, N. and Behan, P.O. (1982). Left-handedness: Association with immune disease, migraine, and developmental learning disorder. Proc. Nat. Acad. Sci. (USA), 79, 5097-5100.

Goldman-Rakic P.S. and Galkin, T.W. (1978). Prenatal removal of frontal association cortex in the fetal rehesus monkey: anatomical and functional consequences in postnatal life. Brain Res., 152, 451-485.

Hier, D.B., LeMay, M., Rosenberg, P.B., and Perlo, V.P. (1978). Developmental dyslexia. Evidence for a subgroup with a reversal of cerebral asymmetry. Arch. Neurol., 35, 90-92.

Hynd, G.W. and Cohen, M. (1983). Dyslexia: Neuropsychological Theory, Research, and Clinical Differentiation, Grune and Stratton, New York.

Kaufmann, W.E. and Galaburda, A.M. (1987). Cerebrocortical microdysgenesis in normal human brains. Soc. Neurosci. Abs., 13, 1601.

Kean, M.L. (1984). The question of linguistic anomaly in developmental dyslexia. Ann. Dyslexia, 34, 137-151.

LeMay, M. (1977). Asymmetries of the skull and handedness. J. Neurol. Sci., 32, 243-253.

McBride, M.C. and Kemper, T.L. (1982). Pathogenesis of four-layered microgyric cortex im man. Acta Neuropath., 57, 93-98.

Nandy, K., Lal, H., Bennet, M., and Bennet, D. (1983). Correlation between a learning disorder and elevated brain-reactive antibodies in aged C57BL/6 and young NZB mice. Life Sci., 33, 1499-1503.

Nowakowski, R.S. (1986). Abnormalities in neuronal migration in the hippocampal formation of the NZB/BINJ mouse. Soc. Neurosci. Abs., 12, 317.

Nowakowski, R.S. and Sekiguchi, M. (1987). Abnormalities of granule cell dendrites and axons in the dentate gyrus of the NZB/BINJ mouse. Soc. Neurosci. Abs., 13, 1117.

Pennington, B.F., Smith, S.D., Kimberling, W.J., Green, P.A., and Haith, M.M. (1987). Left-handedness and immune disorders in familial dyslexics. Arch. Neurol., 44, 634-639.

Prior, M.R., Frolley, M., and Sanson, A. (1983). Language lateralization in specific reading retarded children and backward readers. Cortex, 19, 149-163.

Rakic, P. and Williams, R.W. (1986). Thalamic regulation of cortical parcellation: An experimental perturbation of the striate cortex in rhesus monkeys. Soc. Neursci. Abs., 12, 1499.

Rosen, G.D., Sherman, G.F., and Galaburda, A.M. (1987). Neocortical symmetry and asymmetry in the rat: Different patterns of callosal connections. Soc. Neurosci. Abs., 13, 44.

Scheibel, A.B. (1984). A dendritic correlate of human speech. In Cerebral Dominance: The Biological Foundations (eds. N. Geschwind and A. M. Galaburda), Harvard University Press, Cambridge, USA.

Sherman, G.F., Galaburda, A.M., and Geschwind, N. (1985). Cortical anomalies in brains of New Zealand Mice: A neuropathologic model of dyslexia. Proc. Nat. Acad. Sci. (USA), 82, 8072-8074.

Sherman, G.F., Galaburda, A.M., Behan, P.O., and Rosen, G.D. (1987a). Neuroanatomical anomalies in autoimmune mice. Acta Neuropath., 74, 239-242.

Sherman, G.F., Stone, J., Rosen, G.D., and Galaburda, A.M. (1987b). Neuropeptide architectonics in the brain of the New Zealand Black mouse. Soc. Neurosci. Abs., 13, 1601.

Smith, S.D., Kimberling, W.J., Pennington, B.F., and Lubs, H.A. (1983). Specific reading disability: Identification of an inherited form through linkage analysis. Science, 219, 1345-1347.

Spencer, D.G., Humphries, K., Mathis, D., and Lal, H. (1986). Specific behavioral impairments in association tasks with an autoimmune mouse. Behav. Neurosci., 100, 353-358.

Toran-Allerand, C.D. (1978). Gonadal hormones and brain development: Cellular aspects of sexual differentiation. Amer. Zool., 18, 553-565.

2
Transitory Neuronal Connections in Normal Development and Disease

Douglas O. Frost

INTRODUCTION

The development of the central nervous system (CNS) is a destructive process as well as a constructive one: In many regions of the CNS, there is an overproduction and subsequent elimination of neurons and of the connections between them (reviews in Innocenti, '81a; Cowan et al., '84; Frost, '84; Rakic et al., '86). The different parts of the CNS are highly interdependent during ontogeny. Thus, developmental aberrations at one locus may be cascaded to multiple, distant regions. Furthermore, since CNS development is sensitive to the external environment during the neonatal period (Sherman & Spear, '82; Fregnac & Imbert, '84), defects of the sensory organs (that effectively create anomalous sensory environments) can lead to permanent alterations in CNS morphology and function. Thus, central or peripheral disturbances during development can create abnormal neural pathways due to modulation of the normally occuring reduction or elimination of some sets of immature connections (reviews in Innocenti, '81a; Frost, '86). Here, I describe two series of experiments in our laboratory, in which neural connections that are normally present only at early developmental stages are permanently stabilized. Our results provide new insights into normal developmental mechanisms and the processes that underlie the morphological and functional abnormalities arising in certain disease states.

NORMALLY TRANSIENT RETINAL PROJECTIONS TO NON-VISUAL STRUCTURES

In hamsters, the connections between the eye and brain have just begun to form on the day of birth (day 0 = 15.5 days post-conception; Frost et al., '79; Jhaveri et al., '83). In neonatal hamsters, retinal ganglion cell (RGC) axons project to multiple "non-visual" brain nuclei including the main thalamic somatosensory (ventrobasal, VB) nucleus and the main midbrain auditory nucleus (inferior colliculus, IC; Frost, '84). The projection to VB disappears completely by postnatal day 4; the projection to IC is largely eliminated by the end of the first postnatal week although a remnant persists permanently in a restricted region of IC adjacent to the main midbrain visual nucleus (superior colliculus, SC).

We have examined the ultrastructure of anterogradely labeled, transient, retino-VB and retino-IC axons in neonatal hamsters (Freeman & Frost, '87). Both sets of

17

axons make immature synapses on their target neurons; the synapses are indistinguishable from others in these nuclei, presumably including those made by permanent afferents. Thus, the elimination of transient retino-VB and retino-IC axons is not due to their inability to make synapses. In fact, the formation of synapses by transient retino-VB and retino-IC axons allows the possibility that these axons are eliminated by a mechanism that depends on the pattern or overall level of their synaptic activity (Stent, '73; Changeux & Danchin, '76; Bear et al., '87).

We have also studied the branching patterns of individual, horseradish peroxidase (HRP) filled RGC axons in neonatal hamsters (Langdon et al., '87; Bhide & Frost, unpublished data). We confirmed previous suggestions that RGC axons go through three morphologically distinguishable growth states (Frost, '84; Schneider et al., '85): i) elongation, during which RGC axons extend along the optic tract (OT) from the eye to the mesencephalon, but do not send collaterals into their target nuclei; ii) collateralization, during which unbranched processes extend from the main axonal trunks into the targets of RGC axons; iii) arborization, during which the RGC axons elaborate their terminal arbors within their target nuclei (and form synapses at an accelerated rate [Campbell et al., '84]). Different transient projections are formed by RGC axons in different growth states: The retino-IC projection is due to "exuberant" elongation of RGC axons, which grow caudally across SC and continue into IC. This is not the case for the retino-VB projection. In normal, adult rodents, RGC axons passing to the midbrain on the surface of the brain in the superficial optic tract (SOT) send collaterals to the thalamus (where they terminate in the dorsal lateral geniculate nucleus, LGd); RGC axons that traverse the thalamus deeper, in the internal optic tract (IOT), do not have thalamic collaterals. In neonates, the retino-VB projection arises exclusively from transient IOT axon collaterals. Thus, during development, all RGC axons in the OT form thalamic collaterals, but only the collaterals of SOT axons are maintained; the retino-VB projection is due to "exuberant" collateralization, not elongation.

STABILIZATION OF NORMALLY TRANSIENT RETINAL PROJECTIONS

When two of the principal targets of RGC axons, the SC and LGd, are ablated in newborn hamsters and VB or the auditory (medial geniculate, MG) thalamic nucleus are partially deafferented by ablation of their specific, ascending sensory afferents, RGC axons form permanent connections in VB or MG (Frost, '81, '82, '86). This suggests that the definitive choice of targets by developing RGC axons depends on multiple factors (review in Frost, '86) and can be altered by changes in the axonal environment.

The permanent retino-VB projection arises by the abnormal stabilization and sprouting of the normally transient projection. In normal hamsters, retino-VB projections are absent after day 3; in operated hamsters, they are present at all ages and occupy increasing proportions of VB between birth and 122 days (Frost, '86). (This is not the only mechanism for the formation of abnormal connections. Retino-MG projections arise de novo by rapid, reactive sprouting of RGC axons: they are not present in normal animals at any age, but appear by 48h postoperatively [Frost, '86]).

STABILIZED RETINAL PROJECTIONS AS AN EXPERIMENTAL SYSTEM

We have used the abnormal retinal projections to VB (and MG) in neonatally operated adult hamsters to study the developmental mechanisms underlying several functionally important organizational features of sensory systems.

Morphology of synaptic connections.

Terminals of ascending, specific sensory axons in the thalamus participate in synaptic complexes called "glomeruli" - regions containing numerous neuronal elements engaged in multiple synaptic contacts and isolated from areas of simpler neuropil by sheets of astrocyte cytoplasm. In LGd of normal animals, the morphology of these terminals and the synaptic organization of their glomeruli differ from those in VB and MG with respect to multiple morphological features (review in Campbell & Frost, '88). The surgically stabilized retinal projections to VB and MG provide an opportunity to investigate how terminal morphology and glomerulus synaptic organization are determined. Various features of the terminals and associated synaptic glomeruli of retino-VB and retino-MG afferents can be compared to corresponding features of the normal afferents to LGd, VB and MG. Features of normal retino-LGd afferents that are not shared with the normal, somatosensory- and auditory afferents to VB and MG, respectively, and that are conserved by retino-VB and retino-MG axons, are likely to be determined by the afferent axons. Features of retino-VB and retino-MG axons that more closely resemble those of normal specific sensory afferents to VB and MG, respectively, are likely to be determined by their targets.

We examined normal retino-LGd projections, normal ascending sensory projections to VB and MG, and anomalous retino-VB and retino-MG projections.[1] With respect to all the features examined, retino-LGd axon terminals and their glomeruli differed from those of the normal, specific sensory afferents to VB and MG. We found that for retino-VB and retino-MG axons: i) morphological features of interneuronal contacts (including the type, number and size of interconnected neuronal elements and the loci at which they contact eachother) were typical of normal VB and MG, respectively, and thus are responsive to interactions among interconnected neuronal elements, or to interactions between those elements and their environment (eg., glia, extracellular matrix); ii) features related to intrinsic neuronal functions were typical of normal retino-LGd axons, and thus are not responsive to such interactions. The determination of contact morphology by interactive mechanisms may serve to minimize the amount of genetic information necessary for the assembly of neural circuits.

Receptotopic projections.

In normal, adult hamsters, the entire contralateral retina is represented retinotopically on the surfaces of SC, LGd and the ventral lateral geniculate nucleus (LGv); each point on the retinal surface projects to cylinders of tissue that extend into each of these structures from its surface (Frost & Schneider, '79). We have used the abnormal retinal projections to VB and MG to study how receptotopic organization is normally established. Using anatomical techniques, we mapped the retino-VB and retino-MG projections (Frost, '81). In each nucleus, a given pole of the retina was

---

[1] RGC axon terminals were always identified by anterograde labeling with HRP.

consistently represented at a particular end of the overall retinal projection, and different retinal poles were systematically mapped around the circumference of the projection. Thus, as in the visual nuclei of normal animals, the retino-VB and retino-MG projections are retinotopically organized. This suggests that RGC axons may be "self-organizing": their receptotopic organization may come about by interactions among the developing axons themselves, with only the orientation of the projection within the target nucleus being determined by an interactions between the axons and their targets. For further discussion of this problem see Frost & Schneider ('79) and Frost ('81).

Functional organization of sensory systems.

Using both multiple- and single unit recording, we have studied visually evoked responses in the primary and secondary somatosensory cortices (SI and SII, respectively) of neonatally operated hamsters having retino-VB projections. Visual stimulation of well-defined receptive fields (RF's) reliably evokes multi-unit responses in SI and SII of operated, but not normal hamsters (Frost & Metin, '85). Since the synapses between retino-VB axons and VB neurons are interposed between the retina and the neurons from which we recorded, our data demonstrate that these synapses are functional. The multi-unit cortical responses also show a partially retinotopic organization that is consistent with the anatomical organization of the retino-VB projection and of the normal VB to cortex projection (Frost & Metin, '85).

Single unit recording (Metin & Frost, '88) shows that neurons in SI/SII respond to visual stimulation of distinct RF's and that their response properties resemble, in several characteristic features, those of neurons in primary visual cortex (VI) of normal hamsters. In VI of normal- and SI/SII of operated animals, the same functional categories of neurons occur in similar proportions, and the neurons' selectivity for the orientation or the direction of movement of visual stimuli is comparable. Thirty six percent of visually responsive neurons in SI/SII also had distinct somatosensory RF's.

These data suggest two hypotheses that are not mutually exclusive:

1) Thalamic nuclei and cortical areas at corresponding levels in the visual and somatosensory systems work similar transformations on their inputs. Three lines of evidence support this hypothesis:

a) The visual and somatosensory systems use similar information processing strategies based on similar morphological substrates (review in Metin & Frost, '88).

b) Orientation selective neurons occur with equal frequency and are equally sharply tuned in VI of normal- and SI/SII of operated hamsters[2]. The similar depth distributions of orientation selective units in VI and SI/SII, give further evidence of the similarity of circuitry in these cortical regions.

c) The similarity of the visual and somatosensory response properties of bimodal neurons in SI/SII of operated hamsters to those of single neurons in VI and SI/SII,

---

[2] This datum supports the hypothesis if either of two explanations of cortical orientation selectivity is correct. i) It was originally suggested that the orientation preference of visual cortical neurons is an emergent property of cortical circuitry (Hubel & Wiesel, '62). ii) It is now known that in carnivores, RGC's and LGd neurons show weak orientation biases, although the contribution of these biases to the orientation preferences of cortical neurons is controversial (Vidyasagar, '87). There has been no systematic study in rodents to determine where in the visual pathway different stimulus features are first abstracted. Thus, in rodents, carnivores and other orders, the response preferences of RGC's or thalamic neurons may be sharpened by the cortex.

respectively, of normal hamsters suggests that similar circuits in the visual and somatosensory thalamic nuclei and cortices can generate both visual and somatosensory responses.

2) In sensory thalamic nuclei and cortical areas, the differentiation of some biochemical and morphological features underlying normal function may reflect the modality of the sensory input. While sensory input of the appropriate modality clearly influences the development of sensory systems (Sherman & Spear, '82; Fregnac & Imbert, '84), there are few data on how the differentiation of sensory systems depends on the modality of their input. Available evidence argues against such a dependence: Retino-VB axons participate in synaptic complexes that morphologically resemble those of normal, somatosensory, rather than visual, thalamic afferents (Campbell & Frost, '88).[3] Despite the absence of empirical support for this hypothesis, computer models demonstrate the plausibility of neuronal networks whose connection strengths are modifiable in such a way that the response properties of their constituent neurons develop particular features as a result of their sensory input (Lehky & Sejnowski, '88; Linsker, '88).

NORMALLY TRANSIENT INTERHEMISPHERIC PROJECTIONS

In normal adult cats, retrograde transport of HRP following a large injection in one hemisphere shows that neurons in the visual cortex that send an axon through the corpus callosum (CC) to the contralateral visual cortex (callosal neurons, CN's) have a stereotyped distribution (Innocenti, '80). In the first and second visual areas (VI, area 17 and VII, area 18, respectively) the cortical volume containing callosal neurons (callosal efferent zone, CZ) consists of two radially separated tiers, located in layers III/IV and VI. The III/IV tier is wider and richer in CN's. CN's in areas 17 and 18 are concentrated around their common border, which represents the vertical meridian of the visual field (Tusa et al., '78). Thus, most CN's in area 17 lie in the lateral part, although, particularly rostrally, some extend as far medially as the suprasplenial sulcus.

Some of the callosal connections of the cortex of developing cats are ephemeral: In newborn cats, CN's are distributed in two radially separated tiers, as in adults. The immature tangential (parallel to the cortical surface) distribution of CN's differs from that of adults: In newborn cats CN's are distributed continuously across the entire extent of areas 17 and 18. During the first 3 months of life, CN's gradually become less common medially in area 17 until the adult distribution is attained (Innocenti & Caminiti, '80). Experiments using retrograde transport of long-lasting fluorescent dyes (Innocenti, '81b; Innocenti et al., '86) and electron microscopic counting of axons in the CC (Koppel & Innocenti, '83) indicate that during the first 3 months of life, some immature CN's in area 17 lose their callosal axon but remain in the cortex and form uncrossed, cortico-cortical connections. This does not exclude the possibility that immature CN's die during development; indeed, some immature CN's belong to a special category of neurons that is virtually completely eliminated during normal development (Chun et al., '87).

---

[3] Thus, the morphological features of thalamic synaptic complexes may not determine the parameters of cortical neuronal responses assayed in our visual RF studies.

MODULATION OF THE DEVELOPMENTAL ELIMINATION OF INTERHEMISPHERIC CONNECTIONS

Visual experience early in life affects the stabilization/elimination of immature callosal projections; normal visual experience is necessary for the development of a normal number and distribution of CN's. Some types of abnormal visual experience cause the partial stabilization of immature callosal connections that would normally be eliminated, although there is no form of visual experience known to stabilize all of the callosal connections present in newborn kittens. Rearing kittens with monocular enucleation (ME) from birth, monocular eyelid suture (MD) or bilaterally symmetric (convergent or divergent) strabismus (S) produces an abnormally wide CZ by stabilizing the normally transient callosal axons of immature CN's medially in area 17 (Innocenti & Frost, '79); unilateral strabismus has similar effects (Berman & Payne, '83).

Why do S, ME and MD similarly affect callosal development? Rearing with S, ME or MD causes most neurons in areas 17 and 18 to respond predominantly to stimulation of one eye (reviews in Sherman & Spear, '82; Fregnac & Imbert, '84), whereas in normal cats, most of these neurons respond well to stimulation of either eye (Hubel & Wiesel, '62). To test the relationship between loss of binocularity and stabilization of transient CN's, we reared cats with alternating monocular occlusion (AMO), which also makes most area 17/18 neurons monocular, but unlike S, ME and MD, lacks other physiological effects (Hubel & Wiesel, '65). Cats were raised in total darkness except that for a few hours daily, they explored a normally lit room with one eye occluded; each eye was occluded on alternate days. At age 3 months, in AMO-reared cats, as in cats reared with S, ME or MD, normally transient CN's in medial area 17 were stabilized (Frost et al., '88). Thus, experience-dependent loss of cortical binocular responsiveness and stabilization of normally transient callosal connections are correlated but a causal relationship and the underlying physiological mechanisms remain uncertain.

Other types of abnormal visual experience exaggerate the normally ocurring developmental elimination of immature callosal connections. In area 17/18 of adult cats reared with bilateral enucleation (BE) or bilateral eyelid suture (BD) from birth there are fewer CN's than normal (Innocenti & Frost, '79, '80; Innocenti et al., '85). There are two surprising differences between the effects of BD and BE: i) Although both manipulations reduce the number of CN's in areas 17/18, the effect is greater for BD than for BE, even though enucleation seems to be a more severe form of deprivation. ii) BE produces an abnormally wide CZ in areas 17/18 while BD produces a slightly narrower than normal CZ. These differences might be explained by two obvious differences between BE and BD cats: i) light can evoke responses in RGC's and influence the brain in BD but not BE cats; ii) spontaneous and light-evoked RGC activity reach the brain in BD but not BE cats.

In order to determine the effects of light on callosal connectivity, we examined the visual callosal connections of cats reared in total darkness (Frost & Moy, '88). Dark rearing (DR), like BD and BE, exaggerates the normally occurring partial elimination of immature callosal connections. DR causes a significant reduction in the total number of CN's and slightly narrows the distribution of CN's in areas 17/18. Thus, visual stimulation is not necessary either to initiate the partial elimination of immature callosal connections or to stabilize a large fraction of callosal projections present at birth.

We have begun to study the role of RGC impulse activity on the development of callosal connections by binocularly blocking such activity from birth to 8 weeks with intraocularly administered tetrodotoxin (TTX; Frost & Dubin, unpublished data). In TTX-treated cats, as in cats subjected to neonatal BE, CN's persist in medial regions of area 17 that are acallosal in normal animals of comparable age; the number of CN's in TTX-treated cats remains to be determined. These data indicate that RGC impulse blockade, unlike DR, results in the stabilization of some normally transient callosal connections.

Together, the preceding experiments suggest that the stabilization/elimination of immature callosal connections occurs by mechanisms that depend, in part, on the pattern or overall level of their synaptic activity (Stent, '73; Changeux & Danchin, '76; Bear et al., '87).

CONCLUSIONS

In the systems we have studied, the stabilization/elimination of immature neuronal connections depends on multiple factors that are both intrinsic and extrinsic to the nervous system. These factors probably act by some common mechanisms that reflect the pattern or overall level of synaptic activity. The phenomena described for retinal projections and callosal connections are paradigmatic for those in other neural systems "*in statu nascendi*". For example, ascending auditory, somatosensory and cerebellar afferents transiently grow beyond their definitive thalamic targets during normal development (Asanuma et al., '88); these "exuberant" connections can be permanently stabilized as a consequence of either congenital mutations or experimentally induced lesions, that act primarily on nearby axon systems (Asanuma & Stanfield, '85). We have argued elsewhere (Innocenti & Frost, '80) that the effects of abnormal visual experience on the callosal connections of the visual cortex are paradigmatic for similar effects on local cortical circuits and uncrossed cortical association connections.

Why do transient neuronal connections occur? This question may have different answers in different instances. i) Some transient connections may be epiphenomena of the simplification of developmental rules. For example, it may be more economical (eg., in terms of genetic coding) for all RGC's to follow the same developmental program, elaborate the same types of connections and then have each distinct class of RGC's eliminate inappropriate connections, than it would be to program each class of RGC's to form only appropriate connections from the outset. ii) The overproduction of connections may provide a substrate for ontogenetic or phylogenetic modification of the CNS in response to changes in peripheral receptors or in the environment. For example, interocular distance and ocular alignment change in early postnatal life, so developmental mechanisms must be sensitive to changing visual input in order to assure that the final pattern of cortical connectivity will be appropriately matched to the definitive position and alignment of the eyes. It is attractive to view the modifications we observed in ME, MD, S and AMO cats as partial compensation for the disturbance of the binocular visual field, although the adaptiveness of the changes remains to be demonstrated. Similarly, environmentally controlled narrowing of an initially broad set of neural connections could provide an economical means of adapting one developmental mechanism to the nervous systems of species occupying widely varying ecological niches. iii) Transitory connections may reflect the elimination of erroneous connections arising due to "slop" in the execution of the developmental program. However, in many cases the elimination of immature connections is too massive a phenomenon to believe that such a sloppy developmental program would have survived natural selection.

The above-described phenomena probably underlie neural dysfunction in some disease states arising from the action of mutant genes, teratologic agents or traumatic events during development. For example, congenitally deaf patients exhibit abnormally large visually evoked responses in the auditory cortex (Neville, '88). Finally, our finding that the somatosensory sytem can process visual information in a manner similar to that of the visual system, raises the possibility that novel, surgically induced neural circuits may one day be used to alleviate some types of birth defects.

REFERENCES

Asanuma, C., R. Ohkawa, B.B. Stanfield, and W.M. Cowan (1988). Observations on the development of certain ascending inputs to the thalamus in rats. I. Postnatal development. Dev. Br. Res., 41, 159-170.

Asanuma, C., and B.B. Stanfield (1985). Medical lemniscal axons can innervate the lateral geniculate nucleus in neonatally enucleated and congenitally blind mice. Anat. Rec., 12A, 211.

Bear, M.F., L.N. Cooper, and F.F. Ebner (1987). A physiological basis for a theory of synapse modification. Science., 237, 42-48.

Berman, N.E., and B.R. Payne (1983). Alterations in connections of the corpus callosum following convergent and divergent strabismus. Br. Res., 274, 201-212.

Campbell, G., and D.O. Frost (1988). Synaptic organization of anomalous retinal projections to somatosensory and auditory thalamus: Target-controled morphogenesis of axon terminals and synaptic glomeruli. J. Comp. Neurol., 272, 383-408.

Campbell, G., K.-.F. So, and A.R. Lieberman (1984). Normal post-natal development of retino-geniculate axons and terminals and identification of inappropriately-located transient synapses. Neuroscience., 13, 743-759.

Changeux, J P., and A. Danchin (1976). Selective stabilisation of developing synapses as a mechanism for the specification of neuronal networks. Nature, 264, 705-712.

Chun, J.J.M., M.J. Nakamura, and C.J. Shatz (1987). Transient cells of the developing mammalian telecephalon are peptide-immunoreactive neurons. Nature., 325, 617-620.

Cowan, W.M., J.W. Fawcett, D.D.M. O'Leary, and B.B. Stanfield (1984). Regressive events in neurogenesis. Science., 225, 1258-1265.

Freeman, J.M., and D.O. Frost (1987). Synapse formation by optic tract axons that project transiently to somatosensory and auditory nuclei in the neonatal hamster. Soc. Neurosci. Abstr., 13, 1023.

Fregnac, Y., and M. Imbert (1984). Development of neuronal selectivity in primary visual cortex of cat. Physiol. Rev., 64, 325-434.

Frost, D.O. (1981). Orderly anomalous retinal projections to the medial geniculate, ventrobasal and lateral posterior nuclei of the hamster. J. Comp. Neurol., 203, 227-256.

Frost, D.O. (1982). Anomalous visual connections to somatosensory and auditory systems following brain lesions in early life. Dev. Br. Res., 3, 627-635.

Frost, D.O. (1984). Axonal growth and target selection during development: retinal projections to the ventrobasal complex and other "nonvisual" structures in neonatal Syrian hamsters. J. Comp. Neurol., 230, 576-592.

Frost, D.O. (1986). Development of surgically in induced retinal projections to the medial geniculate, ventrobasal and lateral posterior nuclei in Syrian hamsters: A quantitative study. J. Comp. Neurol., 252, 95-105.

Frost, D.O., and C. Metin. (1985). Induction of functional retinal projections to the somatosensory system. Nature, 317, 162-164.

Frost, D.O., and Y.P. Moy. (1988). Effects of dark rearing on the development of visual callosal connections. Exp. Br. Res., in press.

Frost, D.O., Y.P. Moy, and D.C. Smith. (1988). Effects of alternating monocular occlusion on maturation of feline visual callosal connections. Soc. Neurosci. Abstr., 14, 1112.

Frost, D.O., and G.E. Schneider. (1979). Plastcicity of retinofugal projections aafter partial lesions of the retina in newborn Syrian hamsters. J. Comp. Neurol., 185, 517-568.

Frost, D.O., K.-.F. So, and G.E. Schneider. (1979). Postnatal development of retinal projections in Syrian hamsters: A study using autoradiographic and anterograde degeneration techniques. Neuroscience., 4, 1649-1677.

Hubel, D.H., and T.N. Wiesel. (1962). Receptive fields, binocular interaction and functional architecture in the cat's visual cortex. J. Physiol., 160, 106-154.

Hubel, D.H. and T.N. Wiesel. (1965). Binocular interaction in striate cortex of kittens reared with artificial squint. J. Neurophysiol., 28, 1041-1059.

Innocenti, G.M. (1980). The primary visual pathway through the corpus callosum: Morphological and functional aspects in the cat. Arch. Ital. Biol., 118, 124-188.

Innocenti, G.M. (1981). Transitory structures as substrates for developmental platicity of the brain. Dev. Neurosci., 13, 305-333.

Innocenti, G.M. (1981). Growth and reshaping of axons in the establishment of visual callosal connections. Science, 218, 824-827.

Innocenti, G.M., and R. Caminiti. (1980). Postnatal shaping of collosal connections from sensory areas. Exp. Br. Res., 38, 381-394.

Innocenti, G.M., S. Clarke, and R. Kraftsik. (1986).. Interchange of callosal and association projections in the developing visual cortex. J. Neurosci., 6, 1384-1409.

Innocenti, G.M., and D.O. Frost. (1979). Effects of visual experience on the maturation of the efferent system to the corpus callosum. Nature, 280, 231-234.

Innocenti, G.M., and D.O. Frost. (1980). The postnatal development of visual callosal connections in the absence of visual experience or of the eyes. Exp. Br. Res., 39, 365-375.

Innocenti, G.M., D.O. Frost, and J. Illes. (1985). Maturation of visual callosal connections in visually deprived kittens: a challenging critical period. J. Neurosci., 5, 255-267.

Jhaveri, S., M.A. Edwards, and G.E. Schneider. (1983). Two stages of growth during development of the hamster's optic tract. Anat. Rec., 205, 225A.

Koppel, H., and G.M. Innocenti. (1983). Is there a genuine exuberancy of callosal projections in development? A quantative electron microscopic study in the cat. Neurosci. Lett., 41, 33-40.

Langdon, R.B., J.M. Freeman, and D.O. Frost. (1987) Trajectories and branching patterns of optic tract axons that project transiently to somatosensory thalamus in the neonatal hamster. Soc. Neurosci. Abstr., 13, 1023.

Lehky, S.R., and T.J. Sejnowski. (1988). Network model of shape-from-shading: neural function arises from both receptive and projective fields. Nature, 333, 452-454.

Linsker, R. (1988). Self-organization in a perceptual network. Computer, 21, 105-117.

Metin, C., and D.O. Frost. (1988). Visual responses of neurons in somatosensory cortex of hamsters with experimentally induced retinal projections to somatosensory thalamus. Proc. Natl. Acad. Sci., USA :in press.

Neville, H.J. (1988). Neurobiology of cognitive and language processing: Effects of early experience. In Brain maturation and behavioral development: Biosocial dimensions. (eds. K. Gibson and A.C. Peterson). Aldine Gruyter Press, in press.

Rakic, P., J.-P. Bourgeois, M.F. Eckenhoff, N. Zecevic, and P.S. Goldman-Rakic. (1986)..Concurrent overproduction of synapses in diverse regions of the primate cerebral cortex. Science., 232, 232-235.

Schneider, G.E., S.R. Jhaveri, M.A. Edwards, and K.-.F. So. (1985). Regeneration, rerouting and redistribution of axons after early lesions: Changes with age, and functional impact. In Recent Achievements in Restorative Neurology. Upper Motor Neuron Function and Dysfunction (Adv. Neurol). (eds. M. Dimitrijenc and J. Eccles). Raven Press, New York, pp. 291-310.

Sherman, S.M., and P.D. Spear. (1982). Organization of visual pathways in normal and visually deprived cats. Physiol. Rev., 62, 738-855.

Stent, G.S. (1973). A physiological mechanism for Hebb's postulate of learning. Proc. Natl. Acad. Sci.USA, 70, 997-1001.

Tusa, R.J., L.A. Palmer, and A.C. Rosenquist. (1978). The retinotopic organization of area 17 (striate cortex) in the cat. J. Comp. Neurol., 177, 213-236.

Vidyasagar, T.R. (1987). A model of striate response porperties based on geniculate anisotropies. Biol. Cybern., 57, 11-23.

3
Some Remarks on the Origin of the Phonetic Code

Björn Lindblom

INTRODUCTION: THE ELUSIVE PHONEME

Human languages exhibit **duality** (Hockett 1958) which means that they make combinatorial use of discrete units at two levels of structure: Elements carrying meaning (words, morphemes) are combined to form phrases and sentences according to syntactical rules. Phonemes are combined to form words and morphemes according to phonological rules.

Apparently no other species codes its communicative signals in this combinatorial way. In all languages the building blocks of spoken words are vowel and consonant phonemes. In animal communication systems, on the other hand, meaningful elements cannot be formed by systematic use of discrete units since they lack such units. The signals are Gestalts. Inventories are limited and typically consist of no more than 10-40 holistic patterns (Wilson 1975). By comparison, human vocabularies can become extremely large owing to the combinatorial power of the phonemic principle. Once acquired this "phonetic code" enables the normal child to begin, by its eighteenth month or so, to learn half a dozen new words a day, so that by six years of age it understands seven to eleven thousand phonetic forms, or about ten percent of an adult's vocabulary (Studdert-Kennedy 1983, 1987)

We are thus led to conclude that the property of dual structure is unique to human langauges. It is linguistically universal. And it is the key to their unique expressiveness.

'Slips of the tongue' (spoonerisms and other speech errors) - e g "our queer old dean" for "our dear old queen" - provide strong evidence that the adult language user's production of speech is organized in terms of phonemic segments (Fromkin 1980, MacNeilage,

27

Studdert-Kennedy and Lindblom 1985). Interestingly, 'slips of the hand' are reported to occur in sign language (Klima and Bellugi 1979:126-146). Such facts along with other independent observations confirm the assumption that also sign language uses the method of combining abstract building blocks, i e hand shapes - like phonemes by themselves totally devoid of meaning - to form the complex signs of their vocabularies. Accordingly, duality and the principle of phonemic coding cannot be said to be unique to the vocal-auditory medium (Bellugi and Studdert-Kennedy 1980).

Demonstrably the phonetic code offers an extremely powerful method of coding semantic information. Clearly it would not be possible for a linguist to describe language structure, whether spoken or signed, without the recognition of the phonemic organization of the lexicon. The phoneme represents a major discovery of twentieth-century linguistics (Fischer-Jorgensen 1975).

Yet the phoneme remains elusive to those who study the physical and behavioral aspects of language use. Neither in articulatory movements nor in the speech signal do phonemes appear as beads on a necklace. Their correlates in the signal do not form segments that are sharply delimited along the time axis. And those correlates cannot be unambiguously identified irrespective of context. These difficulties are known as the **segmentation** and **invariance problems** (Perkell and Klatt 1986, Fant 1988, Liberman 1988). Large-scale recognition of human speech by computer still awaits the successful resolution of these classical theoretical issues.

At this point the student of reading would want to intersperse that the **alphabet** which reflects the phonemic segmentation of speech, was developed late in the evolutionary history of language, perhaps no earlier than 3500-4000 years ago. He would also point out that readers tend to vary with respect to their ability to analyze written materials phonologically. Poor readers lack **phonemic awareness** (Liberman 1987, Lundberg, Olofsson and Wall 1980, Lundberg 1987). They have greater difficulties segmenting words into phonemes than good readers.

Accordingly we find that the research interests of those studying speech and those studying reading converge on the baffling but admittedly powerful notion of the phoneme. How could such a complex structure have evolved? The goal of the present paper is to shed some light on that question.

I shall make my presentation in two steps. We begin by first considering how the **phonetic values of phonemes** might have developed. In other words, how do phonetic systems evolve? We then use our tentative

answer to that question to elucidate the origin of the
units themselves? Where did the phonemic principle come
from?

ARTICULATORY AND PERCEPTUAL CONSTRAINTS I: HOW DO
PHONETIC SYSTEMS EVOLVE?

The major dimensions that linguists traditionally
use to describe vowels are: (i) the degree of **rounding**
of the lips and the position of the tongue along (ii) a
front-back and (iii) a **high-low** dimension (Ladefoged
1982). The typological data used in the present paper

FIGURE 1

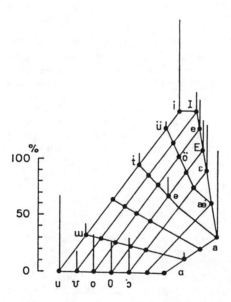

include vowel systems from over 200 languages (Crothers
1978) whose vowel qualities were specified in relation
to a maximal universal set with front, central or back,
rounded or unrounded and seven positions on the high-
low continuum. The most favored inventories are listed
in Table 1.
    Figure 1 shows supplementary data from an
independent investigation of 317 languages (Maddieson

TABLE 1. Most favored vowel systems observed in a corpus of over 200 languages (Crothers 1978).

INVENTORY SIZE	VOWEL QUALITIES	NO OF LG'S
3	i a u	23
4	i a u ɛ	13
4	i a u ɨ	9
5	i a u ɛ ɔ	55
5	i a u ɛ ɨ	5
6	i a u ɛ ɔ ɨ	29
6	i a u ɛ ɔ e	7
7	i a u e o ɨ ə	14
7	i a u ɛ ɔ e o	11
9	i a u ɛ ɔ e o ɨ ə	7

1984). The occurrence of the most frequent symbols have been plotted on a two-dimensional projection of the universal set. Both sources of data converge in demonstrating that only a small subset of the available qualities are brought into play. We further note that there is a clear preference for 'peripheral vowels' such as /i e ɛ a ɔ o u/ and a relative disfavoring of /y o ʌ ɣ ɯ/. Also high-low contrasts are more common than front-back and rounded-unrounded oppositions. These systematic trends represent rather drastic departures from the systems we would generate simply by drawing inventories at random from the maximal set of universal vowel types. How do we explain such patterns?

Here is a brief summary of a theory developed to account for the observed regularities but whose components originally come from several independently motivated research themes. (For an exhaustive description of the research reported in the present and the following sections see Lindblom, MacNeilage and Studdert-Kennedy forthcoming). The theory can be presented in three parts. It provides quantitative definitions of the space of "possible vowels", a constraint on "phonetic discriminability"' and a criterion for selecting the "optimal system".

The point of departure is a physiologically motivated, numerical model (Lindblom and Sundberg 1971) which takes specifications of the position of the jaw, tongue, larynx and the lips as its input and whose output is the shape (area function) of the vocal tract for an arbitrary, but physiologically possible vowel articulation. The acoustic properties of such vocal tract shapes can be ascertained by means of established methods of acoustic theory (Fant 1960). The auditory properties are derived by transforming the acoustic description of a vowel which is given in terms of its harmonic spectrum into an auditory representation. This

last step employs computational models that capture
essential characteristics of the auditory periphery as
revealed by psychoacoustic research (Schroeder, Atal
and Hall 1979). Accordingly, the class of vowels, or
the **vowel space**, generated by this model can be
described in articulatory, acoustic or auditory
dimensions. Since the above-mentioned definitions
quantify general aspects of oral physiology, acoustics
and hearing that are in no way special to speech we can
view the vowel space as a tentative hypothesis about
the a priori range of physical sounds universally
available for the linguistic selection of vowel
contrasts.

The theory analyzes **phonetic discriminability** into
an auditory and a sensori-motor aspect. It can be shown
that it is possible to predict the auditory difference
or distance that a listener assigns to an arbitrary
pair of vowels (Bladon and Lindblom 1981) from

$$AUD_{ij}=c\left(\int_{0}^{24.5} \mid E_i(z)-E_j(z)\mid^2 dz\right)^{1/2} \qquad (1)$$

where c is a constant and $E_i(z)$ and $E_j(z)$ represent
"excitation patterns" calibrated in psychoacoustically
motivated dimensions. The interval $z=0-24.5$, in Bark
units, corresponds to the frequency range of human
hearing (Schroeder, Atal and Hall 1979). There is also
data from experiments using the technique of Direct
Magnitude Estimation (Stevens 1975). These experiments
compared subjects' judgements of movement along the
dimensions of jaw opening and front-back positioning of
the tongue. The DME results indicated that subjectively
jaw movements appeared more extensive than tongue
movements although displacements were equal in terms of
physical measures (Lindblom and Lubker 1985). On the
basis of these findings an articulatory distance
metric, ART_{ij}, was derived for the vowel space
(Lindblom 1986). Taking the product of the articulatory
and the auditory matrices we express phonetic
discriminability as

$$D_{ij} = ART_{ij}*AUD_{ij} \qquad (2)$$

Given the definitions of the space and the
discriminability measure we are in a position to ask:
If vowel systems were seen as evolutionary adaptations
to the idiosyncratic shape of the vowel space and to
selection pressures favoring maximally discriminable
vowel contrasts what would they be like? This question
was addressed in a series of computational experiments
in which **optimal system** was derived by computing:

$$\sum_{i=2}^{k} \sum_{j=1}^{i-1} (1/D_{ij})^2 ----\rightarrow \text{minimized} \qquad (3)$$

TABLE 2.

```
-------OBSERVED----------------------COMPUTED------------
                  INVENTORY SIZE: 3
   i . . . . u                    i . . . . u
    . . . . .                      . . . . .
    . . . .                        . . . .
     . . .                          . . .
       a                              a

       (23)
------------------------------------------------------------
                  INVENTORY SIZE: 4
   i . . . . u                    i . . . . u
    . . . . .                      . . . . .
   ɛ . . .                        ɛ . . .
     . .                            . .
      a                              a

       (13)
------------------------------------------------------------
                  INVENTORY SIZE: 5
   i . . . . u                    i . . . . u
    . . . . .                      . . . . .
   ɛ . . ɔ                        ɛ . . ɔ
     . .                            . .
      a                              a

       (55)
------------------------------------------------------------
                  INVENTORY SIZE: 6
  i . ɨ . . u                    i . . ʉ . u
   . . . . .                      . . . . .
  ɛ . . ɔ                        ɛ . . ɔ
    . .                            . .
     a                              a

       (29)
------------------------------------------------------------
                  INVENTORY SIZE: 7
  i . ɨ . . u                    i . . ʉ . u
   . . . . .                      . . . ʏ .
  ɛ . . ɔ                        ɛ . . .
   . ə .                            . . ɶ
     a                              a

       (14)
------------------------------------------------------------
                  INVENTORY SIZE: 9
  i . ɨ . . u                    i . . ʉ . u
  e . . . o                      e . ə . o
   ɛ . . ɔ                        ɛ . . .
   . ə .                            . . ɶ
     a                              a

       (7)
```

for all possible combinations generated by k=3 through
9 (inventory size) and n=19 (size of universal set).

The results are presented in Table 2. The left column restates the information of Table 1 and is compared with the results of the simulations (right column). In no case does the probability of selecting a correct system by pure chance exceed 10^{-3}. If we make a gross comparison in terms of the number of high-low (vertical) and front-back (horizontal) contrasts there is perfect agreement between the predictions and the data. Looking at the individual qualities we find that certain discrepancies occur in systems with more than six vowels. However, in most cases they are off by no more than a single step on the nineteen-point grid of the universal set.

It appears justified to conclude that the simulations achieve a rather a close agreement with the typological data. Such a result supports the idea that vowel systems can be understood as functional adaptations to articulatory and perceptual constraints.

FIGURE 2

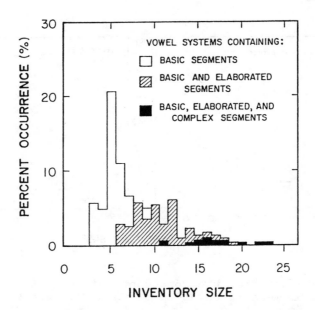

According to the theory presented here the preference for 'peripheral' vowels and the disfavoring of 'interior' vowels originates in an interaction between a "demand" for discriminability on the one hand - which produces a dispersion effect displacing vowels towards the periphery - and the idiosyncratic properties of the vowel space on the other - which leaves more room for high-low contrasts than for front-back and rounding gestures. As we broaden our field of observation the above conclusions tend to be reinforced. The vowel data just examined are limited to systems of so-called 'plain' vowels. Many languages use vowel series that have additional attributes such as apicalization, nasalization, breathy or creaky voice, etc: /iˣ, ẽ, a̤, o̰/ as well as combinations of such additional features: /ãĩ, e̤:/. We classified the vowels of the UPSID database (Maddieson 1984) into those three groups: Basic or plain, Elaborated (with additional features) and Complex (with combinations of elaborated mechanisms). Plotting the distribution of these types as a function of inventory size we obtained the diagram shown in Figure 2. It shows that small systems use Basic segments, medium-sized invoke Basic <u>and</u> Elaborated articulations. Large systems bring all three types into play.

FIGURE 3

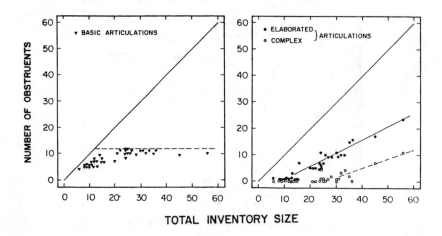

TOTAL INVENTORY SIZE

We classified the consonants of UPSID in a similar manner. Segments such as /p t b d m .../ are treated as Basic; /pʲ t' ɓ ⁿd m̥ .../ represent Elaborated gestures; Articulations that combine Elaborated mechanisms are Complex: /tɬʰ qʷ gc d̤ .../. Examining the occurrence of these consonant categories as a function of inventory size we find patterns closely paralleling those for vowels. Figure 3 presents a representative subset of the UPSID corpus showing data from 47 languages of the Afro-Asiatic and the Indo-Pacific language groups. Each data point refers to a

given language. **The left diagram shows the number of
Basic obstruents as a function of total system size.
The right panel indicates the number of Elaborated and
Complex obstruents as a function of total system size.**
Once more we see that small systems have Basic
articulations, medium systems have Basic **and** Elaborated
gestures and large systems have all three types. Also
note the saturation of Basic elements beyond a certain
system size and the lawful linear growth of the
Elaborated and Complex data.

Our analysis indicates that knowing the size of a
vowel or consonant inventory we can make some fairly
good predictions about its phonetic contents. The
motorically most elaborated and complex phonetic
gestures (e g clicks, vowels simultaneously
diphthongized and pharyngealized etc) are likely to
occur in the largest inventories (as in !Xũ of the
Kalahari desert with its 148 segments) whereas small
systems (n<10, e g Maori and Hawaiian) would not be
expected to contain such sounds but to favor elementary
articulations (p, t, m, e, a etc). This **Size Principle**
makes sense if we assume that in small inventories
Basic articulations achieve sufficient contrast whereas
larger systems place greater demands for intrasystemic
distinctiveness and therefore cause additional
dimensions to be recruited and to be combined to form
more complex segments.

ARTICULATORY AND PERCEPTUAL CONSTRAINTS II: WHERE DOES
THE PHONEMIC PRINCIPLE COME FROM?

In the preceding sections we have argued that the
phonetic values that vowels and consonants exhibit have
evolved in response to universal, non-linguistic
articulatory and perceptual constraints. Let us now see
whether these constraints could have played a role also
in the emergence of the discrete **units** themselves.

Our discussion will be based on a computational
experiment in which we simulate the phonetic growth of
a small vocabulary, a minilexicon. The design of the
experiment is closely analogous to the vowel system
simulations. The point of departure is again the
articulatory model (Lindblom and Sundberg 1971). We use
it to generate a phonetic space consisting in this case
of a set of "possible syllables". A possible syllable
is of fixed duration and is represented as a continuous
trajectory in phonetic space moving from a complete
closure of the vocal tract (whose location ranges from
labial through dental, alveolar, retroflex to palatal,
velar and uvular points of articulation) to an open
configuration. The open configurations are those of the

previously described cardinal vowel set. Figure 4 gives
an example of such a transition with a stylized
frequency-time formant pattern at the top and its
representation in a three-dimensional formant space
below.

The phonetic discriminability of an arbitrary pair
of trajectories was obtained by generalizing the
procedures applied to vowels to the time domain, that

FIGURE 4

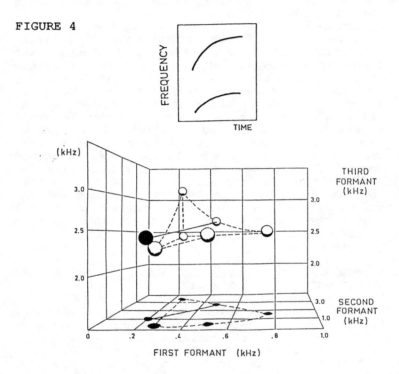

is by representing them as a series of discrete spectra
in time, calculating Eqs 1-3 for each time sample and
then deriving the discriminability measure as the
square root of the sum of the individual samples
squared (cf Eq 3).

Since the reduction phenomena and articulatory
simplifications of on-line speech can in most cases be
explained satisfactorily in elementary biomechanical
terms by representing articulators by damped spring-
mass systems (Lindblom 1983) a rank ordering of every
possible syllable based on articulatory criteria was
also attempted. Such a biomechanical analysis makes us

expect that extreme positions (extreme displacements from habitual rest) and extreme movement rates tend, if possible, to be avoided. That is a fact richly supported by phonetic observations (Lindblom 1983). There is room for only a few examples: Syllables with labial and dental occlusions receive high ranks. They have near-neutral points of closure (cf their high frequency in babbling) whereas a transition with a retracted tongue tip, a retroflex closure, represents a more extreme departure from neutral. The penalty on extreme movement rates leads to a favoring of homorganic, assimilated sequences. Thus a trajectory consisting of a uvular closure followed by a palatal (high-front) open configuration gets a lower score than say a palatal (velar) closure followed by a palatal (velar) open configuration.

Pursuing the analogy with the vowel system simulations further we investigated "optimal systems" of syllables by computing

$$\sum_{i=2}^{k} \sum_{j=1}^{i-1} (a_{ij}/d_{ij})^2 \longrightarrow \text{minimized} \qquad (4)$$

where d_{ij} is the discriminability of an arbitrary transition pair and a_{ij} the articulatory cost of that pair. In words: Find that set of k syllables that simultaneously satisfy the goal of being as easy as possible to say (minimal articulatory cost) and as easy as possible to hear (maximal discriminability). In the present case k=15 and the total inventory was 133. A procedure of cumulative selection was adopted.

TABLE 3

bi	bɛ	ba	bɔ	bu
di	dɛ	da	dɔ	du
gi	gɛ	ga	gɨ	gu

Once an initial syllable had been selected Eq 4 was applied repeatedly until a minilexicon of 15 elements had been obtained. In all there were 133 runs (=initial syllables). The results were pooled which yielded a total of 1995 syllables. The "optimal system" was defined as the 15 forms with the highest frequency in this pooled set. The results are presented in Table 3.

The most significant aspect of this table emerges
when, examining it row by row and column by column, we
observe that trajectory onsets and end-points are
shared. Rows and columns appear to contain
whatlinguists would call "minimal pairs". Why not a
more diverse set of closures and open configurations?

FIGURE 5

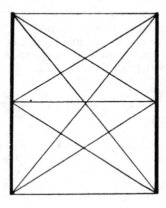

Perhaps the easiest way of obtaining an intuitive
grasp of the causes of the combinatorial structure of
the derived inventory is to invoke a simple geometrical
metaphor. Suppose we consider two vertical line
segments and the task of drawing k lines (trajectories)
from anywhere on the left segment to anywhere on the
right in such away that the area, A, between any pair
of lines will be as large as possible. Mathematically,

$$\sum_{i=2}^{k} \sum_{j=1}^{i-1} (1/A_{ij})^2 \longrightarrow \text{minimized} \qquad (5)$$

Cf Eqs 3 and 4. Figure 5 shows the result for k=9. We
see that trajectory onsets and end-points are shared.
The phonetic space of the simulations is clearly much
more complex but our point is that the convergence of
trajectories in the geometrical exercise is analogous
to the convergence of the optimized phonetic
transitions. The combinatorial pattern appears to be a
consequence of achieving an efficient packing (read:
optimal discrimination) within a bounded space. It can
be shown that the a_{ij} matrix does not influence the
degree combinatorial coding in any major way but it

does play an important role determining the phonetic
values of the derived syllables.

        Suppose we presented Table 3 to a linguist as a
sample from the vocabulary of an unknown language
implying that the forms have different meaning but
being very careful so as not to reveal that they had
been produced as unanalyzed wholes. Undoubtedly he
would note that the table contains numerous minimal
pairs. Assuming that the lexical items are semantically
distinct and following standard linguistic methodology
he would hypothesize that the language in question uses
three consonant phonemes and five vowel phonemes the
minimally contrastive segments being /b d g/ and /i   a
ɛ   ɔ   u/.

FIGURE 6

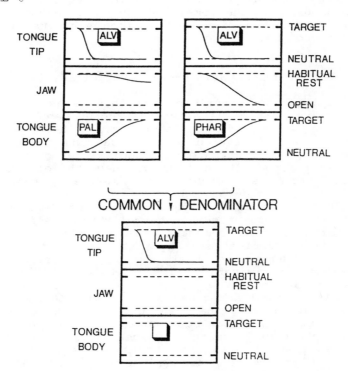

How do we resolve this paradox? For remember: The
syllables are by definition specified as continuous
transitions, as phonetic Gestalts. Their production is
no more segmentally organized than the early
vocalizations of the babbling child. Cf top panels of
Figure 6. Nevertheless, we transcribe such utterances
using segments. Accordingly our use of segments in

Table 3 should be seen as a mere convenience analogous
to the conventional way of describing the phonetic
behavior of the young child.

However, a "phonemic principle" is nevertheless
implicitly present in the derived lexicon since the
existence of minimal pairs implies gestural overlap
among motor scores. This is the point we try to make in
Figure 6 which shows the motor scores of two syllables,
call them /di/ and /da/. The jaw and tongue body time
functions differ whereas the tongue tip curves are
identical. This overlap identifies a common denominator
component. Note that its contents is in a one-to-one
relation with all words linguistically analyzed as
beginning with the phoneme /d/. Were we to examine the
rest of the motor scores of the derived syllables in
the same manner we would obtain analogous common
denominators for the remaining "phonemic segments". We
conclude that the simulated lexicon exhibits **implicit
phonemic coding**.

CONCLUSIONS: THE ELUSIVE PHONEME REVISITED

We began by describing the phoneme as a powerful
but elusive unit of linguistic structure and by asking
how such a complex structure could have evolved.
Although our simulations of lexical growth no doubt
drastically underestimate the complexities of real-life
vocabulary acquisition let us nevertheless briefly
examine what we might have learned from these
preliminary considerations.

The main finding appears to be the demonstration
of the beginnings of **combinatorial structure** in speech-
like signals. The computational experiments tell us
that such combinatorial patterns can arise from
phonetic constraints that favor the selection of
optimally discriminable stimuli. Recall that we first
inferred the presence of such constraints from our
analyses of vowel and consonant systems. In the present
context we have emphasized the role of perceptual
aspects but other factors should also be considered,
for instance learning. Conceivably, articulatory
gestures that a child has already mastered might make
new syllbles also containing those gestures easier to
acquire than totally novel materials. Work now in
progress indicates that such a mechanism would
reinforce the trend towards combinatorial coding even
further and extend it to much larger lexica than the
ones considered here.

Examining the motor scores of the derived
syllables we found gestural components that can be said
to be in a one-to-one relation with phonemic segments.

Note that these subcomponents are not explicit control units in the production process. They are hidden or only implicitly present in the holistic motor scores of the individual words of the lexicon. Making them explicit in the model, that is **turning them into explicit control units is possible but requires additional processing.**

I would like to consider briefly this notion of implicit phonemic coding in the context of reading. Poor readers are reported to lack phonemic awareness. They have greater difficulties processing words phonologically than good readers. Similarly, it has been shown that illiterates score badly on tests involving phonemic segmentation tasks (Morais, Cluyens, Alegria 1984). Phonemic awareness does not seem to develop spontaneously during their language acquisition (Morais, Cary, Alegria and Bertelson 1979). A novel view of the phoneme seems to be emerging out of the present work, namely that the elusive nature of the phoneme - manifest in reading behavior as well as in many other aspects of language use - is related to the fact that the phoneme has implicit rather than explicit status in the mental lexica of language users.

Finally a few remarks on speech development. Psycholinguists assume that unless a child, as it were, "discovers the phoneme" as the building block of the lexicon it will not be able to develop a vocabulary of normal large size. In the computational experiments I have reported the "phoneme" is **not discovered.** Rather minimal pairs identify nodes of "gestural overlap". The notion of gestural overlap may have several interesting consequences worth exploring in future research. It may be an important factor in further learning. Moreover, since by definition overlapping motor scores refer to shared subcomponents of the motor scores they ought to take up less memory space than holistic patterns which require separate individual storage. The simulated phoneme is accordingly not the cause of a large vocabulary. It is the result of the vocabulary growth. It is an emergent consequence of lexical development. The process is automatic. It occurs in a completely self-organizing way as it seems to do in the normal child.

On this view then the reasons why other species lack phonemic organization may have less to do with their ability to produce and receive signals efficiently* than with absence of an urge to communicate and form large vocabularies.

---

* For a different view cf the scenario of Lieberman (1985).

REFERENCES

Bellugi, U and Studdert-Kennedy, M (1980). Signed and Spoken Language: Biological Constraints on Linguistic Form, Deerfield Park, Florida:Verlag Chemie.

Bladon, R A W and Lindblom, B (1981). "Modeling the Judgement of Vowel Quality Differences", J Acoust Soc Am 69:1414-1422.

Crothers, J (1978). "Typology and Universals of Vowel Systems", In: Greenberg, J H, Ferguson, C A and Moravcsik, E A (eds): Universals of Human Language, Vol 2, 99-152, Stanford:Stanford University Press.

Fant, G (1960). The Acoustic Theory of Speech Production, The Hague:Mouton.

Fant, G (1988). "The Speech Code", this volume.

Fischer-Jørgensen E (1975). Trends in Phonological Theory, Copenhagen:Akademisk Forlag.

Fromkin, V A (1980). Errors of Linguistic Performance, New York:Academic Press.

Hockett, C (1958). A Course in Modern Linguistics, New York:MacMillan.

Jakobson, R and Waugh, L (1979). The Sound Shape of Language, Bloomington and London:Indiana University Press.

Klima, E S and Bellugi, U (1979). The Signs of Language, Cambridge, MA:Harvard University Press.

Ladefoged, P (1982). A Course in Phonetics, 2nd ed, New York:Harcourt, Brace and Jovanovich.

Liberman I Y (1987). "Language and Literacy: The Obligation of the Schools of Education", 1-9 in Intimacy with Language, Proceedings of the Orton Dyslexia Society Symposium, Baltimore: Maryland:The Orton Dyslexia Society.

Liberman A M (1988). "Reading is Hard Just Because Listening is Easy", this volume.

Lieberman, P (1985). The Biology and Evolution of Language, Cambridge, MA:Harvard University Press.

Lindblom, B (1983). "Economy of Speech Gestures", 217-245 in MacNeilage, P F (ed): The Production of Speech, New York:Springer Verlag.

Lindblom, B (1986). "Phonetic Universals in Vowel Systems", 13-44 in Ohala, J J and Jaeger, J J (eds): Experimental Phonology, Orlando, Fl:Academic Press.

Lindblom, B (in press). "A Model of Phonetic Variation and Selection and the Evolution of Vowel Systems", to appear in Wang, S-Y (ed): Language Transmission and Change, New York:Blackwell.

Lindblom B, and Sundberg, J (1971). "Acoustical Consequences of Lip, Tongue, Jaw and Larynx Movement", J Acoust Soc Am 50(4):1166-1179.

Lindblom B and Lubker J (1985). "The Speech Homunculus and a Problem of Phonetic Linguistics", 169-192 in V A Fromkin (ed): Phonetic Linguistics, Orlando, Fl:Academic Press.

Lindblom B, MacNeilage P and Studdert-Kennedy M (forthcoming). Evolution of Spoken Language, Orlando, FL:Academic Press.

Lundberg I, Olofsson, A and Wall, S (1980). "Reading and Spelling Skills in the First School Years Predicted from Phonemic Awareness Skills in Kindergarten", Scandinavian Journal of Psychology 21:159-173.

Lundberg I (1987). "Phonologcal Awareness Facilitates Reading and Spelling Acquisition", 56-63 in Intimacy with Language, Proceedings of the Orton Dyslexia Society Symposium, Baltimore: Maryland:The Orton Dyslexia Society.

MacNeilage, P F, Studdert-Kennedy, M and Lindblom, B (1985). "Planning and Production of Speech: An Overview", in Lauter, J (ed): Planning and Production of Speech by Normally Hearing and Deaf People, ASHA reports.

Maddieson, I (1984). Patterns of Sound, Cambridge:Cambridge University Press.

Morais, J, Cary, L, Alegria, J and Bertelson, P (1979).
     "Does Awareness of Speech as a Sequence of
     Phonemes Arise Spontaneously?", Cognition
     7:323-331.

Morais, J, Cluyens, M and Alegria, J (1984).
     "Segmentation Abilities of Dyslexics and
     Normal Readers", Perceptual and Motor Skills
     58:221-222.

Perkell, J and Klatt, D (1986). Invariance and
     Variability in Speech Processes, Hillsdale, N
     J:LEA.

Schroeder, M R, Atal,B S and Hall, J L (1979).
     "Objective Measure of Certain Speech Signal
     Degradations Based on Masking Properties of
     Human Auditory Perception", 217-229 in
     Lindblom, B and Öhman, S (eds): Frontiers of
     Speech Communication Research,
     London:Academic Press.

Stevens, S S (1975). Psychophysics, New York:Wiley.

Studdert-Kennedy, M (1983). "On Learning to Speak",
     Human Neurobiology 2:191-195.

Studdert-Kennedy, M (1987). "The Phoneme as a
     Perceptuomotor Structure", 67-83 in Allport,
     A, MacKay, D, Prinz, W and Scheerer, E (eds):
     Language Perception and Production,
     London:Academic Press.

Wilson, E O (1975). Sociobiology: The New Synthesis,
     Cambridge, MA: Belknap Press.

II
Hemispheric Specializations and Interactions

4
Some Brain Mechanisms for Reading

George A. Ojemann

INTRODUCTION

The importance of lateral perisylvian neocortex of the left
hemisphere in language is well established. That role was
initially defined from observations of aphasias following lesions
there (Broca, 1861; Wernicke, 1874). The deficits following
those lesions, both receptive and expressive, involved reading
and writing, as well as oral language. Subsequently, Penfield
and his associates developed a technique for localizing language
in individual patients during neurosurgical operations under
local anesthesia, using electrical stimulation mapping (Penfield
and Roberts, 1959). Penfield used object naming as the measure
of language. He inferred that the sites where naming was altered
by stimulation identified the essential areas for language
because of their congruence with the sites where lesions produced
aphasia. Later, Ojemann and Dodrill demonstrated that when an
anterior temporal resection for epilepsy encroached on sites with
evoked naming changes, a postoperative increase in many types of
errors on a language test battery occurred that was not present
when the resection margin spared those sites, and could not be
accounted for by the size of the resection, preoperative language
facility or seizure control (Ojemann, 1983). Thus, both
stimulation mapping and lesions seemed to identify the same
cortical areas as essential for language.

Ojemann and his associates then extended this technique to
the localization of essential areas for other language functions,
including naming in multiple languages and reading of simple
sentences, as well as recent verbal memory (Ojemann and Whitaker,
1978a; Ojemann and Mateer, 1979; Ojemann, 1983; Ojemann and
Dodrill, 1985). The first part of the present paper is an
extension of one of those studies, examining the localization of
left lateral perisylvian neocortical sites essential for reading
of simple sentences in 55 patients, establishing the variability

47

in that localization, patient characteristics correlating with
the variability, and contrasting this with the localization and
variability in sites essential for object naming in the same
patients.

Lesions and stimulation identify essential areas for a
function, for the link between a brain area and a behavior is
made only when the behavior fails. Metabolic studies such as
Positron Emission Tomography (PET) or blood flow measures, and
physiologic studies, including electrocorticographic (ECoG) and
single neuron recordings, provide a different type of
information, indicating where neurons change activity with a
behavior, and thus participate in it, but are not necessarily
essential for the behavior. The second part of this paper
reports changes in neuronal activity related to reading of
words, activity recorded from anterior temporal lobe during
neurosurgical procedures under local anesthesia, as part of an
investigation of changes in cortical neuronal activity during
naming, reading and recent verbal memory (Ojemann et al, 1988).
Combining these findings with those from the different
perspective provided by stimulation mapping provides some
insights into the neurobiologic mechanisms underlying reading and
dyslexia.

LOCALIZATION OF SITES ESSENTIAL FOR READING

Methods

These observations were made in 55 patients undergoing left
fronto-temporal-parietal craniotomies under local anesthesia for
the treatment of intractable epilepsy. In 9 patients the
epilepsy was associated with an adult acquired lesion (8
gliomas). Twenty patients were male. Mean age was 28 years
(range 16-55). All were known to have language function in the
left cerebral hemisphere. In 5 there was evidence from
intracarotid amytal testing that there was also some language
function on the right. Preoperative verbal IQ (VIQ) assessment
was available for 52 patients. Mean WAIS VIQ was 99 (Range 126-
81).

Following ECoG, the location of Rolandic cortex and areas
essential for language, based on evoked changes in object naming,
were identified as part of the standard clinical procedure, using
previously described electrical stimulation mapping techniques
(Ojemann, 1983). Then, with the patient's consent, based on
prior review by the University of Washington Institutional Review
Board, the effect of stimulation on reading of single sentences
was assessed at 3-19 (Mean 8.9) of the sites where effects on
naming had been measured. A single sentence was shown on a

monochrome slide, with the patient previously trained to read it
aloud. The patients included in this study were operated on over
an eight-year period. In that time, three different sets of
sentences were used. Each set included single sentences of 8-10
words. Stimulation used trains of 60 Hz 1 msec duration biphasic
square wave pulses delivered in a bipolar manner through
electrodes separated by 5 mm. Trains lasted the duration of time
that a slide with a single sentence was shown, 8-12 secs, with a
uniform time for each sentence set and patient. The stimulation
current was just below the threshold for evoking afterdischarge
in the sampled area of cortex, and was uniform for each patient,
but ranged from 1.5 to 10 mA, measured between peaks of the
biphasic pulse. At least three samples of stimulation effect on
sentence reading were obtained for each site, with interspersed
trials without stimulation providing a measure of nonstimulation
control performance. Error rates on these control trials varied
from 0 to 41% (Mean 9.5%). Sites of stimulation were recorded
photographically.

Performance on sentence reading was analyzed from audio
tapes containing the patient responses and marks for changing of
slides and stimulation. Only major mistakes in sentence reading
were counted as errors: failure to substantially complete
reading the sentence, omission of words or endings, or production
of wrong words or word forms. More subtle changes, such as
alterations in prosody, were not evaluated. Criteria for errors
were explicitly developed for each set of sentences and were
uniform for any one patient, but probably varied some between
patients tested years apart. However, with the analysis spread
over many years, scoring was completely blind to the conclusions
presented in the following section. A site was considered
essential for sentence reading if the error rate evoked by
stimulation exceeded the control error rate with a single sample
binomial probability of .05 or less. Performance during sentence
reading was compared to that during object naming with
stimulation of the same sites and currents. Statistical analysis
of the relation between localization of area essential for
reading and patient characteristics used Fisher's Exact, Chi-
Square or Mann-Whitney U Statistical Test (Seigel, 1956).

Results

Stimulation evoked errors in naming at some site in all
patients. Errors in sentence reading were evoked at 25.5% of the
479 sites where stimulation effects on both naming and reading
were assessed, with at least one site with significant evoked
reading errors in 41 of the 55 patients. This effect could be
quite localized, with sites within 1-1.5 cm showing no evoked
changes in reading. This pattern is similar to that previously
reported by us for sites essential for object naming (Ojemann,

1983). However, essential areas for reading often extended over
a wider area than those for naming (Fig. 1).

    At 52% of the sites with evoked changes in sentence reading,
naming was also significantly altered. These sites, then, would
seem to be essential for some general language function. The
remaining sites with evoked reading changes had intact naming,
suggesting a role more specific to reading, while 11% of sites
without reading changes had significant evoked changes in naming,
suggesting that these sites had a specific role in naming. This
separation of sites essential for naming or sentence reading is
evident in the patient illustrated in Fig. 1.

    Figure 2 demonstrates the individual variability in the
location of these three types of sites in left lateral
perisylvian cortex of the 55 patients. A substantial degree of
individual variability in the location of these sites is evident.
Similar variability for sites essential for naming has been
reported (Ojemann and Whitaker, 1978b; Ojemann, 1983).   Sites
essential for both naming and reading seem to cluster in the
classical posterior inferior frontal "Broca" area and to a lesser
extent, in the posterior superior temporal "Wernicke" area.
Sites related to reading alone extended more widely in frontal
cortex.   In the posterior language area, sites essential for
naming alone predominated in zones immediately surrounding the
posterior superior temporal zone with the largest proportion of
sites related to both reading and naming, while sites related to
reading alone were located in more distant zones especially in
more anterior superior temporal gyrus and inferior parietal
operculum.   Of interest is that no reading or naming errors were
evoked with stimulation of sites in angular gyrus.

    Correlations were sought between several different patient
characteristics and the pattern of localization of sites
essential for naming and/or reading. A rather complex
relationship to preoperative verbal   performance, as measured by
the VIQ was found in posterior language cortex.   This
relationship was most clearly   defined by comparing the 20
patients (10 male) with lowest VIQ's (81-93), to the 20 patients
(9 male) with highest VIQ's (99-126), pooling posterior language
sites in these patients into four regions: parietal, anterior
superior temporal, posterior superior temporal and posterior
middle temporal.   Total number of temporal or parietal regions
with evoked naming and/or reading errors differed little between
these two groups (errors evoked in 52% of sampled regions in high
VIQ group compared to 59% in low VIQ group).   However, regions
with only naming errors were suggestively (p < .1) more frequent
in the patients with low VIQ's (27% of those regions, compared to
14% in high VIQ group), while the high VIQ group had slightly
more regions with only reading errors (24% low vs. 29% high). In
particular, patients with lower VIQ's had sites essential for

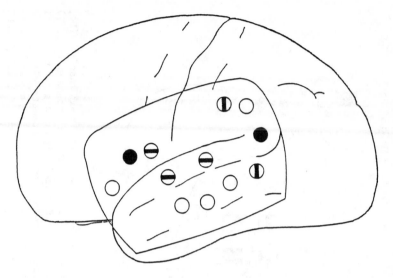

Fig. 1.   Location of left lateral perisylvian sites where
significant errors in naming and/or sentence reading were evoked
during stimulation mapping at 6 mA (between biphasic pulse
peaks), in a 33 year old female with VIQ of 108.   Filled circle –
significant errors in both naming and reading.   Circle with
vertical line – errors in only naming.   Circle with horizontal
line – errors in only reading.   Open circles – no errors.
Control error rates: naming 9.4%; reading 8.8%.

naming alone in superior temporal gyrus, and sites essential for
reading alone in middle temporal gyrus.   The reverse pattern was
present for patients with high VIQ's: sites for reading alone
were in superior temporal gyri and those for naming alone in
middle temporal gyrus.   Fig. 1 is an example.   This complete
pattern was present in 3 of the 20 low VIQ patients and 4 of the
20 patients with high VIQ, with no patients having the reverse
pattern (p<.05, Fisher's Exact Test).   Either the reading alone
or naming alone   halves of the pattern were present for 12
patients with low VIQ's and 10 with high, with 1 and 3 patients
respectively having sites essential for reading alone or naming
alone in the location not predicted by this pattern (p<.005,
Fisher's Exact Test).   The failure to identify the complete
pattern in more patients is most likely due to limited sampling
of cortical areas, a consequence of the time constraints on the
experimental study.   The only relationship between VIQ and site
in posterior language cortex with both naming and reading chan
was a suggestive excess of the few of those sites in par
cortex in patients with low VIQ's.   No differences ba

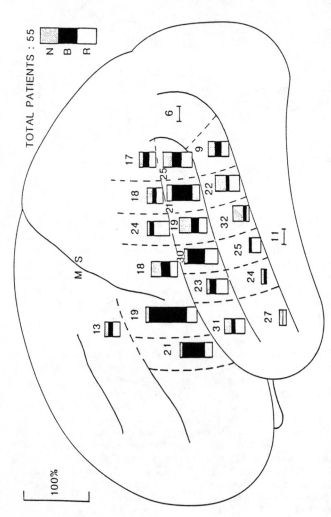

Fig. 2. Individual variability in location of stimulation evoked changes in naming (N), sentence reading (R) or both (B) in the 55 patients of this study. Individual patient maps (Fig. 1) were aligned by motor cortex and end of Sylvian fissure, and sites of stimulation assigned to one of the zones indicated by dashed lines. In each zone is indicated the number of patients with one or more sites in that zone (usually one), and a bar showing the percentage of those sites with significant evoked errors in only naming (stippled), only reading (open) or both (filled). 100% scale for bars is at left above.

patient's age, presence of an acquired or early life lesion, presence or absence of some speech function in the contralateral hemisphere, or sex were apparent in this series. However, in a larger series of 117 patients (that included the present cases) with only assessment of stimulation effect on naming, a sex difference was apparent. For patients with low, but not high VIQ's, males were significantly more likely than females to have parietal sites essential for naming (G. Ojemann et al — forthcoming). In that larger series, the relation between low VIQ and superior temporal gyrus location of sites essential for naming was also clearly shown and the relation between higher VIQ's and middle temporal location of naming sites suggestively present.

LOCATION OF CHANGES IN NEURONAL ACTIVITY RELATED TO READING

Methods

     These data are from the study of Ojemann et al (1988) and represent findings in 17 neuronal populations recorded from left lateral temporal cortex of 13 patients, during craniotomies under local anesthesia. Because of the invasive nature of microelectrodes, recordings were confined to sites in cortex that was subsequently excised as part of the therapeutic resection. However, recordings were made in that portion of the planned resection with the least epileptic activity in the ECoG, and the neuronal populations included in this analysis evidenced little or no burst firings of the kind described for human epileptic neurons (Calvin et al, 1973). Once stable recordings without evidence of injury discharge were obtained, the patients engaged in multiple trials of several tasks where the same visual cues were used for silent reading of words pairs, the same type of silent reading as part of a recent verbal memory measure, and in a spatial matching task. Spatial matching is a function related to the nondominant hemisphere (Benton et al, 1975) and thus served as a behavioral control. In other blocks of trials, a different set of visual cues was used to assess changes in activity with silent naming alone, silent naming as part of a recent memory measure, and a spatial matching task. The detail of those tasks are illustrated in Ojemann et al (1988). In them, the visual cues for reading or naming were shown for 4 sec. Activity recorded during each cue was divided into 3 epochs of 1.2 sec each, and the difference in activity in the analogous (first, second or third) epochs where the same visual cue was used in the different behavioral conditions analyzed statistically. Activity was related to reading or naming when there were significant changes with silent reading or naming both alone and when part of the memory measure, compared to activity in the analogous epoch of the spatial task. Subsequent to the

recording, surface electrical stimulation mapping of the
recording site indicated whether it was essential for naming or
reading.

Results

Changes in activity related to reading were identified in 6
of the 17 neuronal populations. Two of these populations also
showed changes with naming. No population showed only naming
changes. These recordings were obtained at sites that did not
show evoked changes in naming or reading, and no changes in those
functions followed excision of the sites. Thus, these neuronal
populations related to naming and/or reading were recorded at
sites that were not essential for those functions.

In most cases the change in activity related to reading was
an increase throughout all three epochs of reading, suggesting
that this represented a sustained, tonic change in activity with
the process of reading. Figure 3 illustrates two examples. Only
two neuronal populations showed significant greater activity in
the earliest epochs compared to later epochs. Since reading is
completed before the end of the second epoch, these populations
would seem to be related more closely to reading of the specific
words, rather than to the more general change of selective
attention to the reading process identified in the other neuronal
populations. Changes related to naming were also all of the
sustained type suggesting mechanisms of selective attention. No
changes of an inhibitory nature related to naming or reading were
identified in these neuronal populations.

DISCUSSION

Essential areas for sentence reading identified in
individual patients of this study were often localized to one or
more cortical surface areas of 1-2 sq. cms. often with at least
one site in posterior inferior frontal cortex and one or more in
temporoparietal cortex. Approximately half the time these sites
were not essential for naming. When the localization of these
sites is compared across patients, substantial individual
variability is seen. Only the posterior inferior frontal zone,
immediately in front of face motor cortex was essential for
reading in most patients. Elsewhere, including all of posterior
language cortex, no zone had sites essential for reading in over
half of the subjects.

These findings, of discrete localization in individual
patients, different functions often with different essential
sites and substantial individual variation are similar to those
previously reported by us for perisylvian cortex when
stimulation effect for only naming were assessed   (Ojemann and

Whitaker, 1978b; Ojemann, 1979; Ojemann, 1983; G. Ojemann et al, - forthcoming). The same effects were also seen in smaller series with assessment of effect on multiple language functions including sentence reading (Ojemann and Mateer, 1979; Ojemann, 1983) and assessment of recent verbal memory (Ojemann and Dodrill, 1985). Thus, these features seem to be general properties of localization of essential areas for higher human function in this cortical region.

When the zones that are most often essential for naming or sentence reading in the total population are compared, it is apparent that essential areas for reading occupy a wider area than that for naming (Fig. 2). This is also evident in individual patients (Fig. 1). Moreover, more neuronal populations (in non-essential areas) showed change with word reading than with naming. Together these findings indicate that a larger area of cortex must be active with reading than with naming, regardless of whether the measure is the extent of participatory or essential areas, or a simple or more complex reading task. A widespread generalized partial dysfunction of lateral perisylvian cortex, then, as might occur in dyslexia, would interfere much more with reading than naming.

There seems to be a general pattern to zones where naming or reading changes are likely to be found. Zones with a high proportion of sites with changes in both language measures occupy the traditional Broca and Wernicke areas. Extending centripedally from these zones in posterior language cortex are zones with predominately sites for naming alone, and then further away, zones with only reading. As previously noted for a smaller patient series (Ojemann, 1983), zones where only naming changes predominate correspond well to the region where Benson (1975) localized lesions producing anomic aphasia - where the deficit is only in naming. The present study did not examine the detailed nature of evoked reading errors, but in an earlier study of detailed reading errors in a smaller subset of these patients, zones with only evoked reading changes often had a unique error type involving the sentence syntax (Ojemann, 1983).

The area of cortex where neurons participate in reading, as judged by changes in activity during reading tasks, is much larger than the area essential for reading. Similar differences in size of participatory and essential areas were found for naming and recent verbal memory (Ojemann et al, 1988). Within the participating area, neuronal populations often show a sustained, tonic increase in activity, a change suggestive of mechanisms of selective attention (Fig.3). Physiologic features that differentiate essential from participatory areas for reading are presently unknown, but more intense desynchronization of the ECoG recorded during naming differentiates sites essential for naming from surrounding temporoparietal cortex containing neuronal

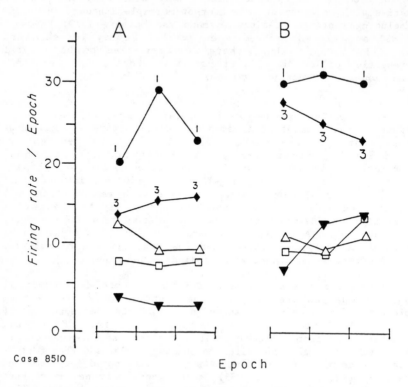

Case 8510

Fig. 3   Frequency of activity in two neuronal populations recorded during separate behavioral assessments, and at different depths (A–2 mm, B–4 mm) but at the same site in left posterior middle temporal gyrus, of a 27 year old female with VIQ of 94, during three successive 1.2 sec epochs when the same visual cues were used for silent word reading alone (filled diamonds), silent word reading as part of a recent verbal memory task (filled circles), and a silent spatial matching task (filled triangles). For comparison, activity recorded from the same population during a different set of visual cues used for silent object naming alone (open triangles) and a silent spatial matching task (open squares) is also shown.   Numbers indicate statistically significant differences in that epoch: 1 – between silent reading as part of the memory task and the spatial task using the same cues; 3 – between silent reading alone and the spatial task.

populations participating in naming (Fried et al, 1981).   This
suggests even more intense activity of mechanism of selective
alerting-attention at essential sites.   These attentional
mechanisms, then, seem to have a major role in the neocortical
physiologic events occurring during language.   Other neuronal
populations demonstrate briefer changes in activity that have
closer temporal relationships to specific language acts,
including perception and expression of speech (Creutzfeldt et al
1987 and this volume), and occasionally word reading (Ojemann et
al 1988). Whether this activity is superimposed on tonic changes
of selective attention, or the temporally related and tonic
changes are characteristics of separate neuronal populations
participating in a language function is presently unknown.

    Of particular interest to the study of dyslexia is the
finding here of a relation between patterns of localization of
essential areas for reading or naming in temporal lobe and
overall verbal performance, as measured by the VIQ.   This
indicates that different neurobiological organizations are
associated with different levels of language ability,   further
evidence that a different brain organization likely underlies
some cases of dyslexia.   The present study indicates that one
location for this difference is temporal neocortex.   The nature
of the difference is puzzling: essential areas for only reading
in superior temporal gyrus and only naming in middle gyrus as a
favorable pattern and the reverse as unfavorable.   This occurs in
a setting where the full extent of essential posterior language
cortex, and of the part of that cortex essential for both naming
and reading are the same for patients with high or low VIQ's.
The area essential for naming alone, however, is suggestively
larger in the low VIQ group.   Independent evidence that the
essential areas for naming may occupy less area when there is
greater facility with a language comes from localization of
naming sites in bilingual patients (Ojemann and Whitaker, 1978a;
Ojemann, 1983).   In those patients, there was a suggestion that
the area essential for naming in the language for which there was
greater competence was smaller (and often at least partly
separated from) the area essential for a language for which there
was lesser facility, even though the actual items used to
determine size of essential areas were named with equal facility
in both languages.   This finding suggests that differences in
size of essential areas may not just reflect the underlying
neuronal substrate. One consequence of having to commit a larger
proportion of a finite essential area for language as essential
for naming may well be that there are not enough neuronal
circuits remaining to adequately subserve the later acquired
language skills such as reading. Whether essential areas shrink
as facility in a language is acquired is unknown, although that
is one interpretation of the difference in size related to
facility in multiple language.   If essential areas do shrink,
this could explain the later acquisition of reading (into areas

formerly essential for naming) in language disabled patients, as
sufficient neuronal circuits to support reading become available.

However, the relation of the pattern of localization to
facile language function is not just one of size of essential
areas, but also involves specific locations for areas related to
reading or naming alone. One theoretical basis for part of this
finding can be derived from several other observations: the
essential role of phonemic awareness in effective reading (Olsen,
Lundberg, this volume), the dependence of phonemic awareness on
a system that links phonemic detection and expression (Liberman
et al, 1967 and this volume) and the demonstration of sites in
superior temporal gyrus that are essential for both phoneme
identification and sequential orofacial speech gestures (Ojemann
and Mateer 1979; Ojemann, 1983). Phonemic awareness in reading,
then, may depend on localization of reading in superior temporal
gyrus adjacent to this common superior temporal cortex for
phoneme identification and speech sound generation. Why sites
essential for naming occupy this location in those with poor
verbal skills remains obscure. Defining differences in the
specific connections of these cortical areas and the activity
there of selective attentional mechanisms during language
processes may also be important leads for investigations into the
different patterns of language organization related to verbal
abilities.

ACKNOWLEDGMENTS

    Supported by NIH grants NS 17111, NS 21724 and NS 20482.
Dr. Carl Dodrill provided IQ data. Drs. H. Whitaker, C. Mateer,
I. Fried, T. Sandquist, O. Creutzfeldt, Mr. E. Lettich and Mr. J.
Ojemann assisted in these studies at various times.

REFERENCES

Benson, D.F. (1979). Neurologic correlates of anomia. Studies
in Neurolinguistics 4, 293-328.

Benton, A., Hannay, H., Varney, N. (1975). Visual perception of
line direction in patients with unilateral brain disease.
Neurology 25, 907-10.

Broca, P. (1861). Remarques sur le siege de la faculte du
language articule, suivies d'une observation d'aphemie (perte de
la parole). Bulletin de la Societe d'anatomie 36,330-57

Calvin, W., Ojemann, G. and Ward, A.A. Jr. (1973). Human
cortical neurons in epileptogenic foci: comparison of interictal
firing patterns to those of "epileptic" neurons in animals.
EEG. Clin. Neurophysiol. 34, 337-351.

Creutzfeldt, .O., Ojemann, G. and Lettich, E. (1987). Single neuron activity in right and left human temporal lobe during listening and speaking. In Fundamental Mechanisms of Human Brain Function. (eds. J. Engel Jr., H. Luders, G. Ojemann and P. Williamson). New York, Raven Press, pp. 69-82.

Fried, I., Ojemann, G. and Fetz, E. (1981). Language related potentials specific to human language cortex. Science 212, 353-56.

Liberman, A.M., Copper, F.S., Shankweiler, D.P. and Studdert-Kennedy, M. (1967). Perception of the speech code. Psychological Review, 73, 431-61.

Ojemann, G. (1979). Individual variability in cortical localization of language. J. Neurosurg. 50, 164-69.

Ojemann, G. (1983). Brain organization for language from the perspective of electrical stimulation mapping. Behav. & Brain Sci. 6,189-230

Ojemann, G.A., Creutzfeldt, O.D., Lettich, E., and Haglund, M.M. (1988). Neuronal activity in human temporal cortex related to short-term verbal memory, naming and reading. Brain in press.

Ojemann, G.A. and Dodrill, C.B. (1985). Verbal memory deficits after left temporal lobectomy for epilepsy. J. Neurosurg. 62,101-107.

Ojemann, G. and Mateer, C. (1979). Human language cortex: Localization of memory, syntax and sequential motor-phoneme identification systems. Science 205,1401-3

Ojemann, G. and Whitaker, H. (1978a). The bilingual brain. Archives of Neurology 35, 409-12.

Ojemann, G. and Whitaker, H. (1978b). Language localization and variability. Brain and Language 6,239-60.

Penfield, W. and Roberts, L. (1959). Speech and brain mechanisms. Princeton University Press, New Jersey.

Siegel, S. (1956). Nonparametric statistics for the behavioral sciences. McGraw-Hill, New York.

Wernicke, C. (1874). Der aphasische symptomen komplex. Cohn & Weigart, Breslau.

5
Reading and Lateralized Brain Lesions in Children

Dorothy M. Aram, Barbara L. Ekelman,
and Letitia L. Gillespie

Introduction

Despite the commonly-held assumption that developmental
reading disorders may be attributable in part to abnormal
structure and/or function of the left hemisphere, little evidence
supports this view. Few studies have addressed reading among
groups of children with documented left or right brain lesions
and the findings reported are inconclusive.

The few studies available provide conflicting data relating
the role of lateralized brain function to reading ability in
children including: whether persistent reading difficulties
follow left hemisphere lesions; whether reading abilities
differentiate among groups of left, right or normal children; and
whether age of lesion onset is related to reading impairment
(Alajouanine and Lhermitte, 1965; Hecaen, 1976, 1983; Kershner
and King, 1974; Kiessling et al., 1983; Vargha-Khadem et al.,
1983).

The contradictory findings of these studies may be attributed
in large measure to three important factors. First, the noncomparability among reading tasks reported, and, in some
instances, the absence of any objective measures. Second, the
inclusion of children with probable bilateral involvement
confounds meaningful attempts to relate reading disorders to
lateralized brain impairment. And third, report of group data
alone limits understanding of factors related to individual
variability. Taken together, few generalizations can be drawn
with any confidence from these studies relating lesion laterality
to resultant reading disorders.

As part of an ongoing study of the language and learning
sequelae of children with unilateral brain lesions, we have
completed two studies of reading ability involving children with
unilateral left or right brain lesions. All lesioned children in

61

these studies met criteria aimed at eliminating children with bilateral or diffuse brain involvement. These criteria include: 1) CT or MRI documentation of a static, unilateral lesion of vascular origin; 2) absence of ongoing seizure disorders; 3) evidence of normal cognitive development prior to lesion onset when the lesion occurred after the perinatal period; and 4) absence of known or suspected genetic or neurological abnormalities beyond the primary lesion. Each lesioned subject was matched by age, sex, race and social class to a normally developing child selected from patients seen at our hospital with congenital heart disorders, since the majority of lesioned subjects presented underlying heart disorders. Arterial blood oxygen saturation level was matched as closely as possible between lesioned and control subject pairs.

In the first study, we reported findings for 20 left lesioned-control and 12 right lesioned-control children on the Woodcock-Johnson Psycho-Educational Battery (WJ) (Aram and Ekelman, in press). On the Reading Achievement Cluster, right lesioned subjects were found to perform significantly lower than control subjects. Despite the absence of significant differences between the left lesioned and left control subjects on the Reading Achievement Tests, half of the left lesioned subjects had experienced difficulty in school in large measure thought to be related to reading problems.

The second study we undertook (Aram et al., under review) addressing reading among children with unilateral lesions aimed to provide more detailed and discriminating analyses of multiple components of reading and to focus upon individual differences in performance rather than solely on group data. In this study, 20 left and 10 right lesioned children were compared to matched controls on an extensive reading battery. All children in the study were assessed by the Wechsler Intelligence Scale for Children-Revised (WISC-R) and had Full Scale IQs within the normal limits. Left lesioned subjects were on the average two years older and two grades more advanced than right lesioned children. No lesioned subject was tested for this study prior to one year post lesion onset.

The reading battery administered was constructed to assess phonetic analysis and segmentation, decoding and comprehension abilities. All tasks were selected from standardized reading tests, thus permitting comparisons in performance across age and grade levels. The tasks included are summarized in Table 1.

Although mean performance on most reading measures were lower for lesioned than control subjects, multivariate results revealed no significant difference between left lesioned and control subjects nor between right lesioned and control subjects in performance on the reading measures. It should be noted, however, that univariate F-test results showed that both left and

TABLE 1

READING DOMAIN AND TESTS	DESCRIPTION
PHONETIC ANALYSIS AND SEGMENTATION	
Sound Analysis (GFW-A)[1]	--- Identify component sounds of nonsense syllables from auditory stimuli, e.g., "What is the last sound in meet?"
Sound Blending (GFW-B)[1]	--- Blend isolated sounds into meaningful words, again with stimuli presented by audiotape recording, e.g., "Tell me what you think this word is: b-r-i-k (brick)."
Phonetic Analysis (St-PA)[2]	--- Recognition of phonemes occurring in words (simultaneously dictated or illustrated or written) and identification of the corresponding graphemes or words including the given phoneme.
DECODING	
Word Identification (WRMT-WI)[3]	--- Oral reading of single words, including both words with regular and irregular phoneme-grapheme correspondence rules.
Word Attack (WRMT-WA)[3]	--- Application of phoneme-grapheme correspondence rules to reading of nonsense words, e.g., knap, darlanker, and ceisminadolt.
COMPREHENSION	
(Youngest Levels) Sentence and Paragraph[2]	--- Comprehension of sentences of various patterns and explicitly stated meanings in short passages.
(Other Levels) Literal (St-LIT)[2]	--- Comprehension of explicitly stated meanings and details.
Inferential (St-INF)[2]	--- Draw conclusions and generalize from explicitly and implicitly stated meanings.

1 = G-F-W Sound Symbol Test
2 = Stanford Diagnostic Reading Test
3 = Woodcock Reading Mastery Tests

right lesioned subjects scored significantly below their control subjects on the Goldman Fristoe Woodcock Sound-Symbol (GFW) Blending subtest with right lesioned subjects also scoring below their control group on the Woodcock Reading Mastery Test-Revised (WRMT) Word Attack subtest.

Individual Variation

Concluding from these data that left hemisphere lesions in children do not impair reading would be erroneous and analogous to basing our understanding of left hemisphere functioning among adult patients on a mean performance derived from averaging across all left hemisphere strokes irrespective of symptomatology or site of lesion. Clearly, the lesioned children are widely heterogeneous in reading ability with performance ranging from poor to superior reading skills. The nonsignificant statistical results between left lesioned and control children (except on tasks of phonemic analysis) obscured the fact that individual lesioned children presented marked reading deficits. Of the subjects 7 years and older, 5 left lesioned subjects fell below the 10th percentile on multiple reading measures, in contrast to only 1 of 30 normal controls who performed at or below the 10th percentile on any reading task.

Group treatment of the reading data also masked the notable individual variability among dyslexic left lesioned children. In an attempt to understand the basis for individual differences, case studies of these five dyslexic left lesioned children will be presented. Each case study will summarize neurological status, reading performance, language skills, visual spatial skills and learning and memory abilities. The order of case presentation begins with the most severely involved child proceeding progressively to the most specific reading disorder. The chapter concludes with a discussion of variables which may be related to these children's contrasting reading performance.

J.K. J.K. suffered a left hemisphere lesion at 6.19 years of age following surgical correction of a congenital heart defect. Prior to lesion onset he was developing normally except for a developmental speech problem which predominantly involved phonology and to a lesser degree expressive syntax. Several measures (PPVT, TACL) documented normal premorbid language comprehension. Right handed prior to the stroke with no family history of left handedness or reading problems, J.K. became left handed consistent with a persistent moderate-severe right hemiparesis greater in the arm than leg or face.

CT scan revealed a large area of decreased attenuation involving both pre- and retrorolandic areas and subcortical nuclei. An MRI scan completed this past month evidenced a large area of left hemisphere cortical damage involving the fronto-parietal lobes, including the pre and post central gyrus and extending subcortically into the anterior and posterior putamen, head of the caudate, the anterior limb of the internal capsule and the globus pallidus. A small right frontal white matter lesion which was not seen previously on CT scan was detected on the MRI scan. This recent finding of a clinically "silent" and previously undetected right white matter involvement demonstrated that J.K. does not present a lesion confined to one hemisphere as previously classified based on CT and clinical findings.

J.K. is the only child in the study who has remained clinically aphasic more than 1 year post lesion onset and who has presented "global" language and learning problems. He has required extensive language therapy and self-contained learning disabilities class. At age 13 years, when tested for the present study, he remained totally dyslexic and presented severe spelling, written language and math limitations, although the latter is his best subject. As summarized in Figure 1, J.K. performed at or below the 10th percentile on all reading measures except for the GFW Analysis subtest, where he scored at the 15th percentile. Speech and language evidenced marked deficits including vocabulary comprehension as measured by the Peabody Picture Vocabulary Test-Revised (PPVT-R), where he scored at the 16th percentile; syntactic comprehension as measured by the Revised Token Test (RTT), where his overall performance fell

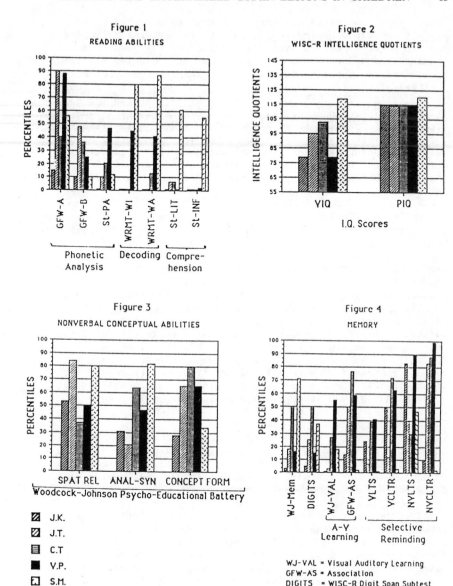

FIGURES 1-4
Left Lesioned Children's Ability Profiles

below the 1st percentile; word retrieval as measured by the
Rapid Automatized Naming Test (RAN), where performance was below
the 1st percentile; and syntactic production assessed by multiple
standardized and experimental measures. Articulation of speech
sounds and diadochokinetic rates for multiple repetition of
/pʌtə kə / also evidenced motor speech problems. WISC-R Verbal IQ
was 79 (Figure 2), with low scaled scores for Information (3) and
Arithmetic (4). In contrast, the WISC-R Performance IQ was 115
with subtests ranging from 7 (Coding) to 17 (Object Assembly).
Several nonverbal subtests on the WJ Battery (Figure 3) evidenced
relatively adequate visual spatial and nonverbal cognitive
abilities including: spatial relations (53rd percentile),
analysis-synthesis (31st percentile) and concept formation (28th
percentile).

     Memory and learning skills (Figure 4) were variable depending
on the task. He performed at the 3rd percentile on the composite
Memory Cluster of the WJ and received a scaled score of 5 on the
Digit Span subtest of the WISC-R. He was unable to learn sound-
symbol relationships for meaningful stimuli (WJ Visual-Auditory
Learning at the 1st percentile) and had difficulty learning
nonmeaningful visual-auditory associations (GFW Association at
the 14th percentile). However, on the verbal portion of the
Selective Reminding Task, which presented meaningful stimuli
auditorily (list of animals), he demonstrated greater difficulty
than normals in storing verbal material (verbal long-term
storage: VLTS), but once stored was comparable to normals in
verbal consistent long-term retrieval (VCLTR). Presented with
visual stimuli for the non-verbal learning task, long-term
storage (NVLTS) was strong, although consistent long-term
retrieval (NVCLTR) was not.

     Overall then, J.K. presented a picture of a profound reading
disorder accompanied by marked language and memory impairments
with strengths in visual spatial and nonverbal conceptual areas.
In sum, he presents a global reading, language and memory
disorder.

     J.T. At 4.33 years of age, J.T. incurred a left middle
cerebral artery occlusion felt to represent fibromuscular
dysplasia. Prior to this time, motor, language and cognitive
development were completely normal in this right handed boy whose
mother is ambidextrous and 2 brothers are left handed. Following
lesion onset, J.T. became left handed and presented with a
reflexive posturing of his right hand and a mild weakness of his
right leg. MRI scan revealed a left subcortical lesion involving
the head of the caudate, the anterior and posterior limbs of the
internal capsule and the globus pallidus. Similar to J.K., J.T.
presents spelling, written language and math problems with math
his strongest academic area. He, too, has received extensive
speech and language therapy and is educated in a learning
disabilities class.

In reading, J.T. is completely unable to decode or comprehend written material despite strengths on phonetic analysis tasks (except when a printed word is the stimulus as on the Stanford Phonetic Analysis task). J.T. presents persistent language problems involving vocabulary comprehension (PPVT-R at the 28th percentile), syntactic comprehension (RTT at the 1st percentile), expressive syntax (multiple measures) and word retrieval (RAN less than the 1st percentile). His speech is judged to be mildly dysarthric. His WISC-R Verbal IQ is 95 with subtest scatter unremarkable, ranging from 8 to 10. Performance IQ of 114 is strong with subtests ranging from 10 (Object Assembly) to 15 (Picture Arrangement). Visual spatial abilities appear generally strong, including the WJ Spatial Relations (84th percentile) and the Concept Formation (65th percentile) subtests, although his performance on the Analysis-Synthesis subtest was at the 21st percentile. J.T. evidenced notable weakness on verbal but not nonverbal memory. He performed at the 18th percentile on the WJ Memory Cluster and received a scaled score of 8 on the WISC-R Digit Span subtest. J.T. demonstrated marked difficulty on the Visual Auditory Learning subtest of the WJ, but average performance on the Association subtest of the GFW (the former presenting meaningful and the latter nonmeaningful forms). On the Selective Reminding Task, both verbal long-term storage and verbal consistent long-term retrieval tasks were notably impaired, although the nonverbal analogues were normal.

In sum, J.T. presents a marked reading disorder accompanied by language and verbal memory limitations. While in some respects he appears to be a less severe variant of J.T., the first child with a global reading and language disorder, he differs from J.T. in presenting good phonetic analysis and strong visual memory skills. J.T. presents a more specific reading, language and verbal memory disorder.

C.T. During infancy C.T. demonstrated a marked preference for his left arm and leg in a family where no immediate members are left handed (the maternal grandmother and uncle are left handed). At 2 1/2 years of age, a CT scan revealed an area of decreased attenuation in the posterior margin of the left sylvian fissure, thought to represent a porencephalic cyst. MRI results conducted this year revealed damage to the post central gyrus and involvement of the posterior periventricular white matter and cortical grey matter. Throughout, C.T. has presented a mild right spastic hemiplegia involving both the arm and leg.

At 9.3 years of age, C.T. presents concomitant spelling and written language deficits, but normal mathematical abilities (68th percentile on Math Cluster of the WJ). C.T.'s reading deficits involve both decoding and reading comprehension while phonetic analysis skills are relatively strong, falling between the 21st and 40th percentiles. He shows some limited ability to apply grapheme-phoneme rules to nonwords on the WRMT Word Attack

subtest (13th percentile), but is almost unable to read
meaningful words (WRMT Word Identification subtest at the 1st
percentile), which severely restricts his reading comprehension.
His WISC-R Verbal IQ is 103 with verbal subtests ranging from 10-
14 except for Information (7). C.T. has difficulty with
syntactic comprehension (RTT-3rd percentile) and word retrieval
(RAN at approximately the 4th percentile). He presents mild
stuttering behavior, characterized by part and whole word
repetitions and occasional prolongations. WISC-R Performance IQ
of 114 reveals no notable scatter. Nonverbal abilities are
generally strong. Memory skills are generally adequate as
evidenced by scoring at the 50th percentile on the WJ Memory
Cluster, receiving a scaled score of 10 on the WISC-R Digit Span
and having no notable problems on either the verbal or nonverbal
Selective Reminding Task. He had no difficulty learning
nonmeaningful visual auditory associations (GFW Association at
the 50th percentile), but performed somewhat lower when required
to learn meaningful visual auditory associations (WJ Visual-
Auditory Learning at the 27th percentile).

    Overall, C.T.'s composite picture is of a child with a
deficit in reading decoding and comprehension and aspects of
language despite intact phonetic analysis, verbal and nonverbal
memory, and nonverbal cognitive functions. He presents a reading
decoding and comprehension disorder along with deficits in
auditory comprehension and word retrieval.

    V.P. Prior to the sudden onset of an idiopathic left
hemispheric stroke at 7.72 years of age, V.P. was a normally
developing child doing well in second grade. A CT scan and
recent MRI revealed left frontal cortical damage and subcortical
involvement including the putamen, globus pallidus, head of the
caudate and anterior limb of the internal capsule. Despite mild
motor limitations on the right side of his body, he remained
right handed. None of his immediate family members are left
handed, although a maternal aunt and two cousins are left handed.
V.P.'s reading problems are confined to reading comprehension
where he consistently fell below the 2nd percentile. He
demonstrated adequate performance on phonetic analysis tasks
(although his performance on the GFW Blending subtest was at the
25th percentile). Decoding, likewise, was normal, achieving the
45th percentile on the WRMT Word Identification and the 41st
percentile on the Word Attack subtests. After acute difficulties
with expressive syntax and word retrieval, most aspects of
language and motor speech have returned to normal except for
persistent word retrieval problems (RAN < 1st percentile) and a
mild to moderate stuttering (fluency) problem which occurred
coincident with the stroke. Verbal IQ of 103 reflects little
subtest scatter. Nonverbal conceptual and spatial abilities are
strong as evidenced by a Performance IQ of 118 and no notable
scatter. Memory skills are generally good, with test scores for
both verbal and nonverbal material at or above average, except

the WJ Memory Cluster, where difficulty repeating sentences and digits backwards contributed to his score at the 16th percentile.

In sum, V.P. presents a severe but very specific disorder of reading comprehension with intact language comprehension, phonetic analysis and decoding skills. He presents a specific disorder of reading comprehension, word retrieval and stuttering.

S.M. At 14.25 years of age, S.M., a high school honor student, presented with sudden onset of a severe headache, language loss and a right hemiplegia. CT scan revealed an arteriovenous malformation which was surgically resected. Follow-up CT scan demonstrated cortical damage predominantly to the parietal lobe with a small posterior frontal infarct and damage to the posterior thalamic region. MRI scan could not be performed due to the presence of surgical clips placed during the AVM resection. Acutely, he presented a pronounced Wernicke's aphasia which recovered rapidly and by 1 month post lesion onset, all scores on the Test of Adolescent Language had returned to normal with scaled scores of 8 (M=10; SD=3) on subtests with verbal memory components. All aspects of language and motor speech presently are considered normal. He has remained right-handed although mild weakness has persisted on the right side of his body, primarily involving the right leg. There is no family history for left handedness. Currently a senior in high school, his school performance has fallen from A's and B's to C's and D's, with particular difficulty in algebra, his most difficult subject prior to the stroke. Nonetheless, he scored at or above the 80th percentile on Math and Written Language aptitude on the WJ. Even though he tested at the 80th percentile range on decoding skills and in the 50-60th percentile range on reading comprehension tests, marked deficits exist in phonetic analysis, scoring at the 10th percentile on the GFW Blending subtest and at the 12th percentile on the Stanford Phonetic Analysis subtest. In addition, he presents marked deficits on verbal and nonverbal memory and learning tasks. His performance on the Selective Reminding Task is one of the poorest observed for our left lesioned children, especially the verbal storage and retrieval tasks. Similarly, his ability to learn new visual auditory associations (e.g., 2nd percentile on the GFW Association Task and the 18th percentile on the WJ Visual-Auditory Learning task) is strikingly poor given his Verbal IQ of 119 and Performance IQ of 120. In sum, S.M. presents a disorder of phonetic analysis and memory for new information.

Discussion

Although group data suggest that left lesioned children perform essentially comparably to controls, these five left lesioned boys present severe yet contrasting reading disorders. How can these boys' deficits and differences in reading be explained?

At the onset, several factors can be dismissed as being
related to the differences presented as these factors are
constant across all five cases and do not differ from the
remaining left lesioned subjects: all are boys; all are white;
all come from at least middle class homes with ample opportunity
to learn; all were right handed premorbidly (presumably C.T.,
whose lesion occurred during prenatal development was destined to
be right handed given the absence of left handedness in his
immediate family); all presented vascular lesions; and all were
tested well after the acute stage. Several variables which are
not constant across cases and may potentially be related to
neuropsychological functioning need to be considered. These
include: premorbid status; age at lesion onset; and lesion
location.

Premorbid Status. An inclusionary criterion for enrollment
in this series of studies is normal premorbid status when the
lesion occurs after the perinatal period. Since C.T. sustained a
perinatal lesion, premorbid status cannot be determined. C.T.,
however, is the only one of these five boys with a family history
for reading disorders. C.T.'s mother was always in the lowest
reading groups and required remedial reading through the 6th
grade. A maternal aunt is retarded ascribed to perinatal
complications and a second maternal aunt also had problems
learning to read. One of three maternal uncles continues as an
adult to be dyslexic. Two natural sisters were slow to read but
now read adequately and a half-brother is in L.D. classes for
reading problems. Of the four sustaining lesions after 4 years
of age, none presented a pre-existing neurological or genetic
disorder and motor and cognitive development were considered
normal. J.K., however, did evidence a pre-existing developmental
speech and language problem which was described as a delayed
rather than a disordered phonological problem with some
expressive syntactic errors. Language comprehension, however,
was documented as normal and he clearly did not present the
pervasive language and learning problems observed following his
stroke. Since a large proportion of children with developmental
speech and language disorders experience reading problems at
school age (estimates range from 40-75%), the possibility exists
that his reading problems may be related in part to a pre-
existing language-learning disorder. While it is unlikely that
the pervasive language-learning problems J.K. presents at 13
years of age can be attributed to his mild premorbid
developmental speech and language problems, the contribution of
his premorbid status on later achievement abilities cannot be
totally discounted.

Age of Lesion Onset. Age of lesion onset varied widely among
these five left lesioned subjects ranging from onset prenatally
(C.T.) to 14.25 years of age (S.M.). Lesion onset for the others
occurred at: 6.19 years (J.K.), 4.33 years (J.T)., and 7.72
years (V.P.). Only V.P. and S.M. had learned to read prior to

lesion onset, which may be a factor associated with their more intact abilities. S.M., who was the oldest at lesion onset, presents with the most circumscribed reading problems confined to phonetic analysis and memory for new information. J.K., who presented the most pervasive problems, falls midway among these five dyslexic left lesioned subjects with two incurring lesions earlier and two later. Thus, later onset may provide an advantage of previously established reading although a simple relationship between age of onset and severity of deficit does not appear to be present for these five subjects or the remaining lesioned subjects. The true effect of age at lesion onset cannot adequately be tested here given the noncomparability of other important factors, notably site of lesion.

Site of Lesion. Site of lesion for the five subjects is summarized in Table 2. With the exception of a CT scan for S.M. who could not undergo MRI scanning, site of lesion is based on MRI scans performed in the last year and read by a neuroradiologist blind to these children's clinical status. As noted, J.K. was found to have a small frontal white matter lesion in the right hemisphere which was not previously visualized on CT scan. He, therefore, has been re-classified as having bilateral damage. He met subject criteria when the reading battery was administered since at this time only his CT scan was available evidencing a left hemisphere lesion. He was presented as a case study for several reasons. First, analysis of factors related to his profound reading disorder may prove significant for other dyslexic individuals. Second, his case is illustrative of the group studies of children thought to present unilateral lesions which, in fact, include children with more diffuse involvement. And third, it is not known whether a small white matter lesion in the right hemisphere has any clinical relevance. Thus, excluding J.K. was considered premature.

Two of the subjects, C.T. and S.M., present predominantly cortical lesions involving the parietal lobes, yet the reading and neuropsychological profiles they present are quite dissimilar. Furthermore, 5 other children in the study presented left parietal infarcts and do not present significant reading disorders. Thus, the contribution of other factors alone or in interaction with left parietal involvement must be considered. For example, the notable difference in age of lesion onset (prenatal for C.T. and 14.25 years for S.M.) may potentially explain more generalized language-learning deficits for C.T. versus the more specific phonetic analysis and verbal memory deficits presented by S.M. Alternatively, the strong family history of reading disorders for C.T. may explain why he but not others with similar parietal lobe lesions exhibits a reading disorder.

The remaining three, J.K., J.T. and V.P., present involvement of the head of the caudate and anterior limb of the internal

TABLE 2

LEFT HEMISPHERE LESIONED DYSLEXIC BOYS

SUBJECT	AGE AT LESION / TEST (YEARS)	HANDEDNESS		PREMORBID STATUS	SITE OF LESION (All left unless otherwise noted)		CLINICAL PICTURE
		PRE	POST		CORTICAL	SUBCORTICAL	
J.K.	6.19 / 13.67	R	L	Speech and language problem	Large left frontal and parietal, small right frontal white matter	Putamen, head of the caudate, anterior limb of internal capsule	Global reading, language and memory disorder
J.T.	4.33 / 9.08	R	L	Normal	None	Head of the caudate, anterior limb of internal capsule	Reading decoding and comprehension disorder accompanied by language and verbal memory deficits
C.T.	Pre-natal / 9.30	?	L	Family history for reading disorders	Parietal	Posterior periventricular white matter	Reading decoding and comprehension disorder accompanied by deficits in language comprehension and word retrieval, and stuttering
V.P.	7.72 / 10.00	R	R	Normal	Frontal	Putamen, head of the caudate, anterior limb of internal capsule	Reading comprehension disorder accompanied by deficits in word retrieval, and stuttering
S.M.	14.25 / 18.33	R	R	Normal	Posterior frontal and parietal	Posterior thalamus	Disorder of phonetic analysis and memory for new information

capsule, along with other areas of the left hemisphere. V.P.'s
and J.K.'s lesions involve frontal and fronto-parietal areas,
although these areas of cortical involvement do not distinguish
them from other left lesioned subjects who do not present reading
disorders. Of potential significance, these three are the only
subjects in this study to have involvement of the head of the
caudate and the anterior limb of the internal capsule. We have
followed three other children not included in this reading study
who had involvement of these same structures. All three
presented significant language and reading problems. The first,
a 7-year old girl originally described as presenting acquired
capsular/striatal aphasia in childhood (Aram et al., 1983)
currently at 13 years continues to present major learning
problems which include reading. A second boy with a prenatal
lesion involving only subcortical structures (putamen, globus
pallidus and external capsule) was 6 years of age when he was
tested with the reading battery and, thus, was considered too
young and without sufficient opportunity to learn to read to be
considered dyslexic. Nonetheless, he is not yet able to read.
Finally, we are following a 2 1/2 year old girl with an extensive
subcortical prenatal lesion also involving these areas. Whether
or not she will present reading problems remains to be seen. The
role of these subcortical structures in development of language
and reading remains speculative, although involvement of these
subcortical structures among adults (Alexander, Naeser and
Palumbo, 1987) and children (Aram et. al., 1983) have been shown
to disrupt previously intact language and reading. We are just
beginning to explore the relationship between specific site of
lesions within a hemisphere and observed behavioral deficits
among the children being followed. Thus, any conclusion at this
point relating site of lesion to reading sequelae is tentative.
However, based on the few cases available to us with left
subcortical involvement, it appears that these structures have a
crucial role in language and reading and that the functions
subserved by these subcortical structures are less able than
cortical areas to reorganize following insult during development.
While as yet this hypothesis has only limited supporting
evidence, it is consistent with all of our current data.

Conclusions and Summary

     Findings based on group studies are inconclusive in regards
to the effect of left hemisphere lesions in childhood upon
learning to read. Group studies, however, obscure marked
individual variation in ability among children with brain
lesions. This chapter presented case studies of five left
lesioned children, all of whom presented severe reading
disorders. Each presented concomitant language and/or memory
problems, although generally intact nonverbal conceptual skills.
The most severely involved, J.K., presents major language,
learning and memory problems. The influence of multiple factors

may explain the severity of his neuropsychological deficits
including: a pre-existing language-learning problem, a
relatively late age of lesion onset although before the onset of
reading, and the presence of a large left hemisphere lesion
involving both cortical and perhaps critically subcortical areas
coupled with a small frontal white matter lesion in the right
hemisphere. J.T., a somewhat less severe variant than J.K. and
with spared phonetic analysis and visual memory, presents only
involvement of subcortical areas with an earlier age of onset
(4.33 years) and no known premorbid factors which would
predispose him to reading problems. C.T., who presents syntactic
comprehension and word retrieval problems in addition to decoding
and reading comprehension limitations, exhibits only cortical
parietal lobe involvement, however a strong family history for
reading disorders may be related to the deficits he presents.
V.P. presents a circumscribed disorder of reading comprehension
coupled with a word retrieval and a stuttering disorder. He
presents no known premorbid factors which would explain his
reading and speech problems, although his lesion was acquired
relatively late after the onset of reading (7.72 years), and
involves subcortical structures hypothesized to play a role in
language and learning. Finally, S.M. presents only memory and
phonetic analysis problems following late onset (14.25 years) of
a cortical lesion involving fronto-parietal areas.

These case studies evidence the need to consider multiple
factors in explaining developmental and acquired reading
disorders in children. While many of us would like to draw
relationships between specific site of lesion and behavior
presented, in children these relationships are not clear cut,
especially for cortical involvement. On the other hand,
subcortical structures appear to be more "fixed" and their
involvement suggests intriguing possible relationships which will
need further exploration and substantiation.

Acknowledgement

This study was supported by the National Institutes of Health:
NINCDS Grant No. NS17366 to the first author.

References

Alajouanine, T.H. and Lhermitte, F.   (1965).   Acquired Aphasia in
     Children. Brain, 88, 653-662.
Alexander, M.P., Naeser, M.A. and Palumbo, C.L.   (1987).
     Correlations of Subcortical CT Lesion Sites and Aphasia
     Profiles. Brain, 110, 961-991.
Aram, D.M. and Ekelman, B.L.   (In press).   Scholastic Aptitude
     and Achievement Among Children with Unilateral Brain Lesions.
     Neuropsychologia.

Aram, D.M., Ekelman, B.L. and Gillespie, L.L. (Under review).
    Reading Abilities in Children with Strokes. Neuropsychologia.
Aram, D.M., Rose, D.F., Rekate, H.L. and Whitaker, H.A. (1983).
    Acquired Capsular Striatal Aphasia. Archives of Neurology,
    40, 614-617.
Hecaen, H. (1976). Acquired Aphasia in Children and the
    Ontogenesis of Hemispheric Functional Specialization. Brain
    and Language, 3, 114-134.
Hecaen, H. (1983). Acquired Aphasia in Children: Revisited.
    Neuropsychologia, 21, 581-587.
Kershner, J.R. and King, A.J. (1974). Laterality of Cognitive
    Functions in Achieving Hemiplegic Children. Perceptual and
    Motor Skills, 39, 1283-1289.
Kiessling, L.S., Denckla, M.B. and Carlton M. (1983). Evidence
    for Differential Hemispheric Function in Children with
    Hemiplegic Cerebral Palsy. Developmental Medicine and Child
    Neurology, 25, 727-734.
Vargha-Khadem, F., Frith, U., O'Gorman, A. and Watters, G.V.
    (1983). Learning Disabilities in Children with Unilateral
    Brain Damage. Paper presented at the Sixth Annual European
    Meeting of the International Neuropsychological Society,
    Lisboa, Portugal.

6
Hemispheric Independence and Interaction in Word Recognition

Eran Zaidel

INTRODUCTION

Hemispheric Independence

The thesis of hemispheric independence posits that each normal cerebral hemisphere has a separate and fairly complete cognitive system capable of processing most environmental information and controlling the behavior of the organism as a whole. Each system contains its own perceptual, mnestic, and linguistic mechanisms; each represents reality differently and processes information using characteristic and complementary strategies. Thus, the thesis of hemispheric independence presupposes the older and widely accepted thesis of complementary hemispheric specialization.

Further, hemispheric independence theory claims that the two normal hemispheres often process information independently and in parallel. This design principle permits a particularly adaptive solution to the implementation of a very complex cognitive system such as the human brain. First, duplication provides redundancy. Second, even when the two hemispheres apply the same information processing strategies, a time delay between the computations permits backtracking and look-ahead for flexible interaction between different levels of processing. Third, hemispheric complementarity in information processing strategies permits effective monitoring and error detection. For example, both hemispheres may compute solutions to the same problem and a discrepancy could signal an error. Or, one hemisphere may compute an answer bottom-up and the other check the answer top-down.

Hemispheric independence can result in competition for resources, mutual interference or conflicting answers. The solutions to some problems are optimized

*This work was supported by NIH grant NS20187, by a gift from the David H. Murdock Foundation for Advanced Brain Studies, and by a Biomedical Research Support Grant to UCLA. Thanks to Jeffrey Clarke, Sarah Copeland, Karen Emmorey, Zohar Eviatar, Kathleen Frederick, and Jill Langley for helpful comments on a draft of the paper, and to Steven Hunt, Kathleen Frederick, and Jeffrey Clarke for computer assistance.

by assigning control to the specialized hemisphere; other problems require interhemispheric cooperation. In both cases, an overall control system is needed to coordinate hemispheric activities, i.e., maintain independence when necessary, effect cooperation when needed, and resolve conflict when it arises.

The concept of hemispheric independence was inspired by research on the split-brain (e.g., Sperry, 1985), but it can be extended to the normal brain in a weak (Bogen, 1986) or a strong (Zaidel, Clarke and Suyenobu, 1988) form. In this paper we illustrate hemispheric independence for lexical analysis in the normal brain. The claim is both new and radical. Its challenge is to integrate linguistic data from hemisphere-damaged patients, split-brain patients and normal subjects. Its promise is to provide a rich model for several central problems in cognitive neuroscience today: (i) alternative systems of representation, (ii) modularity or functional specialization and parallel computation, (iii) intermodular communication, and (iv) monitoring and control.

Corpus Callosum as a Dynamic Communication and Control System

What is the role of the human neocortical commissures in maintaining hemispheric independence and effecting interhemispheric interaction? There is little doubt that the corpus callosum and anterior commissure serve to transmit sensory and motor information between the hemispheres and that different sensory/motor channels are represented in different parts of the callosum. Split-brain studies suggest that simple sensory/motor signals can also transfer noncallosally (Clarke & Zaidel, 1988), that complex semantic-affective (Zaidel, 1976) and conceptual (Cronin-Golomb, 1984) information can transfer subcallosally, and that cross-hemispheric inhibition, i.e., control information, can be relayed in the absence of the neocortical commissures (Zaidel, 1978b). We propose that the normal corpus callosum consists of a series of channels that transfer sensory/motor, processed, and control information, i.e., channels that interconnect homotopic primary, association and tertiary cortex. In particular, we posit that hemispheric independence is sometimes maintained by suppression of callosal transfer (sensory isolation). At other times, callosal channels help maintain dominance by inhibiting computation or arresting response in one hemisphere (Zaidel, Clarke & Suyenobu, 1988).

We further posit that there exist individual differences in regional patterns of callosal connectivity, as a function of gender, handedness and cognitive profile. Greater connectivity in a sensory channel may result in a reduced behavioral laterality effect, whereas greater connectivity in a control channel may result in greater inhibition and thus in an increased behavioral laterality effect. Moreover, greater channel connectivity may improve performance on tasks that require interhemispheric integration but may hinder performance on tasks specialized in one hemisphere. In this paper we investigate the relation between callosal connectivity and hemispheric independence. We index connectivity by anatomical size, assuming a uniform fiber density in any callosal region. Some forms of congenital cognitive deficit may then be attributed to poor callosal mediation of interhemispheric coordination.

Processing Dissociation

Some lateralized tasks are exclusively specialized in one hemisphere. If the stimuli reach the unspecialized hemisphere first, they will have to be relayed through the corpus callosum to the specialized hemisphere prior to critical processing ("callosal relay" tasks). Other lateralized tasks can be processed independently by either hemisphere. If the stimuli reach one normal hemisphere they will be processed in it directly, without callosal transfer ("direct access" tasks). We have developed a set of behavioral criteria for deciding which model applies to a given task and found that linguistic tasks of both kinds exist (Zaidel, 1983). For example, lexical decision of concrete nouns and orthographically regular nonwords is a direct access task whereas dichotic perception of nonsense CV syllables is a callosal relay task, specialized in the LH.

The interpretation of a pattern of results as evidence for direct access or callosal relay rests on the observation that callosal relay often results in substantial increases in latencies and error rates. It is also assumed that stimuli that have similar physical characteristics are relayed at the same rate (e.g., concrete and abstract nouns that have the same length, visual complexity, etc.). Thus, the pattern of results graphed in Figure 1a must reflect independent but equal hemispheric processing since no callosal relay is involved, i.e., the lines have a zero slope. The pattern graphed in Figure 1b is ambiguous. Either the slope reflects callosal relay or it reflects a difference in hemispheric competence. The callosal relay interpretation can only be ruled out if we know the actual effect of cross-callosal transfer for the stimuli in question and if it is different from the observed slope.

The most common pattern of results used to infer direct access or hemispheric independence in a lateralized experiment is a significant statistical interaction between sensory field (e.g., visual hemifield) and some independent

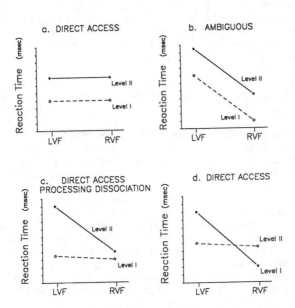

Figure 1. Theoretical patterns of behavioral results in a hemifield tachistoscopic experiment that show direct access or hemispheric independence.

experimental variable with two levels (e.g., noun concreteness in a lexical decision task), when other parameters are counterbalanced. Such an interaction is called "processing dissociation" (Zaidel 1983, 1985; Zaidel, Clarke & Suyenobu, 1988) and is shown in Figure 1c. Unfortunately, this pattern of processing dissociation does not guarantee hemispheric independence. The graph in Figure 1c could be interpreted to reflect independent hemispheric processing of Level I, but callosal relay of Level II. Still, the mere fact that the two levels are differentiated in the left hemifield (LVF) suggests that the right hemisphere (RH) can distinguish between them. Changes in the measurement scale may erase the statistical interaction, unless there is a cross-over condition which argues against callosal relay (Figure 1d). One method of increasing the likelihood that a processing dissociation is evidence for hemispheric independence is the observation of another processing dissociation with an orthogonal independent variable ("Bootstrapping" method; Zaidel, Clarke & Suyenobu, 1988).

Lateralized Lexical Decision

Lateralized lexical decision with orthographically regular nonwords and with word/nonword responses ("Is this a word or not?") consistently yield three main results (Measso & Zaidel, 1988). First, there is an overall advantage of words over nonwords (henceforth the "nonword effect") (cf. Figure 11a). This is a well known result in the psycholinguistic literature, one that proposed models of lexical access attempt to explain first (Garnham, 1985). Forster's "bin lexical search" model accounts naturally for the nonword effect since a nonword decision is reached only if no match is found during an exhaustive lexical search of relevant bins. Becker's "verification" model accounts for the nonword effect if the nonwords share perceptual features with real words (e.g., when they are orthographically regular) so that a verification search is necessary to make more precise matches. Morton's logogen model does not explain the nonword effect naturally but it can be supplemented with a dynamic deadline: If no logogen has reached threshold by the deadline, the response is a nonword.

The second result is an overall right hemifield advantage (RVFA) (Chiarello, 1988), reflecting LH superiority for this linguistic task (cf. Figure 11a). But this result is consistent either with exclusive LH specialization (callosal relay) or with independent processing in each hemisphere (direct access). The latter can be easily accommodated by the three models of lexical access. The RH lexicon may be organized differently and a search through it may be slower than through the LH lexicon (lexical search). The RH may have higher thresholds (logogens), or it may have slower feature extraction or verification (verification model).

The third result is a statistically significant interaction between wordness and VF of presentation (cf. Figure 11a). Usually, there is no hemispheric difference for nonword decisions but RVF superiority for word decisions. Thus, the word-nonword difference is larger in the RVF than in the LVF. Occasionally, the word-nonword difference in the LVF is not significant (Measso & Zaidel, 1988). This pattern fits the processing dissociation criterion for direct access, and suggests that, at the very least, words and nonwords are distinguished (explicitly or implicitly) in the RH and that the RH can process nonwords by itself.

The three models of lexical access can account for a wordness X VF interaction by setting at different values the parameters that account for the nonword effect in each hemisphere. The lexical search model would have to assume a differently organized lexicon in the two hemispheres and the logogen model could assume a similar deadline but slower perception or decision in the RH. However, none of the models can account naturally for equal and above chance performance (in the RH) with words and nonwords (Measso & Zaidel, 1988), let alone for faster or more accurate decision of orthographically regular nonwords than of words (Emmorey & Zaidel, 1988 and see Figure 6a).

CENTRAL VARIABLES

Dual Route Model of Lexical Access

The Dual Route model distinguishes two routes for reading a word aloud. One involves direct lexical access through orthography (lexical route) and subsequent retrieval of the phonological form of the word (addressed phonology), while the other (nonlexical route) involves translating orthography into sound (assembled phonology). This model was used by neurolinguists to account for selective deficits in word recognition by different forms of acquired alexia. Figure 2 illustrates a recent version of the model (cf. Zaidel, 1978a; Shallice, 1988). Although it has been criticized for empirical inadequacy (Humphreys and Evett, 1985), the model does capture a fundamental alleged difference between word recognition in the left and right disconnected hemispheres: The RH has no ability to translate orthography into sound (Zaidel & Peters, 1981). Different stages of processing in this model are indexed by different lexical access tasks or by specific effects of independent variables in word recognition tasks. Thus, length effects in word recognition may implicate an orthographic (or a phonological) decoding process; morphological effects in word recognition appear to implicate an

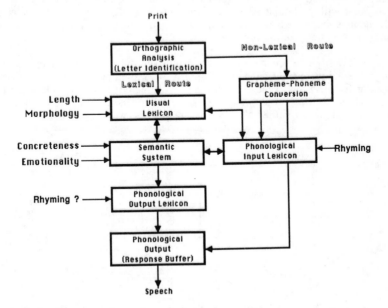

Figure 2. A model of lexical access showing experimental variables that tap some of its stages.

orthographic decomposition; and rhyme judgment indexes grapheme-phoneme conversion, or perhaps a phonological output lexicon retrieved after lexical access, or even an abstract orthographic analysis.

Next, we will describe a series of experiments that show evidence for hemispheric independence in the input, central, output and control stages of lexical analysis of printed words.

Semantic Variables

Here we will present evidence for hemispheric differences in sensitivity to noun concreteness and to emotionality of nouns. Elsewhere, we have shown that the two normal hemispheres also show differential lexical congruity effects (Zaidel, White, Sakurai & Banks, 1988). These include (i) facilitation of lexical decision by associated primes and inhibition of decision by unassociated primes, (ii) congruity effects in symbolic comparative judgment tasks ("Which one is bigger, a mosquito or an ant?"), and (iii) automatic orthographic-semantic facilitation-inhibition effects in an English-Japanese Stroop-like decision task.

Concreteness. Both hemispheres appear to be sensitive to noun concreteness. Only when RH resources are taxed and a change of strategy is required does the RH show selective difficulty with abstract nouns. Hence the conflicting results in the literature (Patterson & Besner, 1984). In the first experiment, the task was lexical decision and the stimuli included concrete and abstract nouns that varied in frequency, as well as "active" and "quiet" verbs (Eviatar, Menn & Zaidel, 1988). Active verbs referred to simple body actions (e.g. kick, shrug) and quiet verbs referred to states or less concrete actions, not associated with particular muscle activation (e.g. wish, sell). The hypothesis was that noun concreteness is characterized by multiple sensory representations and thus can be generalized to active verbs.

Twenty-one female and 11 male undergraduate UCLA students served as subjects. All were right-handed. Stimuli were flashed horizontally on a computer monitor for 80 msec to the LVF or RVF, with the edge closest to fixation falling 1.7 degrees from center and the edge farthest from fixation falling 6 degrees from center. Go/no go rather than verbal responses were used to maximize RH

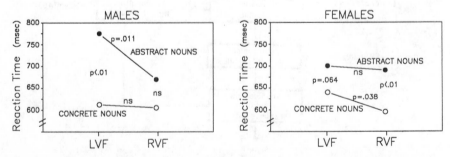

Figure 3. Opposing patterns of concreteness x visual hemifield interactions in lexical decision of nouns by males and by females (Eviatar, Menn & Zaidel, 1988). Significance level of planned comparisons is set at p=.01.

involvement.

Accuracy and latency revealed a RVFA and an advantage of concrete over abstract nouns but no overall concreteness X VF interaction. However, there was a trend toward a sex X concreteness X VF interaction in latency [F(1,30)=3.9, p=.053] with males and females showing opposite patterns of processing dissociation (Figure 3). Males showed the predicted concreteness effect in the LVF [F(1,30)=15.6, p<.001] but not in the RVF; they also showed no VFA for concrete nouns and a strong trend toward a RVFA for abstract nouns [F(1,30)=7.2, p=.011] (Eviatar, Menn & Zaidel, 1988).

Both accuracy and latency showed an overall RVFA and an advantage of active over quiet verbs but no verb type X VF interaction.

Thus, both hemispheres are sensitive to concreteness but that sensitivity reflects individual differences in processing strategies which can but need not vary between the hemispheres. Strictly speaking, we have demonstrated hemispheric independence for concrete nouns in males and for abstract nouns in females (Figure 3).

Emotionality. In another lexical decision experiment, carried out by Z. Eviatar, the length and emotionality of abstract nouns were manipulated in an attempt to reverse RH incompetence for processing abstract words. Seventeen male and 25 female right-handed UCLA undergraduate students participated as subjects in the experiment. The stimuli consisted of 64 words and 64 pronounceable nonwords. The words were either emotional (positive or negative) or neutral, as determined in a separate rating experiment. Stimuli were flashed on a TSD computer monitor (model NDC-15 controlled by a DEC LSI-11/23) to the LVF or RVF for 80 msec and subtended a peripheral width from 2 to 5 degrees away from fixation. A binary unimanual word/nonword response was used and response hand was varied within subjects (Eviatar & Zaidel, 1988).

Both accuracy [F(1,40)=49.5, p<.001] and latency [F(1,40)=9.9, p<.01] revealed an overall RVFA. Accuracy also showed an advantage of emotional over neutral words [F(1,40)=22.9, p<.001]. There was no emotionality X VF

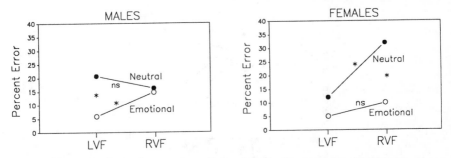

Figure 4. Opposing patterns of emotionality X visual hemifield interaction in lexical decision of abstract nouns by males and by females. Planned comparisons could not be carried out due to the small number of items in each cell (Eviatar & Zaidel, 1988).

interaction (Figure 4) but for accuracy there was a trend toward a significant emotionality X VF X length X sex interaction [F(2,39)=3.06, p=.058]. This interaction is due to complementary emotionality X VF patterns exhibited by males and females to 4-letter words. This time females showed the greater effect of emotionality in the LVF, expected from previous studies, whereas males showed a greater effect in the RVF.

Thus, emotionality, like concreteness, is a "second order" laterality variable in the sense that it is secondary to an overall RVFA: It does not show an unequivocal interaction with VF, but rather interacts with individual differences in hemispheric processing strategies (cf. Graves, Landis & Goodglass, 1981).

Orthographic Variables: Length?

The experiment described above and carried out by Z. Eviatar on hemispheric differences in sensitivity to emotionality also manipulated the length of the words and the nonwords used as stimuli. There were 16 four-letter, 24 five-letter, and 24 six-letter words. Nonwords matched the words in length (Eviatar & Zaidel, 1988). Previous studies showed a selective effect of length on latency of lexical decision of abstract nouns in the LVF (Bub, 1982) and on latency of naming LVF words varying in frequency and imageability (Young & Ellis, 1985).

Our latency data showed a RVFA and a main effect of word length [F(2,34)=4.67, p<.05] but no interactions. Accuracy data revealed a RVFA, a main effect of word length [F(2,39)=11.2, p<.001], and an advantage of emotional over neutral words. In addition, there was a significant interaction between VF and word length [F(2,39)=4.27, p<.05], with 4- and 5-letter words decided more accurately than 6-letter words in the RVF [F(1,40)=11.85, p<.005] and 4-letter words decided more accurately than 5- and 6-letter words in the LVF [F(1,40)=17.57, p<.001] (Figure 5). There was a RVFA for 5- and 6-letter words [F(1,40)=44.42, p<.0001; F(1,40)=19.97, p<.0001, respectively] but not for 4-letter words. The absence of a significant VFA for the 4-letter words suggests that at least short words are processed independently in each hemisphere. Finally, there was a trend toward a significant word length X VF X emotionality X sex interaction in accuracy [F(2,39)=3.06, p=.058], reflecting sex differences in hemispheric sensitivity to emotionality for 4-letter words (Eviatar & Zaidel, 1988).

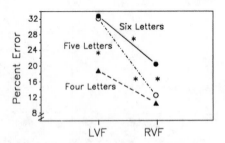

Figure 5. Interaction of length x visual hemifield in lexical decision of abstract nouns (Eviatar & Zaidel, 1988). Henceforth * = significant at the .05 level, ** = .01, *** = .001.

Our accuracy data are generally consistent with Bub's latency results (RVFA for 5- and 6-letter words, no VFA for 4-letter words) but qualify his conclusion that the RVF shows no sensitivity to length. Rather, as the task becomes more complex and resources become limited, the added burden of processing longer words appears to dictate a change of strategy and that strategy shift seems to occur first in the LVF. The fact that the RH is more sensitive to length than is the LH suggests that length effects in word recognition do not reflect phonetic recoding but rather a visual recognition parsing process.

Morphological Variables: Suffix Structure

The next lexical decision experiment was carried out by K. Emmorey and was undertaken to determine whether both hemispheres are equally sensitive to internal word structure (Emmorey & Zaidel, 1988). The word stimuli consisted of 30 verbs and 30 nouns matched for both root and surface frequency and for number of letters. Of the verbs, 15 were inflected (-ed, -ing) and 15 were monomorphemic. Of the nouns, 15 were derived (-er, -age, -ness, -ure, -al, -ty, -ion) and 15 were monomorphemic. Nonwords fell into 4 categories: (i) 15 simple nonwords (clussig), (ii) 15 suffixed nonwords (nasting), (iii) 15 root-initial nonwords (leakma), and (iv) 15 root-suffix illegal combinations (pseudowords) (joyness). Length and pronounceability were controlled or matched.

Stimuli were presented for 150 msec to the left or right of fixation on an Amdek Video-310A monitor controlled by an IBM PC/XT compatible computer. Their closest edge was 2 degrees from fixation and their far edge was from 5 to 7 degrees off fixation. Word/nonword responses were signalled bimanually on a vertically-aligned response panel placed at midline.

Latency results showed a RVFA [F(1,32)=36.48, p<.001], a word advantage [F(1,32)=84.13, p<.001] and a wordness X VF interaction [F(1,32)=53.37, p<.001]. There was a RVFA for words but not for nonwords. The accuracy data showed a RVFA [F(1,32)=43.01, p<.001], no effect of wordness, and a significant wordness X VF interaction [F(1,32)=40.53, p<.001]. Again, there was a significant RVFA for words but not for nonwords (Figure 6a). Furthermore, in the RVF responses to words were more accurate than responses to nonwords [F(1,32)=7.68, p<.01] but in the LVF responses to nonwords were more accurate than responses to words [F(1,32)=5.53, p=.025]! These patterns suggest

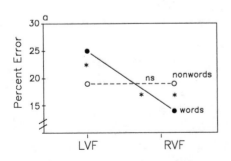
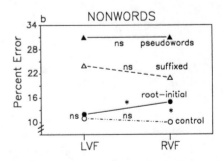

Figure 6. Effect of morphology on lexical decision in the two hemifields (Emmorey & Zaidel, 1988).

RH independence at least in processing the nonwords, and we will therefore restrict our attention to morphological effects in nonword decisions (Figure 6).

Latency of nonword decisions disclosed no VFA and a main effect of nonword category [F(3,96)=37.53, p<.001], but no significant interactions. Planned comparisons revealed no difference in latency between control nonwords and root-initial nonwords but a significant advantage of control nonwords over suffixed words [F(1,32)=34.58, p<.001] and over root-suffix illegal nonwords [F(1,32)=63.17, p<.001]. Accuracy data too showed no VFA, a main effect of nonword category [F(3,96)=52.07, p<.001] and no nonword category X VF interaction (Figure 6b). Planned comparisons revealed that control nonwords were more accurate than root-initial nonwords [F(1,32)=9.11, p=.005], more accurate than suffixed nonwords [F(1,32)=28.47, p<.001] and more accurate than root-suffix illegal nonwords (pseudowords) [F(1,32)=132.11, p<.001]. Only the root-initial nonwords showed a VFA with more accurate performance in the LVF (F(1,32)=4.98, p=.03) (Emmorey & Zaidel, 1988).

Thus, both hemispheres showed a similar sensitivity to internal nonword structure and the RH appeared to perform automatic nonword decomposition similarly to the LH. In particular, the RH could recognize a true suffix attached to the end of a nonword (garnly) so that suffixed nonwords were rejected more slowly and less accurately than control nonwords. Furthermore, the RH appeared to be more misled by this suffix than the LH since we found a RVFA in latency for suffixed nonwords. Both hemispheres performed equally poorly on root-suffix illegal nonwords which were recognized worst of all nonword categories. These nonwords are most difficult to reject because both the root and suffix can be recognized as separately legal and it is only their combination that must be rejected as illegal.

Phonological Variables: Rhyming

The disconnected RH is known to have no grapheme-phoneme translation rules and thus to be incapable of rhyme judgment of written words or nonwords (Zaidel & Peters, 1981). The present experiment, carried out by J. Rayman, involved rhyme judgments of orthographically dissimilar lateralized words and was intended as a callosal relay task exclusively specialized to the LH (Rayman & Zaidel, 1988). It was originally used in order to compare the effects of unilateral and bilateral presentations on the laterality effect.

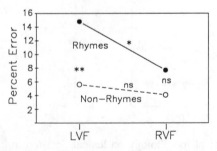

Figure 7. Rhyme decision in the two hemifields (Rayman & Zaidel, 1988).

Forty right-handed UCLA undergraduates, 19 females and 21 males, participated in the experiment. Subjects saw a central word followed by a 100 msec test word in either the LVF or RVF and had to decide whether the test word rhymed with the central word. On half of the trials two test words appeared, one in each VF, and an arrow at fixation indicated the one to be judged. The central words were monosyllabic and 3-6 letters long. Test words were 3 letters and 1 syllable long. Stimuli were presented on an Amdek Video 310A CRT monitor controlled by an IBM AT-compatible computer. Responses were signalled bimanually on a vertically-aligned panel placed at midline.

Results showed a RVFA in accuracy [F(1,38)=16.32, p<.001] and an insignificant RVFA of 15 msec in latency. Subjects responded more accurately [F(1,38)=29.36, p<.001] but not faster on nonrhyme trials. Surprisingly, there was a significant rhyme class X VF interaction in accuracy (Figure 7) [F(1,38)=5.55, p=.022]. The RVFA was significant only for the rhyming word pairs [F(3,114)=9.66, p<.05]; rhyming and nonrhyming trials differed significantly only in the LVF [F(3,114)=16.07, p<.01]. Moreover, for rhyming pairs the length of the central word was positively correlated with item difficulty (r=.387, p<.01) but frequency of the test word was not correlated with difficulty (r=.007). For nonrhyming pairs the opposite pattern occurred: Frequency of the test word correlated with item difficulty (r=-.469, p<.005) but length of the central word did not (r=-.002) (Rayman & Zaidel, 1988). This pattern of correlations was found in both VFs.

Thus, the results reveal hemispheric independence at least for nonrhyming pairs. Moreover, the correlations with difficulty suggest that judgment of rhyming and nonrhyming pairs is accomplished by different processes and that a similar nonrhyme decision process is available to both hemispheres.

Grammatical Variables: Faciliation by Functor-Noun/Verb Agreement

This experiment involved a noun-verb decision task and was carried out by L. Menn. Half of the words were flashed with a congruent function word above them (my child, to bring) and half were flashed with a neutral cue above consisting of XXX. The question was whether the function word-content word agreement provided a facilitating cue to noun/verb decisions in both VFs (Menn & Zaidel, 1988).

Stimuli were all 4- to 6-letter monosyllables. They included 32 pure nouns (child), 32 pure verbs (bring) and 36 words which could be either nouns or verbs (walk), all matched for frequency. The 32 pure nouns were further subdivided into 16 abstract and 16 concrete nouns. Two blocks of trials required the subject to answer "Is this a noun?" and two blocks required him/her to answer "Is this a verb?". Yes and No responses were signalled unimanually. Noun-congruent cues included the possessive pronouns "my," "his" and "your" and the article "the." The verb-congruent functors were the pronouns "we," "you" and "they" and the preposition marker "to." Subjects were 29 male and 26 female undergraduate students at Tufts University. Stimuli were flashed for 100 msec on the CRT of a PDP-11 computer.

Latency scores showed an advantage of verb over noun decisions and a main effect of cue type. Nouns also showed a significant concreteness X VF interaction [F(1,47)=4.11, p=.042] with a RVFA for abstract nouns but not for

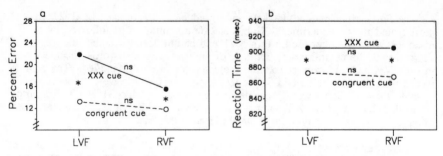

Figure 8. Effect of function word-verb agreement on accuracy and latency of noun/verb decisions in the two hemifields (Menn & Zaidel, 1988).

concrete nouns. This processing dissociation suggests hemispheric independence at least in processing the concrete nouns. There was no overall cue type X VF interaction. Accuracy showed an overall RVFA [F(1,54)=3.97, p=.051] and a main effect of cue, with the congruent cue condition yielding more accurate responses than the neutral cue condition. There was no interaction between cue type and VF.

Restricting our attention to verbs (Figure 8) we see that latency shows no VFA with neutral cues and suggests hemispheric independence in that condition (Figure 8b), whereas accuracy shows no VFA with congruent cues and suggests hemispheric independence in that condition (Figure 8a). Moreover, both hemispheres are sensitive to the grammatically congruent function words and their verb decisions are facilitated by the congruent relative to neutral cue condition in both dependent variables. Surprisingly, then, RH independence extends to simple grammatical context effects.

INPUT, OUTPUT AND CONTROL VARIABLES

Input Variables: Medium of Presentation

Changes in the perceptual characteristics of stimuli affect the hemispheres differentially (e.g. Sergent and Hellige, 1986), and yet different media for presenting lateralized stimuli that vary in stimulus contrast, persistence, size and spatial frequency are used interchangeably in the experimental literature. In the next experiment, carried out by S. Copeland and A. David, we have compared the laterality effects in a lexical decision task using three common presentation media: (i) a Gerbrands three-field projection tachistoscope with high contrast negative slides as stimuli, (ii) an IBM AT-compatible computer with an Amdek video 310A monochrome monitor in which the stimuli are amber letters on black background, and were specially designed to approximate the font used with the tachistoscope (Helvetica Medium 24), and (iii) the same computer presentation but in reverse video with black letters on amber background. Reverse video presents the stimulus by illuminating the background and turning off the pixels that correspond to the stimulus. The stimulus is, in turn, terminated by turning the corresponding pixels on so that the effect of phosphor persistence is eliminated.

Thirty UCLA undergraduate students served as subjects. The stimuli

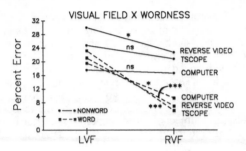

Figure 9. Effect of medium of presentation on lexical decision in the two hemifields (Copeland, David & Zaidel, 1988).

consisted of 136 letter strings, each 4-6 letters long. Half were concrete and imageable English nouns and half were orthographically regular nonwords, matched for length, phonological complexity and orthographic regularity. Stimuli were flashed horizontally for 40 msec either to the LVF or to the RVF with their closest edge two degrees of arc from fixation and their distant edge at most six degrees from fixation. Medium of presentation was varied between subjects.

Accuracy revealed a classic overall RVFA, an overall advantage of words over nonwords and an overall wordness X VF interaction (computer: p=.044; T-scope: p=.022; reverse video: p=.119) (Figure 9). There was no main effect of presentation medium, no interaction of medium with VF or wordness, nor a medium X wordness X VF interaction. However, the word advantage in the RVF, though significant in all three conditions, was significantly smaller in the standard computer condition than in either the tachistoscope condition (p=.029) or the reverse video condition (p=.038). There was no word advantage in the LVF with any medium. The RVFA was smaller in the computer condition (p>.05) than in either the reverse video or tachistoscope condition. Medium affected accuracy for nonwords but not for words (computer nonwords worse than reverse video nonwords, both overall and in the LVF). Thus, presentation medium, i.e., early visual perceptual components, seemed to affect hemispheric processing strategies and had different effects on word and on nonword processing. In particular, computer presentation appears to diminish the RVFA and reverse video presentation seems to enhance it, relative to the projection tachistoscope.

Latency scores accentuate the advantage of words but deemphasize the RVFA or the wordness X VF interaction. The computer condition revealed no laterality effect (for words or nonwords), whereas the tachistoscope condition showed a RVFA (p=.001). At the same time, the computer condition had a wordness effect which was greater in absolute value than the wordness effect in the tachistoscope condition (computer: 164.33 msec; T-scope: 124.9 msec; both significant at p<.001). Thus, standard computer presentation does tend to obscure laterality effects relative to more traditional modes of presentation, perhaps because it emphasizes RH contribution to early visual information processing.

Output Variables: Response Programming

The next experiment, carried out by G. Measso, manipulated the response programming requirements of a lateralized lexical decision task (Measso & Zaidel, 1988). The stimuli were a subset of those used for studying the effects of medium of presentation above. The 4-5 character long strings were presented for 80 msec on an Amdek Video-310A CRT monitor controlled by an IBM PC/XT-compatible. The horizontal strings subtended from 2 to 3 degrees with the innermost edge 2 degrees away from fixation. Three manual response conditions were included: (i) go/no go with words as targets, (ii) go/no go with nonwords as targets, and (iii) word/nonword two-choice responses. The positions of the response buttons were counterbalanced between subjects. The experimental question was whether changes in response programming affect the basic laterality effects in lexical decision.

Somewhat different results were obtained for latency and for accuracy (Measso & Zaidel, 1988). The latency data showed a word advantage [$F(1,60)=36.1$, $p<.001$] and an interaction between wordness and VF [$F(1,60)=12.9$, $p<.001$] but no RVFA [$F(1,60)=1.2$, $p=.272$] (Figure 10b). The accuracy data showed a word advantage [$F(1,60)=14.4$, $p<.001$] and a RVFA [$F(1,60)=16.3$, $p<.001$] but no interaction between wordness and VF [$F(1,60)=1.98$, $p=.161$] (Figure 10a). For neither dependent variable did the significant effects (RVFA, wordness advantage or wordness X VF interaction) interact with response condition [latency: $F(1,60)=.18$, $p>.5$; accuracy: $F(1,60)=.08$, $p>.5$].

There was no VF difference for nonword decisions in any condition in either dependent variable and there was no VF difference in latency for words in the go/no go condition, suggesting a uniform hemispheric independence for nonword decisions and at least sometimes for word decisions. Thus, the data suggest that similar response programming processes operate in both normal hemispheres and affect decision in each hemisphere similarly. Put differently, it appears that response programming does not play an important role in hemispheric asymmetries during lexical analysis.

Control Variables: Error Correction

The same lexical decision procedure and stimuli which were used for studying the effects of input and of output variables and which revealed a direct access pattern were employed in an attempt to compare the error correction ability of each hemisphere. Stimuli were presented for 40 msec in a random order to the

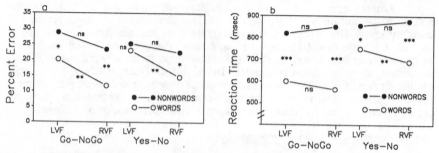

Figure 10. Effect of response programming on accuracy and latency of lexical decision in the two hemifields (Measso & Zaidel, 1988).

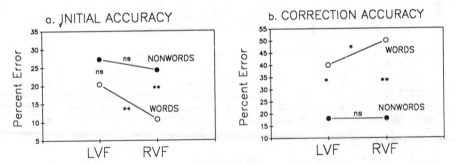

Figure 11.   Accuracy of initial lexical decisions and of manual self-corrections in the two hemifields (Stein & Zaidel, 1988).

left and right of fixation using a projector tachistoscope in an attempt to yield a relatively high error rate. Word/nonword responses were signalled on a two-way toggle switch (the direction of word responses was counterbalanced) and subjects were instructed to be both fast and accurate but to correct themselves as soon as possible by pushing the switch in the opposite direction to the initial response if they thought that they had made an error. A special scoring system rewarded self-corrected errors and penalized uncorrected errors. The experiment was carried out by R. Stein and the results are reported in Stein and Zaidel (1988) and summarized in Zaidel (1987).

Hemispheric independence in lexical decision does not guarantee hemispheric independence in error correction. Accuracy of initial decisions revealed the classic RVFA (RVF=82.4%, LVF=76.2%, F=20.6, p=.0001), the advantage of words over nonwords (words=84.4%, nonwords=74.2%, F=14.4, p=.001), and the wordness X VF interaction (F=4.46, p<.05), suggesting hemispheric independence for initial accuracy (at least for nonwords) (Figure 11a). Twenty-one percent of the trials were errors and 12% of the trials led to self corrections. There was a significant negative correlation between initial accuracy and correction accuracy in both visual hemifields. Correction accuracy revealed no VFA and an advantage of nonwords over words (nonwords=82.2%, words=60.4%, F=26.58, p<.0001).   These differences from initial accuracy confirm that error correction and initial decisions are carried out by separate processes.

There was also a significant wordness X VF interaction in self-correction accuracy (F=6.9, p=.01) with no VF difference for nonwords but a LVFA for words (!), suggesting direct access in error correction (definitely for nonwords) and showing RH independence in monitoring (Figure 11b). Thus, our data suggest that each normal hemisphere has separate modules for initial decisions and for response monitoring. The results show that the LH is superior in lexical decision whereas the RH is superior in correcting erroneous decisions.

ANATOMICAL CORRELATES

Here we will report preliminary findings from an ongoing study carried out by J. Clarke in which behavioral scores on a lateralized lexical decision task with associative priming are correlated with anatomical measures of the sizes of different regions of the corpus callosums as determined by midsagittal Magnetic Resonance Images (MRI) (cf. Clarke, Zaidel & Lufkin, 1988).

Midsagittal magnetic resonance images were obtained from a 0.3 tesla FONAR Beta 3000 Magnetic Resonance Imager using the spin echo technique (TR=500 msec, TE=28 sec). Images of the corpus callosum (CC) were digitally enlarged to 2x life size and were transferred to film. The CC was traced, a line representing the maximum anterior-posterior length of the CC was drawn, and the following subdivisions were made: (i) the anterior half of the CC, (ii) the region between the anterior half and the posterior third of the CC (i.e., the posterior body), (iii) the region between the posterior body and the posterior fifth of the CC (i.e., the isthmus), and (iv) the posterior fifth of the CC (i.e., the splenium). The areas of the total CC and each of the four regions were measured using a Microcomp Planar Morphometry digitizing system.

The lexical decision task consisted of lateralized concrete nouns and orthographically regular nonwords. Targets were presented for 60 msec on a computer-controlled monochrome monitor at an eccentricity of 2 degrees, subtending widths ranging from 2 to 3 degrees of visual angle. The targets were similar to the ones used in the input, output and error correction experiments above where they exhibited a direct access pattern. Targets were preceded by lateralized primes presented for 100 msec with an ISI of 500 msec. The targets were either associated with the primes (as determined by free association norms) or unassociated; they were counterbalanced for frequency, imageability, length and orthographic regularity.

The behavioral data from 35 subjects indicated that subjects were more accurate when targets were presented in the RVF (81.1% correct responses) then when they were presented in the LVF [68.7%, $F(1,31)=14.9$, $p<.001$]. Subjects were more accurate when targets and primes were associated (79.1%) then when they were unassociated [70.6%, $F(1,31)=14.5$, $p<.001$]. There was no significant effect of visual hemifield of prime, suggesting that the corpus callosum permitted effective visual interhemispheric transfer so that the lexicon in each hemisphere was accessed independently regardless of prime hemifield. The correlation between overall LVF and RVF scores across subjects was low ($r = .13$). There was no main effect of handedness, but there was a significant statistical interaction of handedness X association X target hemifield [$F(1,31)=10.3$, $p<.01$]. In right handers (N=15) related targets facilitated detection accuracy in the LVF (80% vs. 60.4%) but not in the RVF (85.0% vs. 79.6%). The reverse was true for left handers (N=20): Related targets facilitated detection in the RVF (84.4% vs. 75.9%) but not in the LVF (68.8% vs. 66.3%). In either case, the interaction of association with VF is consistent with a direct access pattern.

A more extensive earlier experiment presented the same test on a projection tachistoscope to right-handed subjects and included a baseline condition requiring lexical decision of the targets alone. The results showed both greater facilitation of decision by associated primes and greater inhibition by unassociated primes, relative to baseline, in the LVF than in the RVF (Zaidel, White, Sakurai & Banks, 1988).

Seventeen of the 35 subjects with behavioral data have undergone MRI to date (10 females, 10 right-handers). Behavioral-anatomical correlations revealed that total corpus callosum area was negatively correlated with accuracy of decision

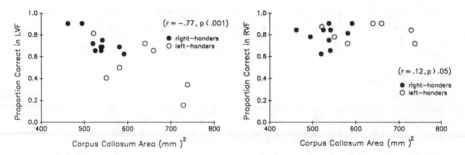

Figure 12.   Correlation between size of the corpus callosum and accuracy of lexical decision in the left and right hemifields (Clarke, Zaidel & Lufkin, 1988).

of targets in the LVF (r=-.77, p<.001), but uncorrelated with targets in the RVF (r=.12, p>.05) (Figure 12).   There were significant negative correlations (p<.05) between LVF accuracy and all callosal divisions except for the posterior body. It therefore appears that in this task the corpus callosum serves to maintain hemispheric independence: A larger callosum implies worse RH performance on this direct access task, perhaps due to greater LH interference. Thus, individual differences in size of callosal anatomy may have as much to do with maintenance and modulation of interhemispheric independence as with transfer of information between the hemispheres.

    What are the implications of this result to the relationship between reading ability and callosal size?   That would depend on whether we regard normal RH contribution to lexical analysis as critical for effective reading. Let us presuppose that competence in lexical decision is an index of competence in reading.   Suppose further that the normal LH controls effective reading and that the RH interferes with effective reading.   Then out result suggests that a larger corpus callosum would inhibit RH competence, minimize its interference and optimize reading.   In that case, we would expect congenital dyslexics to have smaller-than-usual callosums.   On the other hand, suppose that normal RH contribution to reading is important.   Then our result suggests that a larger corpus callosum would inhibit RH competence, minimize its contribution, and impair reading.   In that case, we would expect congenital dyslexics to have larger-than-usual callosums.   This latter result is in fact what has been observed (B. Pendleton, personal communication).   Indeed, we have seen that the normal RH has substantial lexical competence and we believe that this competence is adaptive for effective reading.

    Our result could also be interpreted to mean that a larger corpus callosum is associated with greater hemispheric specialization for reading, i.e., a greater RVFA for lexical decision.   The interpretation follows from the observation that a larger callosum has no effect on the RVF score but predicts lower LVF scores and thus a greater RVFA.   This association contrasts with the usual claim that greater callosal size in left handers or women is associated with greater interhemispheric connectivity and thus with reduced laterality effects.   Our results argue also against the ontogenetic hypothesis of Galaburda and his collaborators that progressive hemispheric specialization is mediated by decreasing callosal connectivity (cf. Sherman, Rosen & Galaburda, this volume). Our argument rests on the assumption that callosal size correlates positively with callosal connectivity or with number of callosal fibers, given a uniform density of such fibers in a cross section of the corpus callosum (Aboitiz et al., 1988).

CONCLUSION

Duality

The most parsimonious explanation for the behavioral and anatomical evidence of direct access or independent word recognition in the two hemifields of normal subjects is that the two hemispheres have separate lexicons which are organized or accessed differently. It is possible but not parsimonious to argue that the two hemispheres share a lexicon but have separate and differently structured access routes to it. In that case, the diverse hemispheric differences described in this paper would apply to a rich structural characterization of lexical access routes which is accompanied by an austere characterization of the structure of the lexicon itself. Theoretically, it is probably impossible to distinguish characterizations of lexical access that put the structural burden on the representation of the lexicon from those that put the structural burden on access routes to it.

Hemispheric independence in lexical access is probably useful for higher level processes that depend on lexical information. It is particularly adaptive for lexical monitoring operations and perhaps also for linguistic operations that involve maintaining two competing semantic interpretations of an incoming message. It is an empirical question whether hemispheric independence in the normal brain extends to operations that last one or two orders of magnitude longer than lexical access, which itself lasts less than one second.

The finding that there is hemispheric independence in lexical access is important not only for psycholinguistics and for neuropsychology but also as a general cognitive neuroscientific model for brain utilization of high level parallel processes. We presented evidence that each hemisphere utilizes parallel processes in two different two-choice word decision tasks: Word/nonword and rhyme/no rhyme. Similar results have been reported for yes/no decisions in lateralized semantic membership tasks (D. Zaidel, personal communication) and in lateralized same/different judgments (Bagnara, Boles, Simion & Umilta, 1982). Generally, there is no hemispheric difference for nonword, nonrhyme, non-membership and different decisions, but a hemifield advantage for word, rhyme, membership or same decisions. In all these cases a logical design would be to check the fit of the stimulus to one category (e.g., Is it a word?) and if the check fails, conclude that the stimulus belongs to the other category (It is a nonword). Instead, it appears that separate checks for each category are initiated in parallel. This is what we would expect from a heuristic process that cannot guarantee a solution and that makes decisions in the absence of complete information.

Thus, we see parallel implementations at diverse levels of cognitive organization in the brain, both between and within the hemispheres. It would appear that parallel implementations are ubiquitous in brain organization. There remains the question of coordinating the two processes by some priority mechanism. In the case of interhemispheric coordination, priority may depend on the nature of the task, the individual, or the set, and it may be mediated by cross-callosal inhibition.

Challenges

One specific challenge that emerges from the data on hemispheric independence in word recognition is the frequent discrepancy between latency and accuracy measures of hemispheric competence. (Note that if the two choices in a decision task are processed by two separate processes, then the signal detection measure of sensitivity may be inappropriate if it presupposes a single monotonic scale along which both the signal and the noise distributions can be represented.) Lateralized tasks that emphasize both speed and accuracy are more likely to yield laterality effects in accuracy than in latency. But, occasionally, speed and accuracy interact with an experimental variable (dependent variable incongruence, Eviatar & Zaidel, 1988). Such incongruencies are difficult to interpret in the absence of more detailed hemispheric processing models. The articulation of processing models and the resolution of conflicts between effects in latency and in accuracy hold promise for both methodological and theoretical advances in cognitive neuropsychology.

The second challenge is a more general, theoretic one. It involves the convergence of data on right hemisphere language from hemisphere-damaged patients, from split-brain patients and from normal subjects. Syndromes of aphasia obscure some language competence observed in the disconnected RH. Similarly, data from the RH damage leads us to underestimate the language capacity of the disconnected LH. Moreover, the data reported here suggest that the linguistic profile of the disconnected RH underestimates the contribution of the normal RH to language functions. The first part of the challenge of convergence then is to separate aphasic syndromes into (i) residual processes in the damaged LH, (ii) LH inhibition of RH competence, and (iii) compensatory RH takeover. The second part of the challenge is to find the scope of RH independence in language operations and the extent of its actual contribution to natural language processing.

REFERENCES

Aboitiz, F., Zaidel, E., & Scheibel, A.B. (1988). Variability in fiber composition in different regions of the posterior corpus callosum in humans. American Association of Anatomists 1988 Meeting. Abstract.

Bagnara, S., Boles, D.B., Simion, F., & Umilta, C. (1982). Can an analystic/holistic dichotomy explain hemispheric asymmetries? Cortex, 18, 67-78.

Bogen, J.E. (1986). Mental duality in the intact brain. Bulletin of Clinical Neurosciences, 51, 3-29.

Bub, D.N. (1982). The nature of half field assymmetry for word processing as a function of hemispheric specialization. Unpublished Doctoral Dissertation, University of Rochester, Rochester, New York.

Chiarello, C. (1988). Lateralization of lexical processes in the normal brain: A review of visual half-field studies. In Contemporary Reviews in Neuropsychology. (ed. H.A. Whitaker). Springer Verlag, New York, pp. 36-76.

Clarke, J.M., & Zaidel, E. (1988). Simple reaction times to lateralized light flashes: Varieties of interhemispheric communication routes. Brain. In press.

Clarke, J.M., Zaidel, E., & Lufkin, R.B. (1988). Visuospatial performance is related to the size of the splenium of the corpus callosum in normal subjects. Abstract. Journal of Clinical and Experimental Neuropsychology, 11. In press.

Copeland, S., David, A., & Zaidel, E. (1988). Effects of computerized tachistoscopic presentation on laterality effects in lexical decision. Manuscript in preparation.

Cronin-Golomb, A. (1984). Intrahemispheric processing and subcortical transfer of non-verbal information in subjects with complete forebrain commissurotomy. Unpublished Doctoral Dissertation, Division of Biology, California Institute of Technology, Pasadena.

Emmorey, K., & Zaidel, E. (1988). Morphological complexity and hemispheric specialization. Manuscript in preparation.

Eviatar, Z., Menn, L., & Zaidel, E. (1988). Right hemisphere contribution to lexical analysis. Manuscript submitted for publication.

Eviatar, Z., & Zaidel, E. (1988). The effects of word length and emotionality on hemispheric contribution to lexical decision. Manuscript submitted for publication.

Garnham, A. (1985). Psycholinguistics. Methuen, London.

Graves, R., Landis, T., & Goodglass, H. (1981). Laterality and sex differences in visual recognition of emotional and nonemotional words. Neuropsychologia, 19, 95-102.

Humphreys, G.W. & Evett, L.J. (1985). Are there independent lexical and nonlexical routes in word processing? An evaluation of the dual-route theory of reading. The Behavioral and Brain Sciences, 8, 689-740.

Measso, G., & Zaidel, E. (1988). The effect of response programming on laterality effects in lexical decision. Manuscript submitted for publication.

Menn, L., & Zaidel, E. (1988). Grammatical priming and hemispheric specialization. Manuscript in preparation.

Patterson, K., & Besner, D. (1984). Is the right hemisphere literate? Cognitive Neuropsychology, 1, 315-341.

Rayman, J., & Zaidel, E. (1988). Rhyming in the right hemisphere. Manuscript submitted for publication.

Sergent, J., & Hellige, J.B. (1986). Role of input factors in visual-field assymmetries. Brain & Cognition, 5, 174-199.

Shallice, T. (1988). From Neuropsychology to Mental Structure. Cambridge University Press, Cambridge.

Sperry, R.W. (1985). Consciousness, personal identity and the divided brain. In The Dual Brain. (eds. D.F. Benson & E. Zaidel). Guilford, New York, pp. 11-26.

Stein, R., & Zaidel, E. (1988). Hemispheric error correction in lexical decision. Unpublished manuscript, Department of Psychology, UCLA.

Young, A.W., & Ellis, A.W. (1985). Different methods of lexical access for words presented in the left and right visual hemifields. Brain and Language, 24, 326-358.

Zaidel, E. (1976). Auditory vocabulary of the right hemisphere following brain bisection or hemidecortication. Cortex, 12, 191-211.

Zaidel, E. (1978a). Lexical organization in the right hemisphere. In Cerebral Correlates of Conscious Experience. (eds. P. Buser & R. Rougeul-Buser). Elsevier, Amsterdam, pp. 177-197.

Zaidel, E. (1978b). Concepts of cerebral dominance in the split brain. In Cerebral Correlates of Conscious Experience. (eds. P. Buser & A. Rougeul-Buser). Elsevier, Amsterdam, pp. 263-284.

Zaidel, E. (1983). Disconnection syndrome as a model for laterality effects in the normal brain. In Cerebral Hemisphere Asymmetry: Method, Theory and Application. (ed. J. Hellige). Praeger, New York, pp. 95-151.

Zaidel, E. (1985). Callosal dynamics and right hemisphere language. In Two Hemispheres--One Brain?. (eds. F. Lepore, M. Ptito, & H.H. Jasper). Alan R. Liss, New York, pp. 435-459.

Zaidel, E. (1987). Hemispheric Monitoring. In Duality and Unity of the Brain. (ed. D. Ottoson). Macmillan, Hampshire, pp. 247-281.

Zaidel, E., & Peters, A.M. (1981). Phonological encoding and ideographic reading by the disconnected right hemisphere: Two case studies. Brain and Language, 14, 205-234.

Zaidel, E., White, H., Sakurai, E., & Banks, W. (1988). Hemispheric locus of lexical congruity effects: Neuropsychological reinterpretation of psycholinguistic results. In Right Hemisphere Contributions to Lexical Semantics. (ed. C. Chiarello). Springer, New York, pp. 71-88.

Zaidel, E., Clarke, J., & Suyenobu, B. (1988). Hemispheric independence. In Neurobiological Foundations of Higher Cognitive Function. (eds. A. Scheibel and A. Wechsler). Guilford Press, New York. In press.

7
Relative Interactive Hemispheric Dominance in Reading

Theodor Landis and Marianne Regard

An apparent discrepancy exists between the astonishing
language competence of the isolated right cerebral hemisphere (RH)
in some split-brain patients (for review see Zaidel, 1985), or in
patients who underwent left hemispherectomy during adulthood
(Smith, 1966) or late adolescence (Patterson and Vargha-Khadem,
1989), and the sometimes complete lack of language competence in
aphasic patients despite an intact RH. There is one major
difference between the two conditions. In split-brain patients and
patients with hemispherectomies the largest interhemispheric
communication channel, the corpus callosum and the cerebral
commissures are disrupted, while in aphasic patients with damage
to the left, language dominant hemisphere the intact RH is still
connected to its damaged partner. This had led modern investigators (Rubens and Benson, 1971; Moscovitch, 1973, 1976) to
reconsider the old idea, expressed by Wigan (1844) over a century
ago, that the dominant controlling hemisphere inhibits the
potential function of its opposite fellow.

It is not possible, of course, to test this dynamic,
interactive hypothesis in the disconnected split-brain patients or
in hemispherectomized patients. The investigation of normal
subjects with methods of lateralized stimulus presentation or the
testing of selected patients with unilateral cerebral damage might
be a fruitful approach. Considering hemispheric interaction in
reading several questions arise. 1) Is it possible to show
quantitative or qualitative reading differences between the two
cerebral hemispheres in normal subjects? 2) Do they correlate with
the reading pattern observed in patients with unilateral damage to
the language dominant left hemisphere (LH)? 3) Are there special
conditions in which differences in the reading pattern of each
hemisphere can be elicited? 4) Are there situations in which a
shift in reading ability can be examined with respect to the
hemisphere involved in information processing?

Concerning the questions one and two, we know that the two
hemispheres' appreciation of lexical meaning dissociate with
respect to concreteness and imageability of nouns (e.g. Ellis and
Shepherd, 1974; Day, 1977; Richardson, 1975); and that there exist
a number of highly selected aphasic patients, usually with very
large LH lesions (Marin, 1980), the so-called "deep dyslexics"
(Marshall and Newcombe, 1973) in whom the reading pattern is
strikingly similar to that observed in the RH of split-brain
patients (for review see Coltheart et al., 1980).

In recent years the RH has been associated with a "dominant"
processing of emotional information (Carmon and Nachson, 1973,
Tucker et al., 1976, Suberi and McKeever, 1977. Landis et al.,
1979; Bryden et al., 1982; for review see also Bear, 1983, Heilman
and Satz, 1983). When defining reading as the process of gathering
meaning from visually presented language information, we wondered
if the superior ability of the RH to deal with emotional
information would not extend to words. We therefore created two
sets of nouns, one with "high-emotional" (e.g. "LOVE") and one
with "low-emotional" content (e.g. "FACT") of matched frequency.
We conducted two experiments, one with unselected aphasic patients
with damage to their language dominant LH (Landis et al., 1982)
and one with healthy subjects (Graves et al., 1981). Aphasic
patients were simply asked to read these words aloud, while we
presented them tachistoscopically to either the left visual field
(LVF) or the right visual field (RVF) together with pronounceable
English non-words. The subjects' task in this lexical decision
experiment was to press response keys whenever they saw an English
word.

As shown in figure 1a, aphasic patients are significantly
better in reading emotional than non-emotional nouns. Normal
subjects (figure 1b) detect both word classes better when
presented to the LH than when shown to RH, but make no
distinctions between the two classes. When presented to the RH,
only high-emotional words are detected, the low-emotional words
are not reliably recognized as real words. The experiment with
normal subjects suggests that depending upon the hemisphere
stimulated, two different reading processes are at work, the one
in the RH being especially sensitive to the emotional aspect of
the lexical meaning of words. An item analysis comparing the
correct readings of aphasic patients with the performance in
lexical decision of the left and right visual field of normal
subjects respectively revealed a highly significant correlation
($p = 0.003$) between the aphasics' performance and that of the LVF
(RH) in normals but no significant correlation ($p > .05$) with the
performance of the RVF (LH) of normals (Goodglass et al., 1980).
This result suggests that for the emotional meaning of words the
same reading process we observed in the RH of normal subjects was
used by aphasic patients with damage to the LH.

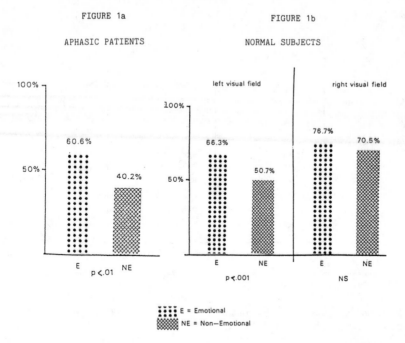

Figure 1a,b: Percent accuracy of aphasic patients in reading aloud
emotional (E) and non-emotional (NE) nouns (Fig. 1a) and lexical
decision of the same words in LVF and RVF of normal subjects (Fig.
1b).

A hallmark of the reading pattern of deep dyslexic patients,
whose reading has been associated with right hemisphere processing
(Coltheart, 1980a) is their unusually high production of semantic
paralexias (e.g. reading "FLOWER" for "DAISY"). We therefore
expected semantic paralexias to occur more often in the RH of
normal subjects. We tachistoscopically presented 40 German
4-letter nouns to the RVF-LH and the LVF-RH of healthy right
handed subjects at brief exposure durations (mean 9 msec) to allow
only some 25 % correct reading (Regard and Landis, 1984).

As shown in figure 2 almost four times as many semantic
paralexias were produced when the nouns were flashed to the RH
than to the LH, while other errors or correct readings did not
differ signifiantly between the two hemispheres. An informal
qualitative analysis of the semantic paralexias (Landis, 1987)
showed semantic paralexias occurring subsequent to RH stimulation
not only to be more frequent but also to have a different
"flavour", that of wider semantic distance between target and
response than those elicited subsequent to LH stimulation.

FIGURE 2

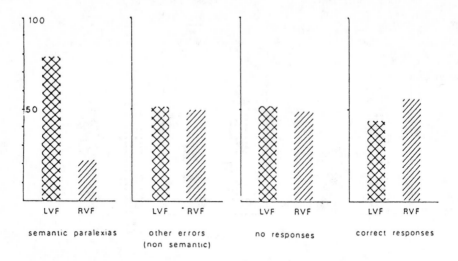

Figure 2: Percentage of experimentally induced reading errors and correct responses by visual field (LVF, RVF).

To test this observation formally we created two sets of pairs of nouns matched for frequency and length. One set contained pairs with a narrow semantic distance (e.g. "SALARY" - "WORK") and one pairs with a more distant semantic relationship (e.g. "AUTUMN" - "AGE"). The pairs of this latter set also have poetic connatations, sometimes referred to as topoi. These pairs were presented tachistoscopically for 100 msec to either the LVF or the RVF of 46 healthy right handed subjects, who had to press response keys whenever they felt that the two words were related in meaning. The results of this experiment (Rodel, 1989) are presented in figure 3.

As one can see in figure 3, there is a significant ($p < .001$) interaction between the hemispheres involved and the semantic distance. Again this shows that the two hemispheres appreciate word meaning differently and implies the presence of two different reading strategies proper to each hemisphere.

A condition in which the reading capacity of the non-dominant hemispheres could be expected to show up is the classical clinical "disconnection" syndrome of pure alexia, in which the right visual cortex is anatomically disconnected from the left hemisphere language zones by a left infero-medial occipito-temporal and a splenial lesion (Dejerine, 1892; Geschwind, 1965; for review see Greenblatt, 1977; Damasio and Damasio, 1983). Clinically, however,

FIGURE 3

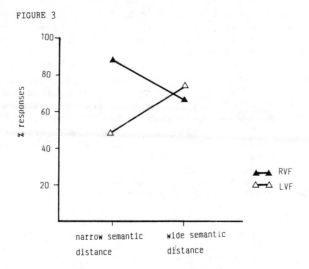

Figure 3: Percent responses of pairs of nouns acknowledged as related in meaning with respect to visual field of presentation (LVF, RVF) and semantic distance in normal subjects.

only a few of these patients have shown some reading ability when tested with multiple choice word-object or object-word matching or with matching of spoken names to a written word (Kreindler and Ionasescu, 1961; Caplan and Hedley-Whyte, 1974; Stachoviak and Poeck, 1976; Assal and Regli, 1980). Pure alexic patients did not, as would be predicted, behave like some split-brain patients (Benson and Geschwind, 1969; Benson, 1985), who can retrieve with the left hand an object which corresponds to an object name flashed in the left visual field, while unable to read the word and verbally unaware of its presence (Zaidel, 1978; Sperry et al. 1969). A few years ago, we saw a pure alexic patient who under special conditions showed the expected "split-brain like" performance (Landis et al., 1980). This patient, a typical letter-by-letter reader with a complete right hononymous hemianopia, was tested tachistoscopically subsequent to the removal of a left occipito-temporal glioblastoma. Words were flashed in his LVF, which projects to the healthy RH. The threshold for reading single letters was at 50 msec exposure duration. Only at exposure durations which allowed for letter-by-letter reading, generally well above 1000 msec, was he able to read whole words of 4 and 5 letters. We presented him with names of familiar objects below his threshold for single letter reading and asked him to point to the corresponding object in a large display of familiar objects. Although he was unable to read these names or to recognize their single letters he pointed to his own astonishment correctly to the corresponding object. When we retested the patient later in exactly the same manner his alexia

was clinically unchanged, but his threshold for reading single
letters was now in the range of normals. Thus he was able to read
some individual letter of these briefly exposed names, but now he
was unable to point above chance to the corresponding object.
Concerning our third question, this patient shows that under
specific conditions different reading abilites can be accessed.
When able to recognize a single letter he was bound to use a
letter-by-letter reading strategy, but when presented with words
so briefly that he could not recognize individual letters, he
apparently could extract the meaning of a whole word by correctly
performing a word-object match without being aware of having seen
or read the projected name. This second reading strategy is
identical to the reading pattern of the RH observed in split-brain
patients, who show a complete figural-verbal disconnection. In our
patient the anatomical connection was incomplete, since he was a
letter-by-letter reader, but we suggest that complete functional
disconnection was induced by the short exposure duration. In our
patient the two reading processes observed, that is letter-by-
letter reading and the recognition of whole word meaning appeared
to be disconnected from each other since single letter recognition
prevented access to lexical meaning.

    The findings observed in the isolated hemispheres of
split-brain patients have led to the idea of basic differences
between the two cerebral hemispheres in information processing
(Levy, 1974; for review see Hellige, 1983). The LH has been
associated with a rather sequential, the RH with holistic
processing. Short exposure duration supposedly interferes more
with sequential processing than with holistic processing. Since we
could elicit access to whole word reading identical to that
observed from the right hemisphere in split-brain patients by
means of short tachistoscopic word presentation in the above
mentioned alexic patient and since reduction of exposure time
reduces LH performance in face processing associated with RH
dominance (Rizzolatti and Buchtel, 1977; Sergent, 1982) we
wondered if healthy subjects too could access RH reading by a
reduction of exposure duration. We designed a lexical decision
experiment with German function words. Function words are known to
be the most difficult class of words for aphasic patients to
process and therefore constitute a class of stimuli which strongly
favour a LH mode of processing. We presented tachistoscopically to
healthy right handed subjects two 4-letter strings, one to the LVF
and one to the RVF simultaneously. They saw either to the right or
to the left of the point of fixation a German function word and on
the other side a pronounceable German non-word or they saw two
pronounceable German non-words. We asked the subjects to press
response keys whenever they saw a real German word. According to
the above hypothesis we ran the experiment at three different
exposure durations at 150 msec, at 100 msec and at 50 msec
(Regard, Landis and Graves, 1985). The results of this experiment
are shown in figure 4a.

FIGURE 4a   FIGURE 4b

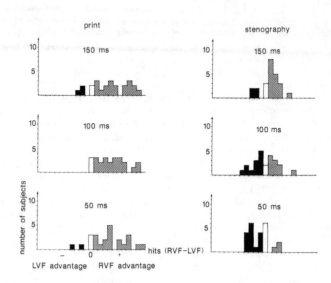

Figure 4a,b: Distribution of the subjects with respect to the difference scores between number of correct responses per VF (RVF - LVF) for the three conditions 150, 100, 50 msec, i.e. negative differences represent a LVF advantage (RH), positive differences represent a RVF advantage (LH). Fig. 4a (print) and Fig. 4b (stenography).

As shown in figure 4a reduction of exposure duration could not alter the strong advantage the LH has in recognizing function words as real German words. Apparently reduction of exposure duration alone for this word class is not sufficient in healthy subjects to access the non-dominant right hemisphere's ability to deal with lexical decisions as shown in split-brain patients by Zaidel (1983). We thought of two possible reasons for this failure, one reason could have been that in the intact connected healthy brain the dominance of the language leading LH was strong enough to prevent or inhibit any concomitant lexical decision by the RH or that function words with their lack of concreteness and lack of imageability were a class of words the RH was simply not able to deal with.

The latter reason could be experimentally tested if we were able to find a way of altering words so that they remained German function words but would gain appeal for a right hemispheric mode of processing. The history and findings of pure alexia in two patients who prior to the event were proficient stenographers provided the basis of our experiment. The stenography system explored is a phonetic shorthand writing system predominantly syllabic in nature in which meaning is altered by spatial variations. The first patient was a right handed woman who subsequent to a stroke in the territory of the right posterior cerebral artery developed a left hononymous hemianopia and a complete alexia without agraphia for stenography but only a mild and fluctuating alexia for print (Gloning et al., 1955). The second patient was a retired right-handed architect, and as a proficient stenographer member of the editorial board of the Swiss Journal of the Association of Stenographers, in which he published articles in stenography until the occurrence of a right homonymous hemianopia, severe alexia without agraphia for print and a very mild anomic aphasia due to a large left occipital metastasis of a recto-sigmoid carcinoma. When tested for reading he was himself astonished that while he was completely unable to read a single printed letter or word he continued to fluently read and write stenography at his premorbid level (Regard et al., 1985). These two cases, one with a right posterior and the other with a left posterior lesion show a double dissociation of function with respect to the reading of stenography versus print, the right posterior patient being severely alexic for stenography but much less so for print, the left posterior patient being completely alexic for print but unimpaired at reading stenography. Although reading and writing of stenography can be impaired in aphasic patients with left, language dominant lesions (Leischner, 1950) this dissociation suggests some affinity of the right non-dominant hemisphere for the reading of stenography.

We therefore designed a lexical decision experiment with function words identical to that reported above, except that function words as well as German pronounceable non-words were now written in stenography. The same subjects as in the previous experiment, all proficient stenographers participated in this study and again three exposure durations (150, 100, 50 msec) were used (Regard, Landis and Graves, 1985). Results of this study are presented in figure 4b. Similarly to the lexical decision of functions words written in print, the detection of the same function words written in stenography is a property of the LH when presented at long exposure durations. Presented however at short exposure durations a shift to an equally strong right hemisphere advantage is shown. Reduction of exposure duration therefore is one means of accessing RH capacity for lexical decision. Moreover the failure to induce RH lexical decisions of function words with printed material cannot be attributed to an inability of the right hemisphere to deal with function words per se, but may rather reflect an insufficient inhibition of left hemisphere language dominant processing by reduction of exposure duration.

The clinical and experimental data gathered from patients with reading disturbances due to lesions in the language dominant with reading dirsturbances due to lesions in the language dominant left hemisphere and from normal subjects point to the presence of two different kinds of reading abilities in each hemisphere and to an interaction between the two when it comes to demonstrating access to lexical semantics by the non-dominant right hemisphere. According to Wigan's view (1844) this interaction is inhibitory, that is the reading dominant hemisphere prevents the non-dominant hemisphere from expressing its reading abilites.

To verify directly this model of right hemisphere release under the condition of left hemisphere inhibition the unique situation would be needed in which the reading performance of both hemispheres could be monitored during a transient dysfunction of the dominant hemisphere. A prolonged left non-convulsive limbic status epilepticus is a condition in which such an interaction could be investigated. Complex partial status epilepticus is an exceedingly rare condition in which no overt seizure may occur and the symptomatology may be restricted to psychosensory or vegetative signs (Wieser et al., 1985). If such a situation occurs in patients with medically intractable seizures who undergo depth electrodes recording (SEEG) with a view to an eventual amygdalahippocampectomy (Wieser and Yasargil, 1982) the seizure activity as a model of a transient localized dysfunction could be monitored together with transient behaviour changes. We investigated such a patient, a 26 year old ambidextrous nurse who had suffered for 3 years from frequent complex partial seizures resistant to all therapy (for details see Regard et al., 1985). Beside these seizures she had experienced several episodes of gustatory sensations, lasting up to 10 days. During depth electrode recordings she frequently experienced these sensations, thus being during the whole experimental investigation in a more or less pronounced limbic aura status. During SEEG recordings we performed two long-term lateralized tachstistoscopic experiments. One consisted of the lexical decision task with function words already described, the other of a similarly designed experiment for associative matching of facial emotional expressions, a task showing a right hemisphere advantage in normal subjects (Landis et al., 1979). In the SEEG an active left limbic focus was found and its activity classified into 5 patterns of varying severity. The result of these two experiments with respect to the focal SEEG pattern during which the patient responded are shown in figure 5a,b.

The clinically and experimentally relevant SEEG pattern nr 4, during which the patient experienced her gustatory sensation consists of high frequency spike activity in the left hippocampus. As can be seen in figure 5a the performance of lexical decision on function words made during these high frequency left limbic discharges following LH stimulation drops to chance level while those following RH stimulation reach the best performance.

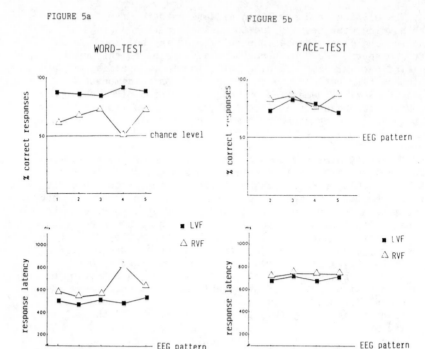

Figure 5a,b: Results in percent correct responses (top) and
response latencies in msec (bottom) for each visual field (LVF,
RVF) with respect to the five electric activity pattern for a
lexical decision (Fig. 5a) and a facial matching task (Fig. 5b).

Figure 5b shows that the limbic seizure activity in the LH does
not interfere with the facial task associated with RH processing.
Three points can be made from these results. First, deep limbic
seizure activity which is clinically manifested only by a
transitory sour-bitter taste interferes with a higher cortical
language function, e.g. lexical decision of function words.
Second, this interference is specific for place and cognitive
task, since it impairs only the LH and lexical decisions of
function words associated with an advantage of the language
dominant hemisphere and not the RH nor the face task. Third, the
loss of the ability to detect function words presented to the LH
occurring together with the best performance of the RH in the same
task may best be explained by a model of functional inhibition and
release.

     There are, however, two points which detract from the
strength of this last statement: The patient was ambidextrous and
could well have had bilateral language representation as is

frequently the case in temporal lobe epileptics (Millner, 1974; Rausch and Walsh, 1984) and she showed an overall RH-advantage in lexical decision.

In order to further clarify interhemispheric interaction in reading we investigated a similar patient but with clear left hemisphere language dominance. The right handed man with no left handedness in his family had suffered for 18 years from complex partial seizures of increasing frequency resistant to all therapy. These seizures were always followed by a prolonged period of postictal aphasia of some 10 to 20 minutes duration. He underwent depth electrode recordings during which he was presented with the long-term tachistoscopic lexical decision experiment for function words previously described. During the experiment he experienced one of his typical seizures which left him aphasic for some 10 minutes. During the postictal period of aphasia he was able to continue the experiment which was ran until the aphasia cleared and the SEEG pattern returned to the preictal state. SEEG monitoring demonstrated the onset of the seizure with high frequency spike activity to be in the left hippocampus. Seizure activity never spread to the right hemisphere, but there was a marked slowing confined to the electrodes placed in the left hemisphere during his aphasic state. The performance in lexical decision of both hemispheres before the seizure, during the postictal aphasic state and after the aphasic state are summarized in table 1 with respect to the number of experimental runs performed (Regard et al., 1986).

Table 1   Percentage correct responses in the lexical decision task task showing a RVF (LH) advantage in the preictal phase (run 1), a shift into a LVF (RH) advantage in the postictal phase (run 2), and gradual recovery·in runs 3 to 5

	run 1 preictal	SEIZURE	run 2 postictal	run 3 aphasia	run 4	run 5
RVF (LH)	92		58	50	75	92
LVF (RH)	50		83	58	50	58
overall correct	69		67	66	71	77

As shown in table 1 the patient showed preictally a performance identical to that of normal subjects, that is a good performance in lexical decision in the LH and a chance performance in the RH. This LH dominance for lexical decision shifted to an RH dominance during the period of postictal EEG slowing and aphasia and returned to the previous LH dominance with normalization of the clinical and SEEG state.

The starting point of the investigations presented here was the discrepancy between the sometimes astonishing reading ability of the isolated RH and a frequently very poor reading ability of severely aphasic patients in whom the RH is intact but connected to the damaged LH. In particular we were interested in testing the hypothesis that the reading dominant controlling LH inhibits the potential reading function of its opposite partner which had been proposed to explain this discrepancy. This interaction can of course only be tested while the two hemispheres are anatomically connected. In the hope of obtaining a maximum of converging evidence from different sources we tested healthy subjects by means of lateralized tachistoscopic stimulus presentation, aphasic patients with unilateral LH lesions, selected patients with pure reading disturbances and patients with transitory cognitive dysfunction due to focal seizures originating from deep LH structures.

We now try to answer the four questions formulated in the introduction. Question 1 concerns quantitative or qualitative reading differences between the two cerebral hemispheres in normal subjects. We found quantitative as well as qualitative differences in reading with respect to the emotional tone of nouns, the quality of semantic paralexias and the kind of writing system used, such as function word detection of print versus stenography. These results suggest the presence of two different reading strategies in the two cerebral hemispheres. The second question was concerned with a possible correlation between the reading pattern in patients with damage to the reading dominant LH and the reading performance of the RH in healthy subjects. We demonstrated a correlation between the reading ability of unselected aphasic patients and the RH performance in healthy subjects concerning the emotional tone of nouns. Furthermore, we have shown that the reading of stenography in selected patients and the lexical decision about function words written in stenography in healthy subjects have an affinity for the RH. These findings suggest a link between the reading ability of patients lesioned in the reading dominant hemisphere and the reading pattern associated with RH processing in normal subjects. In the third question we asked about conditions in which a right hemisphere reading pattern may be elicited experimentally. Using short exposure duration we could show access to lexical meaning in a letter-by-letter reader with left posterior damage and again using short exposure durations we found in normal subjects a shift from a LH to a RH advantage in lexical decision about function words written in stenography. We conjecture that brief exposure duration, disfavouring LH sequential processing in combination with a specific LH damage or a specific affinity of the RH for the stimulus type (stenography) impairs dominant LH reading and releases a hitherto hidden RH reading ability. In the fourth question we asked for a condition in which a transient hemispheric shift in reading dominance could be directly tested. Our investigation in two patients with deep left limbic seizure

activity correlated with a transitory cognitive dysfunction of the
LH provides such a model; especially the second patient
demonstrated a shift for lexical decision about function words
from the LH to the RH induced by postictal SEEG slowing restricted
to the LH and aphasia.

To conclude, despite the differences in population studied,
and the experimental methods used, we found converging evidence
for a reading potential of the "non-dominant" RH and of an
interaction of the two hemispheres in reading. Although both
hemispheres are potentially able to read, they seem to weight
lexical meaning differently, arrive at different meaning via
different paths of information processing and they may be
attracted by different attributes of the same written information.
Moreover, reading impairment of the left "dominant" hemisphere was
shown in some circumstances to lead to a release of the reading
capacity of the "non-dominant" RH. We believe that these results
are best interpreted by a model of relative interactive
hemispheric dominance in reading due to interhemispheric
inhibition and release of function, as proposed by Wigan (1844)
over a century ago.

References

Assal, G. and Regli F. (1980). Syndrome de disconnexion
  visuo-verbale et visuo-gestuelle. Rev. Neurol., 136, 365-376.
Bear, D.M. (1983). Hemispheric specialisation and the neurology
  of emotion. Arch. Neurol. 40, 195-202.
Benson, D.F. (1985). Alexia. In Handbook of Clinical Neurology,
  45. (eds. G.M. Bruyn and H.L. Klawans). North-Holland,
  Amsterdam.
Benson D.F., and Geschwind, N. (1969). The alexias. In Handbook of
  Clinical Neurology, 4. (eds. P.J. Vinken and G.M. Bruyn).
  North-Holland, Amsterdam.
Bryden M.P., Ley R.G. and Sugarman J.H. (1982). A left ear
  advantage for identifying the emotional quality of tonal
  sequences. Neuropsychol. 20, 83-87.
Caplan L.R. and Hedley-Whyte T. (1974). Cuing and memory
  dysfunction in alexia without agraphia. Brain 97, 251-262.
Carmon A. and Nachshon I. (1973). Ear asymmetry in perception of
  emotional non-verbal stimuli. Acta Psychol. 37, 351-357.
Coltheart M. (1980). Deep dyslexia: a right hemisphere hypothesis.
  In Deep Dyslexia. (eds. M. Coltheart, K. Patterson and J.C.
  Marshall). Routledge and Kegan Paul, London.
Coltheart M., Patterson K. and Marshall J.C. (1980). Deep
  Dyslexia. Routledge and Kegan Paul, London.
Damasio A.R. and Damasio H. (1983). The anatomical basis of pure
  alexia and color "agnosia". Neurol. 33, 1573-1583.
Day J. (1977). Right-hemisphere language processing in normal
  right handers. J. Exp. Psychol.: Hum. Perc. Perf. 3, 518-528.
Dejerine J. (1892). Contribution à l'étude anatomo-pathologique et
  clinique des différentes variétés de cécité verbale. C.R.
  Séances Mém. Soc. Biol. 44, 61-90.

Ellis H.D. and Shepherd, J.W. (1974). Recognition of abstract and concrete words presented in the left and right visual fields. J. Exp. Psychol. 103, 1035-1036.

Geschwind N. (1965). Disconnexion syndromes in animals and man (part I). Brain 88, 237-294.

Gloning I., Gloning K., Seitelberger F. and Tschabischer H. (1955). Ein Fall von reiner Wortblindheit mit Obduktionsbefund. Wien. Z. Nervenheilkd. 12, 194-215.

Goodglass H., Graves R. and Landis T. (1980). Le role de l'hémisphère droit dans la lecture. Rev. Neurol. 136, 669-673.

Graves R. Landis T. and Goodglass H. (1981). Laterality and sex differences for visual recognition of emotional and non-emotional words. Neuropsychol. 19, 95-102.

Greenblatt S.H. (1977). Neurosurgery and the anatomy of reading: A practical review. Neurosurg. 1, 6-15.

Heilman K.M. and Satz P. (1983). Neuropsychology of Human Emotion. Guilford Press, New York.

Hellige J.B. (1983). Cerebral Hemisphere Asymmetry. Praeger, New York.

Kreindler A. and Ioanescu V. (1961). A case of "pure" word blindness. J. Neurol. Neurosurg. Psychiat. 24, 275-280.

Landis T. (1987). Right hemisphere reading: A clinico-experimental approach to the dual brain interaction. Habilitationsschrift, Universität Zürich.

Landis, T., Assal, G. and Perret E. (1979). Opposite cerebral hemispheric superiorities for visual associative processing of emotional facial expressions and objects. Nature 278, 739-740.

Landis T., Graves R. and Goodglass H. (1982) Aphasic reading and writing: possible evidence for right hemisphere participation. Cortex 18, 105-112.

Landis T., Regard M. and Serrat A. (1980). Iconic reading in a case of alexia without agraphia caused by a brain tumor: A tachistoscopic study. Brain Lang. 11, 45-53.

Leischner A. (1950). Über Störungen des Stenographierens. Arch. f. Psychiat. Z. Neurol. 185, 271-290.

Levy J. (1974). Psychobiological implications of bilateral asymmetry. In Hemispheric Function in the Human Brain. (eds. J.S. Dimond and J.G. Beaumont). Paul Elek, London.

Marin O.S.M. (1980). CAT scans of five deep dyslexic patients. In Deep Dyslexia, appendix I. (eds. M. Coltheart, K. Patterson and J.C. Marshall). Routledge and Kegan Paul, London.

Marshall J.C. and Newcombe F. (1973). Pattern of paralexia: a psycholinguistic approach. J. Psycholing. Res. 2, 175-199.

Milner B. (1974). Hemispheric specialisation: Scope and limits. In The Neurosciences. Third Study Program. (eds. F.O. Schmitt and F.G. Worden). MIT Press, Cambridge, Mass.

Moscovitch M. (1973). Language and the cerebral hemispheres: Reaction-time studies and their implications for models of cerebral dominance. In Communication and Affects: Language and Thought. (eds. P. Pliner, L. Krames and T.M. Alloway). Academic Press, New York.

Moscovitch M. (1976). On the representation of language in the right hemisphere of right-handed people. Brain Lang. 3, 47-71.

Patterson K. and Vargha-Khadem F. (1989). Reading with one hemisphere. Brain (in press).

Rausch R. and Walsh G.O. (1984). Right-hemisphere language dominance in right-handed epileptic patients. Arch. Neurol. 41, 1077-1080.

Regard M. and Landis. T. (1984). Experimentally induced semantic paralexias in normals: A property of the right hemisphere. Cortex 20, 263-270.

Regard M., Landis T. and Graves R. (1985). Dissociated hemispheric superiorities for reading stenography vs print. Neuropsychol. 23, 431-435.

Regard M., Landis T. and Hess. K. (1985). Preserved stenography reading in a patient with pure alexia. Arch. Neurol. 42, 400-402.

Regard M., Landis T., Wieser H.G. and Hailemariam S. (1985) Functional inhibition and release: unilateral tachistoscopic performance and stereoencephalographic activity in a case with left limbic status epilepticus. Neuropsychol. 23, 575-581.

Regard M., Stodieck S.R.G., Landis T. and Wieser H.G. (1986). Temporary shift from left to right hemisphere dominance in lexical decisions caused by seizure. J. Clin. Exp. Neuropsychol. 8, 127.

Richardson J.T.E. (1975). The effect of word imageability in acquired dyslexia. Neuropsychol. 13, 281-287.

Rizzolatti G. and Buchtel. H.A. (1977). Hemispheric superiority in reaction time to faces: a sex difference. Cortex 13, 300-305.

Rodel M. (1989). Unterschiedliche Struktur- und Verarbeitungs- prinzipien von Sprachzusammenhängen in den beiden Hirnhemisphä- ren. Unpublished doctoral thesis, University of Zürich.

Rubens A.B. and Benson D.F. (1971). Associative visual agnosia. Arch. Neurol. 24, 305-316.

Sergent J. (1982). Theoretical and methodological consequences of variations in exposure durations in visual laterality studies. Percept. Psychophys. 31, 451-461.

Smith A. (1966). Speech and other functions after left (dominant) hemispherectomy. J. Neurol. Neurosurg. Psychiat. 29, 467-471.

Sperry R.W., Gazzaniga M.S. and Bogen J.E. (1969). Inter- hemispheric relationships: The neocortical commissures; syndromes of hemispheric disconnection. In Handbook of Clinical Neurology, 4. (eds. P.J. Vinken & G.W. Bruyn). North-Holland, Amsterdam.

Suberi M. and McKeever W.F. (1977). Differential right hemispheric memory storage of emotional and non-emotional faces. Neuropsychol. 15, 757-768.

Stachowiak F.J. and Poeck K. (1976). Functional disconnection in pure alexia and color naming deficit demonstrated by deblocking methods. Brain Lang. 3, 135-143.

Tucker D.M., Watson R.T. and Heilman K.M. (1976). Affective discrimination and evocation in patients with right parietal disease. Neurol. 26, 354.

Wieser H.G., Hailemariam S., Regard M. and Landis. T. (1985). Unilateral limbic epileptic status activity: Stereo EEG, behavioral and cognitive data. Epilepsia 26, 19-29.

Wieser H.G. and Yasargil M.G. (1982). Selective amygdalo-
    hippocampectomy as a surgical treatment of mesiobasal limbic
    epilepsy. Surg. Neurol. <u>17</u>, 445-457.
Wigan·A.L. (1844). <u>Duality of the Mind</u>. Longman, Brown, Green and
    Longmans, London (reprinted by Joseph Simon Publ. 1985).
Zaidel E. (1978). Lexical organization in the right hemisphere. In
    <u>Cerebral Correlates of Conscious Experience</u>. (eds. B.A. Buser
    and A. Rougeul-Buser). Elsevier, Amsterdam.
Zaidel E. (1983). Disconnection syndrome as a model for laterality
    effects in the normal brain. In <u>Cerebral Hemisphere Asymmetry:
    Method, Theory and Application</u>. (ed. J. Hellige). Praeger, New
    York.
Zaidel E. (1985). Right hemisphere language. In <u>The Dual Brain</u>.
    (eds. D.F. Benson and E. Zaidel). Guilford Press, New York.

8

Spatial Constraints on the Distribution of Selective Attention in the Visual Field

G. Berlucchi, S. Aglioti, M. Biscaldi, L. Chelazzi,
M. Corbetta and G. Tassinari

INTRODUCTION

The term selective attention refers to those intrinsic
mechanisms by which an animal becomes temporarily more reactive to
some aspects of its sensory environment while at the same time its
responsiveness to other components of the same environment
diminishes. These opposite changes in reactivity occur both between
and within sensory modalities. Selective attention is traditionally
distinguished from arousal, which alludes to the modulation of the
overall reactivity of the organism without selection between
stimuli, and with intention, defined as the preparation to move
(see Heilman, Watson, Valenstein and Goldberg, 1987). While the
distinction between selective attention and arousal is necessary
and feasible in both physiological and behavioral terms, the
usefulness and the legitimacy of a complete conceptual separation
between selective attention and intention are more questionable.
Normal behavior undoubtedly suggests that in any situation the
brain can choose one or more among many of its sensory inputs for
further processing, as well as select one of several possible motor
outputs for appropriate action. However, since the selection of a
sensory input will ultimately become manifest in behavior through a
motor output, one wonders whether the selection process involves a
specific increase in the response of the brain sensory systems to
the selected stimulus, or rather a facilitated access of the
sensory activity evoked by that stimulus to the motor systems for
translation into action. In the latter case the differentiation
between selective attention and intention would become difficult if
not downright impossible.

Inspired by an action-based view of cerebral organization for
perception proposed by Sperry (1952), we have recently suggested
that selective attention may be regarded as an operational
adjustment of the brain which primes or facilitates all motor
responses potentially triggered or guided by the selected stimulus
(although the degree of facilitation may vary from one response to

another), to the disadvantage or exclusion of motor reactions to other stimuli (Tassinari, Aglioti, Chelazzi, Marzi and Berlucchi, 1987). Which response is eventually emitted to the attended stimulus depends on a variety of internal and external conditions which are relevant to the responder's goals at that moment and which are too numerous and heterogeneous to be jointly categorized as "intention". For present purposes it is sufficient to say that under otherwise identical conditions the same motor response will be elicited more promptly and easily by an attended than an unattended stimulus, mainly if not exclusively because of a facilitated linkage between the sensory input representing the attended stimulus and the motor output controlling the response.

From the physiological point of view this suggestion is consonant with the notion that the limited and specific changes in neuronal activities required by a process of selective attention are seen not in primary sensory areas of the cortex, but rather in areas such as the posterior parietal cortex which can more directly channel sensory input into a variety of motor outputs (see Wurtz, Goldberg and Robinson, 1980; Heilman et al., 1987). By contrast, attention (or intention?) can be focussed at will on a single muscle by facilitation processes which are likely to occur in the primary motor cortex or even more peripherally (Gandevia and Rothwell, 1987). From the psychological point of view our suggestion is compatible with late-selection theories of attention (see e.g.Duncan, 1981), according to which attention acts not on the first level representation of the stimuli, but rather on their capacity-limited (and therefore selective) entry into a second-level representation which makes them available for conscious awareness and behavioral output.

In the following we describe and discuss the results of some experiments which bear on this issue. We will deal with a much studied form of selective attention, e.g.attention to a specific visual field location (visuospatial attention). In ordinary photopic human vision, targets of selective attention are normally processed faster and more accurately than non-attended targets mainly because they are positioned on the region of highest acuity of the retina (the fovea) by appropriate saccadic or pursuit eye movements. However, it has long been known from everyday experience, as well as from ingenious but non-systematic experimental observations made in the past century (Helmholtz, 1867), that by a conscious and voluntary effort it is possible to turn attention to any chosen portion of the entire visual field without moving the eyes to it. These anecdotal claims of a possibility to dissociate selective visuospatial attention from the direction of gaze have recently been validated with quantitative methods that allow a precise cost-benefit analysis of the effects of directed attention. The employment of the reaction time (RT) method in investigating attentional influences on both detection and discrimination of targets presented in different locations of the visual field has been particularly useful for this purpose

(Ericksen and Hoffman, 1972; Posner, 1978; Jonides, 1980). We shall concern ourselves chiefly with the attentional modulation of RT for the detection of a simple suprathreshold luminous target presented alone in a nearly empty visual field.

SPEED OF RESPONSE TO LIGHT TARGETS AS A FUNCTION OF SPATIALLY ALLOCATED ATTENTION

The pioneering experiments on this topic are those of Posner and his colleagues (see Posner, 1978, 1980; Posner, Cohen and Rafal, 1982). While maintaining fixation, subjects show decreases in reaction time (RT) for detecting targets at deliberately attended extrafoveal positions, and RT increases for targets at unattended extrafoveal positions, compared with a neutral or baseline condition in which there is no motivation or instruction to allocate attention to any specific target position. Spatial allocation of attention is controlled in these experiments by a central cue (e.g. an arrow) that precedes the target and provides valid or invalid information about the probability of target occurrence at each possible location. The probability of target occurrence is high for the cued position (e.g.80% probability of target occurrence at the position indicated by the arrow) and low for the other positions (e.g.20% altogether). The condition in which the target appears at the cued position is called valid, whereas the condition in which the target appears at non-cued positions is called invalid. In additional trials the cue is replaced by a signal (e.g. a cross) that indicates an equal probability of stimulus occurrence at all positions (neutral condition).

These findings have suggested the existence of a covert orienting mechanism that can shift the focus of attention over the visual field independent of ocular movements and can be metaphorically described as a continuously orientable spotlight (Posner, 1978, 1980). According to this view benefits from valid cues result from the spotlight being correctly aimed at the target location before the presentation of the target itself, whereas costs from invalid cues are linked with the necessary reorientation of a misdirected spotlight after target appearance. Other interpretations have instead supported the notion that spatially directed visual attention involves the total or partial concentration of processing resources at the selected visual field location, as opposed to the even distribution of resources among all possible target locations which is thought to be typical of the neutral, attentionally uncommitted state (Jonides, 1983; Eriksen and Murphy, 1987; Murphy and Eriksen, 1987). These accounts stress the advantage that directed attention may confer to performance by improving the extraction of information from the attended position, but do not consider the possibility that enhanced performance may derive from facilitated sensory-motor integration. We shall examine this possibility by assessing the spatial distribution of the costs and benefits of directed attention.

SPATIAL PATTERNS OF THE EFFECTS OF DIRECTED ATTENTION

Our method for analyzing the costs and benefits of the
voluntary allocation of attention to a visual field location
differs in important respects from the precuing paradigm typically
employed by Posner and coworkers. Their paradigm may be
unnecessarily complicated, first, because on each trial the subject
must interpret the cue before responding to the target, second,
because sampling errors may arise from the fact that there are many
more responses to attended than to unattended locations, and third,
because the performance of the subject may be guided more by
probabilistic operant conditioning than by a voluntary control of
attention.
We studied RT for detecting small flashes of light under
conditions of equal probability of stimulus occurrence at all
possible locations, in the complete absence of pre-stimulus cues.
There were five possible stimulus positions, aligned along either
the horizontal or the vertical meridian of the visual field. One
position coincided with the fixation point, while the other
positions lay 10 and 30 degrees of visual angle on either side of
the fixation point. The constant response task involved a speeded
manual key-press to a flash of light appearing at any position; the
variable attentional task changed from one block of trials to the
next, with five blocks of trials requiring a deliberate and
sustained allocation of attention to each of the five positions in
turn, one position per block, and another block destined for an
even distribution of attention among the five positions (diffuse-
attention condition). Fixation of the central position was
maintained troughout each trial. For each stimulus position
benefits were measured as differences between median RT in the
diffuse-attention condition and median RT in the attended
condition; costs were measured as differences between median RT in
the non-attended condition (that is when attention was directed
elsewhere) and median RT in the diffuse-attention condition.

Figure 1 illustrates the main aspects of the outcome of this
experiment and shows that the overall pattern of results did not
depend on the horizontal or vertical alignment of the stimuli. With
both stimulus arrangements we found the following:
1) all positions showed significant benefits from directed
attention. These were smallest for the central position,
intermediate for the intermediate position, and largest for the
most peripheral position, with no significant differences in
benefits between the right and left fields, and between the upper
and lower fields. There was however an overall RT superiority of
the lower field over the upper field;
2) when attention was allocated to an extrafoveal position (e.g.
right internal or low internal), there were significant and equal
costs for both positions in the opposite field (i.e. both left or
both upper positions), but not for the other position in the same
visual hemifield (i.e. right external or upper external);
3) paying attention to the central stimulus induced costs in all

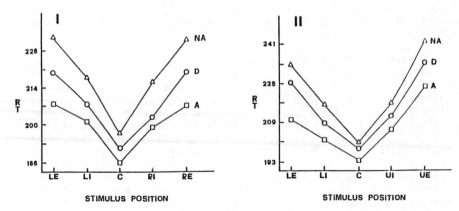

Figure 1. Benefits and costs of voluntary selective attention. Reaction time (RT, msec) is shown as a function of stimulus position and attentional condition. In I and III the stimulus array was horizontal (LE = left external position; LI = left internal position; C = central position; RI = right internal position; RE = right external position) while in II and IV it was vertical (LE = lower external position; LI = lower internal position; C = central position; UI = upper internal position; UE = upper external position). I and II show both benefits and costs of directed attention (A = attention directed to stimulated position; NA = attention directed to positions other than the stimulated position; D = diffuse attention, i.e. attention distributed among all possible positions); III and IV show a break-down of costs as a function of the positional relationship between locus of attention and target location (AD = attended location and target location are within the same hemifield; S = attended location and target location are symmetrically placed across the vertical or horizontal meridian; NS = attended location and target location are non-symmetrically placed across the vertical or horizontal meridian; D = diffuse attention). RT for the central position is not shown in III and IV. The increase in RT associated with the eccentricity of the target and the difference in RT between upper and lower fields are explained by retinal factors. Note the similarity of the patterns of costs and benefits of directed attention between horizontal and vertical arrays, and the limitation of costs to the hemifield opposite the one containing the attended location in both conditions.

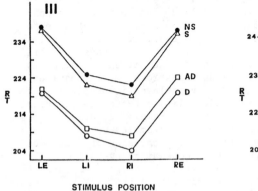

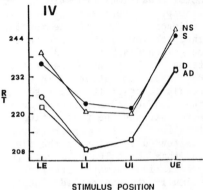

other positions, and these were significantly greater for the more
peripheral positions.

Possibly because of the elimination of the aforementioned
complications implicit in the precuing technique these results
compound partially contrasting findings from other cost-benefit
analyses of directed attention using that technique. Thus our
finding of benefits limited to the attended position agrees with
Downing and Pinker (1985) and Rizzolatti, Riggio, Dascola and
Umilta' (1987), but not with Hughes and Zimba (1985, 1987) who
found virtually no benefits from directed attention. The finding
that costs affect locations in the hemifield contralateral to the
hemifield containing the attended location, but not unattended
positions in the ipsilateral hemifield is in agreement with the
results of Downing and Pinker (1985) and Hughes and Zimba (1985,
1987), but not with those of Rizzolatti et al. (1987) who found
ipsilateral costs which however were vastly smaller than
contralateral costs. Taken together all these investigations concur
in supporting the claim that the main meridians of the visual field
act as dividers between a homogeneous cost area and a
dishomogeneous benefit area where benefits affect a restricted
location rather than the entire hemifield. When cost areas and
benefit areas are separated by the vertical meridian one might
surmise that this spatial pattern is the result of interactions and
differentiations between the activities of the two cerebral
hemispheres, each of which receives its primary visual input from
the contralateral visual field. However, the fact that the
description of this spatial pattern applies to the right and left
hemifields as much as to the upper and lower visual fields rules
out the possibility of an exclusive hemispheric interpretation,
since the upper and lower visual fields are represented in both
hemispheres (Hughes and Zimba, 1985, 1987; Rizzolatti et al., 1987;
Tassinari et al., 1987).

Our explanation of these results is as follows. When attention
is selectively turned to a location, the head-start afforded to
motor reactions to stimuli from that location is associated with
widespread contrasting effects on allied and opposed response
tendencies. Even if the response under examination is not directed
in space (such as, for example, a key-press), it will nonetheless
be planned and executed within a general motor set whose spatial
frame of reference is the location of the attended stimulus.
Responses to stimuli in non-attended locations will require a
readjustment of the motor set and will be delayed in proportion to
the degree of difference or incompatibility between the required
motor set and the preexisting set. If for example one attends to a
location in the upper visual field and a stimulus occurs at an
unattended location in the lower field, the emission of a response
to this stimulus will call for a time-consuming reversal of the
preexisting upward directional motor bias. However, responses to
stimuli at unattended locations within the upper visual field
should require no directional respecification and only a vastly

less time-consuming amplitude respecification of the preexisting motor set. Respecification of amplitude is indeed known to be much faster than direction respecification in programs for saccadic movements of the eyes (Hou and Fender, 1979) as well as for rapid movements of the hands (Rosenbaum, 1980). According to this view, the horizontal and vertical meridians of the visual field would serve as dividers between cost areas and benefit areas of directed attention simply because they are the main polar axes for specifying direction. This view can be examined further by analyzing the spatial distribution of the inhibitory after-effects of covert orienting.

INHIBITORY AFTER-EFFECTS OF EXTERNALLY CONTROLLED COVERT ORIENTING

In the precuing studies cited in the previous section, positional expectancies for extrafoveal target positions were induced by foveal cues that were remote from the cued positions and therefore where apt to signal them solely by reference to a predetermined system of symbolic relations connecting each cue to a specific position. Positional expectancies thus generated are thought to produce corresponding attentional shifts by a conscious and voluntary effort. The "symbolic" cues resulting in voluntary control of attention allocation have been contrasted with "spatial" cues engendering positional expectancies because of their spatial coincidence or contiguity with the cued position. It has been suggested that under these conditions attention is attracted automatically to the cued position without requiring a conscious effort of the will, and that these automatic attentional shifts can occur either overtly as orienting movements of the eyes, or covertly when eye position remains fixed. In the latter case attentional shifts should be revealed by improved detection or discrimination performance at the cued position (Jonides, 1983). Discrimination or detection of structured visual targets is indeed facilitated by spatial cues (Ericksen and Hoffman, 1972; Jonides, 1983).

However Posner and Cohen (1984), Maylor (1985) and Maylor and Hockey (1985) have reported an apparently paradoxical increase in RT (inhibition) for detecting simple luminous targets at the cued position. We have extended their results by studying the spatial spread of this inhibition in the visual field (Tassinari et al., 1987; Berlucchi, Tassinari, Marzi and Di Stefano,1988). In our experiments subjects made a speeded manual key-pressing response to the second of two successive light flashes in a pair, the cue and the target, while maintaining fixation. Each of the two flashes could appear at random in one of four positions, two in the right and two in the left visual field, or two in the upper and two in the lower visual fields. The stimulus-onset-asynchrony (SOA) between cue and target was varied randomly between 0.2 and 4 or 5 sec.

Our results confirmed the increase in RT to targets preceded by

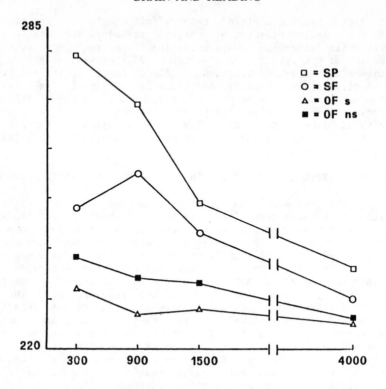

Figure 2. Reaction-time (RT, msec) to targets preceded by cues at the same position (SP), by cues at a different position within the same visual hemifield (SF) and by cues in the opposite hemifield, at a symmetrical (OF s) or non-symmetrical position (OF ns), at different cue-target SOAs (msec). Cues and targets appeared 10 or 20 degrees from the fixation point, in the right and left hemifield. At the first three SOAs RT on SP combination is significantly longer than RT for SF combinations, and this in turn is significantly longer than the RTs for the two OF combinations which do not differ from one another. From Berlucchi et al., Neuropsychologia, 1988.

a cue in the same position relative to RT to targets preceded by cues at other positions. However, our results additionally showed that inhibition affected not only targets presented at cued locations, but also targets occurring in the visual half field containing the cue. Inhibition from ipsilateral cues was long lasting since it was seen with cue-targets asynchronies ranging from 0.2 to 1.5 sec or more (Figure 2). Inhibition from ipsilateral cues occurred between right and left fields as well as between upper and lower fields, both across fixation and across points of the vertical and horizontal meridians away from fixation, and independently of the eccentricity of target and cue positions over the explored range (from 1 to 30 degrees from the main meridians). We have described this inhibition as an effect which irradiates from the cued location and arrives at the horizontal and vertical meridians without crossing them (Tassinari et al., 1987; Berlucchi et al., 1988). Thus, as in the case of deliberately allocated attention, the spatial spread of these RT effects appears to be limited by the main meridians of the visual field.

We have interpreted these effects in accord with the previously described concept of directed attention as a mechanism acting at the sensory-motor interface. Suddenly appearing extrafoveal luminous signals are strong stimuli for eliciting saccades toward their location, but this oculomotor tendency must be suppressed in experiments on covert orienting because fixation must be maintained. This suppressive action is bound to have consequences for more general motor adjustments. Important for our purposes is the directional conflict between the command that inhibits the natural ocular reaction toward a cue and the manual response to a subsequent target occurring in the same hemifield. It is conceivable that by a process of generalization in the overall motor set the oculomotor command opposing movements toward the cue can also retard manual responses to closely following targets from that same direction. Ipsilateral inhibition is a toll to be paid for being allowed to dissociate the direction of attention from the direction of gaze.

INFLUENCE OF EYE MOVEMENTS ON THE DISTRIBUTION OF ATTENTION

The essential functional significance of ocular motility is that of aligning the fovea with the focus of visuospatial attention. While, as we have seen in the foregoing, the focus of attention can shift over visual space in spite of a complete stillness of the eyes, it would seem reasonable that ocular movements cannot occur without corresponding attentional shifts. There is considerable evidence to support this association. For example, according to Posner at al. (1987) and Rafal et al. (1988) brain lesions that impair the ability to move the eyes to a target also slow down covert shifts of attention toward that target; and Shepherd, Findlay and Hockey (1986) have shown that in neurally intact subjects the preparation to make a voluntary saccadic eye movement inevitably involves the allocation of attention to the target for the saccade. In fact by facilitating motor reactions to the attended stimulus directed attention is likely to be a factor in the control of eye movements to that stimulus.

On the above assumption that attending to a stimulus at a location on, say, the right tends to facilitate responses to stimuli from other right locations as well and to inhibit responses to stimuli from the left, it can be suggested that a voluntary

movement of the eyes to an extrafoveal stimulus is preceded by an
attentional shift that may expedite motor responses not only toward
that specific stimulus, but also toward regions of the visual space
in the general direction of both stimulus and related ocular
movement. Stated differently, the directional (hemifield) patterns
of the spatial distribution of the costs and benefits of directed
visual attention should also be apparent upon an attentional shift
causing a corresponding eye movement. The development of a similar
directional pattern during the programming of a saccade would
strongly argue for a cause-effect link between the attentional
shift and the ocular movement. This suggestion was tested in
studies carried out in our laboratory on normal subjects according
to the following experimental paradigm.

    The task required that a voluntary saccade be made from a
central fixation point toward a continuously present visual target
upon hearing a 1000 Hz binaural tone delivered through earphones.
In two experiments the target was to the right of the fixation
point in half experimental sessions, and to the left in the other
sessions. In another experiment the saccade was made to a target
positioned above or below the fixation point, again in separate
experimental sessions. In all cases the distance between the
fixation point and the saccade target was 10 degrees of visual
angle. The task also required a manual key-press immediately after
seeing a small flash of light, presented at different time
intervals after the auditory tone, either ipsiversively or
contraversively to the direction of the saccade. Ipsiversive and
contraversive were defined by reference to the current fixation
point and the direction of the intended ocular movement. The eyes
were to remain on the target for the saccade until after making the
key-press response. The SOA between each auditory tone and the
subsequent flash could randomly take one of five values: 0.1, 0.3,
0.5, 0,7 (or 0.9) and 1 (or 1.5) sec. These values were chosen on
the expectation that at the first SOA (0.1 sec) the flash would
appear at a time when the saccade was being programmed but had not
yet begun, whereas at the other SOAs the flash would appear after
the saccade had been terminated. The occurrence of ipsiversive and
contraversive flashes was equiprobable, and the flash position was
expected to be such that on each trial the two types of flashes
would occur equidistantly from the current fixation point, i.e. the
initial fixation point on the before-saccade trials and the final
fixation point on the after-saccade trials. Electrophysiological
monitoring of saccadic time-course through electro-oculographic
recordings confirmed these expectations save for the 0.3 sec SOA
at which in a non-negligible number of cases the saccadic movement
had not yet been completed and thus the eyes were not yet on
target. When equidistancy of ipsiversive and contraversive flashes
from current fixation point was ensured, in all trials with long
SOAs and in some trials with a 0.1 sec SOA the distance between the
current fixation point and the flash was set at 20 degrees, so that
ipsiversive flashes occurred well beyond the target for saccade; in
some other trials with a 0.1 sec SOA this distance was set at 10

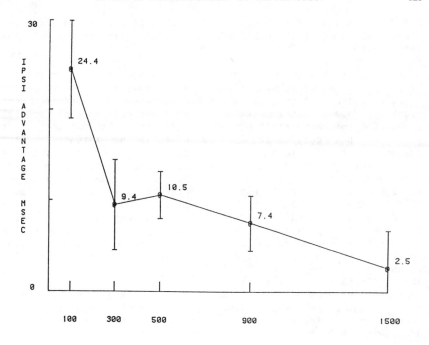

Figure 3. Advantage for ipsiversive over contraversive manual RT as a function of SOA between the command for making a saccade and target. RT and SOA in msec; vertical bars indicate standard deviations. The advantage becomes insignificant at the 900 msec SOA.

degrees, in which cases the position of ipsiversive flashes coincided with that of the actual saccade target.

Our working hypothesis predicted that ipsiversive flashes would be consistently responded to faster than contraversive flashes, thus indicating a shift of the focus of attention in the general direction of the saccade before and after the saccade itself. The results presented in Figure 3 generally corroborate this prediction. There was a highly significant ipsiversive advantage which depended on SOA, since it was maximal at the 0.1 sec SOA and declined with increasing SOA to disappear completely at the 0.7 sec SOA in one experiment and at the 0.9 sec SOA in another. The following features of the results are most relevant to our purposes: 1) the ipsilateral advantage seen when the flash position coincided with the position of the saccade target was comparable to that seen when the flash occurred in the direction of the saccade,

but well beyond its target; and 2) the pattern of results was the
same regardless of the horizontal or vertical arrangement of the
target array.

   The fact that voluntary saccades are preceded and accompanied
by changes in speed of manual responses to stimuli as a function of
their position in the visual field is consistent with the idea that
saccades cannot occur without a rearrangement of the spatial
allocation of attention. Our results show that attention is
allocated not only to the location which is the target for the
saccade, but also to other locations in the general direction of
the target. To the extent that an upward saccade speeds up manual
responses to stimuli in the upper visual field, and a rightward
saccade speeds up manual responses in the right visual field, these
effects are comparable to those observed in our experiments on
voluntary and externally controlled covert orienting. Our account
of these effects is that an allocation of attention to a point in
space - i.e. a facilitation of motor responses to stimuli from that
location - precedes and plays a causal role in the generation of a
voluntary saccade to that location. Both the actual eye movement
and the facilitation of manual responses to stimuli in the attended
location (and from points in its general direction) are expressions
of the motor set which is essential to directed attention.
Oculomotor readiness does not precede directed attention (see
e.g.Klein, 1980) but rather is a component of it.

REFERENCES

Berlucchi, G., Tassinari, G., Marzi, C.A., and Di Stefano, M.
(1988). Spatial distribution of the inhibitory effect of peripheral
non-informative cues on simple reaction time to non-fixated visual
targets. Neuropsychologia 26, in press.

Duncan, J. (1981). Directing attention in the visual field.
Percept.Psychophys. 30 90-93.

Ericksen, C.W., and Hoffman, J.E. (1972). Some characteristics of
selective attention in visual perception determined by vocal
reaction time. Percept.Psychophys. 11, 169-171.

Ericksen, C.W., and Murphy, T. (1987). Movement of the attentional
focus across the visual field: a critical look at the evidence.
Percept.Psychophys. 42, 299-305.

Gandevia, S.C., and Rothwell, J.C. (1987). Knowledge of motor
commands and the recruitment of human motoneurons. Brain 110, 1117-
1130.

Heilman, K.M., Watson, R.T., Valenstein, E., and Goldberg, M.E.
(1987). Attention: behavior and neural mechanisms. In Handbook of
Physiology Section 1, Volume V, Part 1 (V.B.Mountcastle, F.Plum,
S.R.Geiger Eds.). American Physiological Society, Bethesda.

Helmholtz, H. (1867). Handbuch der Physiologischen Optik. Voss, Leipzig.

Hou, R.L., and Fender, D.H. (1979). Processing of direction and magnitude by the saccadic eye-movement system. Vision Res. 18, 1421-1426.

Hughes, H.C., and Zimba, L.D. (1985). Spatial maps of directed visual attention. J.Exp.Psychol.: Human Percept.Perform. 11, 409-430.

Hughes, H.C., and Zimba, L.D. (1987). Natural boundaries for the spatial spread of directed visual attention. Neuropsychologia 25, 5-18.

Jonides, J. (1980). Towards a model of the mind's eye 's movements. Can.J.Psychol. 34 103-112.

Jonides, J. (1983). Voluntary versus automatic control over the mind's eye's movement. In Attention and Performance IX (J.Long and A.Baddeley Eds.). Erlbaum, Hillsdale N.J.

Klein, R. (1980). Does oculomotor readiness mediate cognitive control of visual attention? In Attention and Performance VIII (R.S.Nickerson Ed.). Erlbaum, Hillsdale N.J.

Maylor, E.A. (1985). Facilitatory and inhibitory components of orienting in visual space. In Attention and Performance XI (M.I.Posner and O.F.Marin Eds). Erlbaum, Hillsdale N.J.

Maylor, E.A. and Hockey, R. (1985). Inhibitory component of externally controlled orienting in visual space. J.Exp.Psychol.: Human Percept.Perform. 11, 777-787.

Murphy, T.D., and Ericksen, C.W. (1987). Temporal changes in the distribution of attention in the visual field in response to precues. Percept.Psychophys. 42 576-586.

Posner, M.I. (1978). Chronometric Explorations of Mind. Erlbaum, Hillsdale N.J.

Posner, M.I. (1980). Orienting of attention. Q.J.Exp.Psychol. 32, 3-25.

Posner, M.I., and Cohen,Y. Components of visual orienting. In Attention and Performance X (H.Bouma and G.G.Bouwhuis Eds.). Erlbaum, Hillsdale N.J.

Posner, M.I., Cohen, Y., and Rafal, R.D. (1982). Neural systems control of spatial orienting. Phil.Trans.R.Soc.B 298, 187-198.

Posner, M.I., Inhoff, A.W., Friedrich, F.J., and Cohen, A. (1987).
Isolating attentional systems: a cognitive-anatomical analysis.
Psychobiology 15 107-121.

Rafal, R.D., Posner, M.I., Friedman, J.H., Inhoff, A.W., and
Bernstein, E. (1988). Orienting of attention in progressive
supranuclear palsy. Brain 111 267-280.

Rizzolatti, G., Riggio, L., Dascola, I., and Umilta' C. (1987).
Reorienting attention across the horizontal and vertical meridians:
evidence in favor of a premotor theory of attention.
Neuropsychologia 25, 31-40.

Rosenbaum, D.A. (1980). Human movement initiation: specification of
arm, direction and extent. J.Exp.Psychol.: Gen. 109, 475-495.

Shepherd, M., Findlay, J.M., and Hockey, R.J. (1986). The
relationship between eye movements and spatial attention.
Q.J.Exp.Psychol. 38A 475-491.

Sperry, R.W. (1952). Neurology and the mind-brain problem. Am.Sci.
40, 291-312.

Tassinari, G., Aglioti, S., Chelazzi, L., Marzi, C.A., and
Berlucchi, G. (1987). Distribution in the visual field of the costs
of voluntarily allocated attention and of the inhibitory after-
effects of covert orienting. Neuropsychologia 25, 55-71.

Wurtz, R.H., Goldberg, M.E., and Robinson, D.L. (1980). Behavioral
modulation of visual responses in the monkey. Progr.
Psychobiol.Physiol.Psychol. 9, 43-83.

9
Dynamics of Information Processing of the Somatosensory Cortex

B. L. Whitsel and O. G. Franzén

For a long time it seemed as if in
natural science the problem of
language played only a secondary
rôle.

W. Heisenberg, 1960

Language, the symbolic representation of thought and action, is one of the most valuable mechanisms we possess through which man communicates with other people and leaves records of past experiences. It is intricately intertwined with our perception, memory and emotional life - all vivid expressions of the dynamic actions of specifically interconnected, large-numbered structures concerned with the analysis of complex sensory and cognitive processes.

A long trip begins with the first step and it goes without saying that disturbances in the machinery of the brain, however subtle they may be, can have far-reaching consequences for the developing human being. Of considerable importance to our understanding of the brain mechanisms underlying language is the fact that many children less than two years of age and with damage to the language areas of the left hemisphere can go on to develop satisfactory language ability. This observation implies that specialization of the brain mechanism responsible for language function is not completed at that age and that the plasticity of these complex neural networks permits their adaptive reorganization. In contrast, the majority of teenagers who experience comparable brain damage never recover normal language function (Fischer and Lazerson, 1984).

Also of great significance to an appreciation of the nature
of the mechanisms involved in language is the emerging view that
developmental dyslexia is a condition in which the distributed
functional systems of the cerebral neocortex that subserve reading
seem to interconnect and operate abnormally, indicating that the
cerebral cortical dysfunction observed in this learning disability
is global rather than local and that it has an anatomical substrate. The evidence supporting this view derives from very
different types of studies: for example, (i) neuroanatomical
studies of the brains of dyslexics have detected multiple telen-
cephalic anomalies in the development of laminar architecture
manifested as abnormal layering and orientation of cells which is
attributable to defects in neuronal migration and selection
(Geschwind and Galaburda, 1984, 1985), (ii) neurophysiological
studies have detected abnormal cerebral cortical neuroelectrical
activity in wide-spread areas of the brain of dyslexic subjects
(Duffy et al., 1980) and (iii) behavioral studies have reported
that dyslexic subjects exhibit an interaction between foveal and
peripheral vision which interferes with reading in the foveal
field (Geiger and Lettvin, 1987). Thus, dyslexia is a complex
disability in the use of language that involves a constellation of
factors (Franzén, 1982). These developmental abnormalities may
have as their cause an abnormal perinatal hormonal environment.
This is assumed to be a critical factor in determining the functional development of the brain and even if only temporarily
disturbed, can result in permanent changes at all levels of the
nervous system with repercussions in the organism's adult life
(Geschwind and Galaburda, 1984, 1985).

Neither the neurophysiological nor the behavioral consequences of connectional abnormalities comparable to those observed
in the brains of subjects with developmental dyslexia can be
stated with any degree of certainty until fundamental studies
using animal subjects have allowed (i) characterization of the
poorly understood "dynamic processes" which are presumed to
underlie the appreciable information processing capabilities of
normal cerebral cortical neural networks, and (ii) determination
of the effects on information processing capabilities of controlled manipulations of the multiple afferent drives that access
all cerebral cortical networks. While the currently available
evidence falls far short of that required to "explain" such a
high-order disability as dyslexia, there is much room for opti-
mism, because recent work has led to substantial progress in our
appreciation of the dynamic processes governing the representations of sensory surfaces in cerebral cortex (this is especially
evident in the recent literature dealing with the somatosensory
cerebral cortex), has provided a wealth of new information about
the cellular actions and receptor systems for the various cortical
neurotransmitter substances, and has permitted identification of
the connectional pattern representative of each of the different

classes of neurons that can be identified within neocortical cell columns.

The findings obtained in the field mapping studies of Merzenich and his colleagues (see Merzenich et al., 1988 for review) have exerted a particularly strong influence on current ideas about the mechanisms underlying cortical functional plasticity in normal subjects and the defective cerebral mechanisms in e.g. dyslexia and a variety of other disorders of cerebral cortical information processing. Specifically, the studies of Merzenich et al. (1988) have demonstrated that the spatial distribution of mechanoreceptive cutaneous input to the somatosensory cortex of adult animals can change in response to experimental manipulation of the normal pattern of peripheral sensory innervation. Among those manipulations which have been shown to lead to changes in the somatosensory cortical maps of the skin surface are amputation of a body part, transection of a peripheral nerve, surgical rearrangement of the normal neighborhood relations among skin areas, and prolonged exposure of a skin area to natural or electrical stimulation. Comparable findings obtained in studies of the effects of manipulations on the functional organizations demonstrable with neurophysiological mapping methods in the auditory and motor cortices led Merzenich et al. (1988) to propose a general theory of neocortical operation. The chief ingredients of this general theory are (i) the assumption that the functional connectivity of the entire neocortex is dynamically maintained throughout adult life, (ii) the suggestions that a principal factor in the determination of the functional connectivity exhibited by any neocortical field is the extent to which spatially distributed inputs the network receives over its multiple afferent channels, are temporally correlated, and (iii) the idea that the weight of synaptic connections between thalamic axons and cortical neurons remains modifiable to greater or lesser extent throughout the entire lifespan of the organism.

Work carried out in our laboratories at the University of North Carolina has led to view of dynamic cerebral cortical processes which, at least in some details, differs sharply from that expressed by the general theory of neocortical operation advocated by Merzenich et al. (1988). This view is illustrated schematically in Figure 1., and its details are based on experimental observations provided in C-14-2-deoxyglucose metabolic and receptive field mapping studies of the somatosensory cortex (Juliano and Whitsel, 1987; Juliano et al., 1988; Favorov and Whitsel, 1988a, b), and also on the data provided in studies on the effects of repetitive tactile stimuli on the responsiveness of individual somatosensory cortical neurons in unanesthetized animals (Diamond et al., 1986; Whitsel and Kelly, 1987; Whitsel et al., 1988). Two fundamental experimental observations exerted prominent influence on the nature of the model: first, our disco-

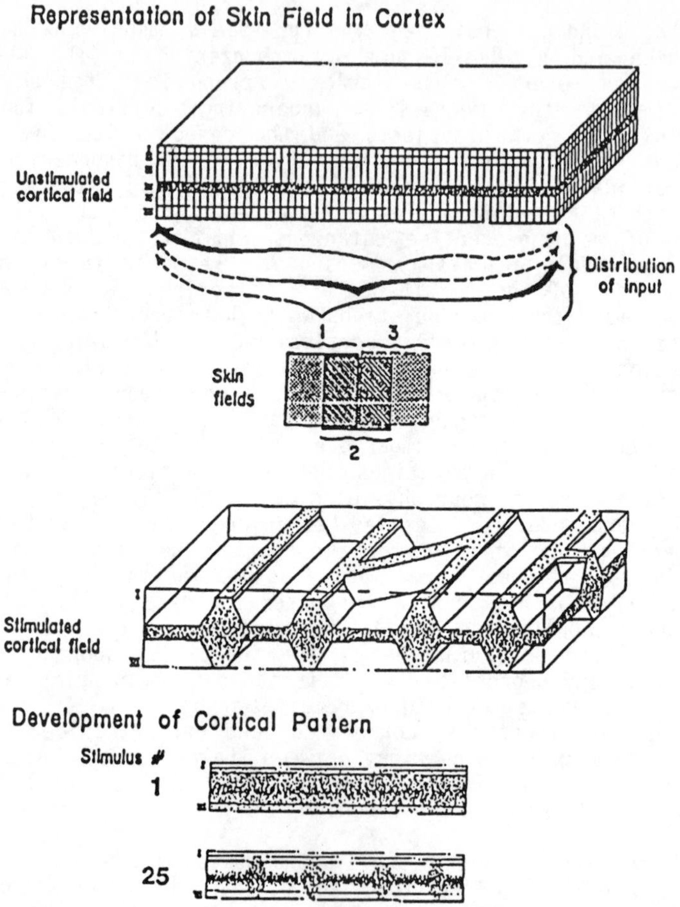

Representation of Skin Field in Cortex

Figure 1   At the top: the S-I cortical area receives its input from all regions of the skin field accessing the entire cortical field (illustrated by the diverging arrows between the skin and cortex). The schematic view of the unstimulated cortex shows the distribution of metabolic activity being low in all layers with the exception of layer IV. In the middle: the inhomogeneous spatial pattern of metabolic labeling set up by skin stimulation (note the strip-like above-background pattern). At the bottom: postulated time course of development of the strip-like pattern of activity of the S-I cortex evoked by the first stimulus (1) and by the 25th stimulus (25).

very (in receptive field mapping experiments) that the low-threshold mechanoreceptors from a restricted region of skin always project to an extensive sector of the S-I or S-II cortex (this is indicated by the widely-diverging and overlapping brackets drawn between the different parts of the skin and the cortex), and second, we have been guided by our consistent finding (in C14-2DG metabolic mapping experiments) that stimulation of any skin region with either natural or electrocutaneous stimulation never activated the total S-I or S-II cortical region which receives input from the stimulated field. Instead, repetitive stimulation of the skin field always fractionated the cortical territory that received input from the stimulated skin region into an inhomogeneous, strip-like activation pattern (Tommerdahl et al., 1987).

Additional evidence obtained in our experiments suggested an explicit mechanism for the nonrandom fractional activation of the cortical field evoked by repetitive tactile stimulation. Specifically, based on the effects of bicuculline on stimulus-evoked metabolic labeling patterns (bicuculline is a drug that blocks the inhibitory actions of gamma-amino-butyric acid, GABA, on cerebral cortical neurons) we now believe that (i) the effectiveness of the thalamic input which accesses the middle layers of the cortex is regulated by intrinsic dynamic or "adaptive" mechanisms involving GABAergic inhibitory connections, and that these regulatory influences occur chiefly in the vicinity of the principal thalamic recipient layer (layer IV and the basal part of layer III), and (ii) when the inhibitory neurons in the middle layers are strongly activated, they prevent thalamic excitatory input from activating upper- or lower-layer cortical neurons in neighboring columns which receive less strong excitatory drive, i.e. the intercolumnar intrinsic GABAergic inhibitory circuitry is proposed to act as a gate that prevents excitatory thalamocortical input from activating superficial and deep layer neurons in columns neighboring those which receive the most powerful thalamocortical drive - an outcome which identifies this as a cortical "opponent" mechanism. As a result of this type of gating, the network-wide distribution of stimulus-evoked activity in those neuron populations located above and below the middle cortical layers of the somatosensory cortex fails to correspond to that present in the middle layers (see Figure 1). This non-correspondence was a routine observation in our C14-2DG mapping studies (see Whitsel et al., 1988).

The dynamic processes which we believe govern the formation of the spatial activity patterns evoked by natural stimuli in somatosensory cortex exhibit a pronounced time-dependency. This aspect of our model of cortical stimulus representation is depicted schematically by the two unfolded sections shown at the bottom of Figure 1. According to the model, following a prolonged period in which no stimuli are delivered, the first tactile stimulus evokes activity distributed relatively homogeneously

throughout the entire somatosensory cortical territory that
receives input from the stimulated skin site (e.g., see the
activity pattern evoked by hypothetical stimulus number 1 at
bottom of Figure 1). However, with repetition of the same stimulus, dynamic cortical processes are recruited into action, leading
to the development (in the superficial and deep cortical layers)
of a spatio-intensive pattern of activity which uniquely reflects
the parameters of the physical stimulus and perhaps the context in
which the stimulus was delivered.

It is important to recognize that the view of dynamic cortical processes indicated by the model summarized in Figure 1
departs significantly from that advocated in the general theory of
neocortical operation of Merzenich et al. (1988). First, the view
of Merzenich regards the cortex as functionally two-dimensional
(i.e., it sees the variations in the receptive field and response
properties of neurons sampled at different levels of the same
cortical column as so minor that they can be ignored), while it is
our position that the laminar variations in single neuron receptive field and response properties are substantial and are highly
meaningful for somatosensory cortical information representation
and processing. Second, it is our view that the functional plasticity of the somatosensory cortex is regulated on a moment-to-
moment basis (i.e., we believe it can change drastically over the
course of a few tactile stimuli extending over only a few seconds), and that such rapid changes are affected by a mechanism
(thalamocortical gating) quite unlike that which is widely assumed
to be operative in neocortical development (i.e., Hebbian-type
synaptic weight modification). In general, our model appears consistent with the idea that variability and complexity are important and fundamental characteristics of biological systems capable
of dynamically responding to constantly changing internal and
external challenges (Goldberger et al., 1988a, b; Goldberger,
1988).

On the basis of the available evidence, one cannot reject the
possibility that both thalamocortical gating and the Hebbian
synaptic weight modifying mechanisms may be operative in the adult
cortex, and that both cooperate (i) in the moment-to-moment
regulation of the cortical response to repetitive tactile stimuli
(which we have emphasized in our studies), and (ii) in the topographic remodeling of the somatic cortex that occurs in adults
after prolonged and drastic afferent activity pattern manipulations of the type studied by Merzenich and his colleagues. Evaluation of the relative role(s) of the two mechanisms in mediating
the plasticity of the normal and partially deafferented somatosensory cortex will require further experimentation.

The process of transmitting a message from one individual to
another dominantly utilizes the auditory and visual sensory

systems of the brain, as well as the higher brain regions with which they are interfaced. From this standpoint, therefore, it seems clear than an improved understanding of the neural dynamics operative in sensory information processing is likely to lead to an improved understanding of dyslexia and related disorders. We have chosen the mechanoreceptive system as a vehicle to approach the basic problem of understanding the dynamic neural mechanisms underlying sensory perception in the tacit belief that such mechanisms are common to all sensory systems.

In support of our belief that common dynamic mechanisms underlie cerebral cortical sensory information processing is the fact that the fingertip serves as the fovea of the blind. Reading Braille is indeed a marvelous example of a complex tactile task which requires the simultaneous participation of a variety of cortical neural mechanisms subserving tactile motion sensitivity, including those mediating direction sensitivity, perceived traverse length and subjective velocity. Their optimal conduct falls within the range of stimulus velocities between 5 - 20 cm/sec where the ability to distinguish opposing directions of motion across the skin is greatest, and subjective estimates of distance traversed are most veridical and nearly constant. Together they operate to assure that proper spatio-temporal features of the tactile characters of the Braille system are presented in high fidelity to the higher-order brain regions which subserve touch (Essick, Franzén and Whitsel, 1988). In view of the presumed global nature of the cortical neural disturbances in dyslexia it would be of fundamental interest to determine if the weak visual imagery and tendency to make reversals in the right-left orientation in reading words in dyslexic subjects is paralleled by analogous deficiencies in the tactile sense.
The future challenges for the interdisciplinary neural mechanisms research we are pursuing, are (i) to learn more about the complex somatosensory information channel and to establish additional and more objective experimental bases for the participation of dynamic processes in neocortical function, (ii) to determine the roles of the different cortical neurotransmitter and receptor systems in these processes, and ultimately, (iii) to ascertain if and to what extent defects in cortical dynamic processes we are studying, contribute to disorders such as developmental dyslexia.

Supported by NIH Program Project Grant DE07509.

REFERENCES

Diamond, M., Favorov, O., Tommerdahl, M., Kelly, D. and
Whitsel, B.L. (1986). The responsivity of S-I-cortical
neurons changes systematically with repetitive tactile
stimulation. Neurosci. Abs., 12, 1431.

Duffy, F.H., Denckla, M.B. and Sandini, B. (1980). Dyslexia:
regional differences in brain electrical activity by topographic mapping. Ann. Neurol. 7, 414-420.

Essick, G.K., Franzén, O. and Whitsel, B.L. (1988). Discrimination and scaling of velocity of stimulus motion across
the skin. Somatosens. Res. In press.

Favorov, O. and Whitsel, B.L. (1988a). Spatial organization
of the peripheral input to Area 1 cell columns: I. The
detection of "segregates". Brain Res. Revs., 13, 25-42.

Favorov, O. and Whitsel, B.L. (1988b). Spatial organization
of the peripheral input to Area 1 cell columns: II. The
forelimb representation achieved by a mosaic of segregates.
Brain Res. Revs., 13, 43-56.

Fischer, K.W. and Lazerson, A. (1984). Human development.
From conception through adolescence. Freeman. New York.

Franzén, O. (1982). Final discussion of International Symposium on Dyslexia, p. 159. (ed. Y. Zotterman) Dyslexia:
neuronal, cognitive and linguistic aspects. Pergamon Press,
Oxford.

Geiger, G. and Lettvin, J (1987). Peripheral vision in
persons with dyslexia. N. Engl. J. Med., 316, 1238-1243.

Geschwind, N. and Galaburda A.M. (1984). Cerebral dominance.
The biological foundation. Harvard University Press, Cambridge, Massachusetts and London, England.

Geschwind, N. and Galaburda A.M. (1985). Cerebral lateralization. Biological mechanisms, associations, and pathology:
I. A hypothesis and a program for research. Arch. Neurol.,
42, 428-459.

Goldberger, A.L. (1988). Chaos and fractals in physiology and
medicine. Workshop on the biomedical implications of chaos
theory. The Johns Hopkins University, Laurel, Maryland, USA.

Goldberger, A.L., Bhargava, V., West, B.J. and Mandell, A.J. (1988a). On a mechanism of cardiac electrical stability: the fractal hypothesis. Biophys. J., 48, 525-528.

Goldberger, A.L. and Rigney, D.R. (1988b). Sudden death is not chaos. (eds. J.A.S. Kelso, A.J. Mandell and M.F. Shlesinger). Dynamic patterns in complex systems. World Scientific Publishers. Singapore. 248-264.

Juliano, S. and Whitsel, B.L. (1987). A combined 2-deoxyglucose and neurophysiological study of primate somatosensory cortex. J. Comp. Neurol., 263, 514-525.

Juliano, S, Whitsel, B.L., Tommerdahl, M and Cheema, S. (1988). Determinants of patchy metabolic labeling in the somatosensory cortex of cats: a possible role for intrinsic inhibitory circuitry. J. Neurosci. In Press.

Merzenich, M.M., Recanzone, G., Jenkins, W., Allard, T. and Nudo, R. (1988). Cortical representational plasticity. In Neurobiology of the Neocortex. Dahlem Konferenzen. (eds. P. Rakic and W. Singer). J. Wiley Sons, New York, N.Y.

Tommerdahl, M., Whitsel, B.L., Cox, E., Diamond, M. and Kelly, D. (1987). Analysis of the periodicities in somatosensory cortical activity patterns. Neurosci. Abs., 13, 470.

Whitsel, B.L. and Kelly, D. (1987). Knowledge acquisition ("learning") by the somatosensory cortex. In Brain Structure, Learning, and Memory. (eds. J.L. Davis, R.W. Newburgh, and E.J. Wegman). AAAS Selected Symposium 105, Westview Press, Wash., D.C.

Whitsel, B.L., Favorov, O., Tommerdahl, M., Diamond, M., Juliano, S. and Kelly, D. (1988). Dynamic processes govern the somatosensory cortical response to natural stimulation. In Organizational Principles of Sensory processing: The Brain's View of the World. (ed. J.S. Lund, Oxford University Press, New York, N.Y.

10
Disordered Right Hemisphere Function in Developmental Dyslexia

John Stein, Patricia Riddell and Sue Fowler

Majority opinion at present holds that specific reading disability is a result of disordered language processing (Vellutino, 1978); and that, contrary to many people's beliefs, seldom, if ever, can it be explained by impaired visual perception. To those who accept the 'motor' theory of speech comprehension (Lieberman et al., 1967) such difficulties with learning to read are only to be expected. Understanding written script depends upon being able to segment the continuous sounds of spoken language into separate phonemes, which can then be represented in print as graphemes. However, the very existence of the 'phoneme' is questionable. The concept is somewhat arbitrary and artificial, because there is no exact correspondence between what we describe as separate phonemes and the continuous sequence of articulatory gestures which we use to generate speech. Hence whilst a child learns to speak almost automatically with no special teaching, reading is much more difficult. It usually requires a lengthy period of teaching; and many children fail. Those who believe that dyslexia has a purely linguistic basis hence often go further and argue that it must be caused by disordered function of the dominant left cerebral hemisphere.

The idea that dyslexia is exclusively a linguistic problem does not survive close study however. Although many dyslexics find it difficult to segment the sounds in speech into their constituent phonemes, by no means all do so. Measures of this ability in young children do indeed correlate significantly with their rates of reading progress; but they predict less than 10% of the variance in subsequent reading ability (Bradley & Bryant, 1983). It is likely therefore that linguistic problems are only a partial explanation for dyslexia; and that other difficulties, such as impaired visuospatial perception, may be involved as well.

Likewise the evidence that in dyslexics the left hemisphere is specifically disorganised, is weak. Although some do have abnormal left hemispheric function, it should be noted that in blood flow,

139

EEG and neuroanatomical studies the right hemisphere has been found
to be involved as well. This accords with modern concepts of
complimentary specialisation of both hemispheres (Code, 1987) rather
than absolute dominance of the left. The right hemisphere has as
important a role to play in visuospatial function, as the left has
for speech; and both are required for reading.

In this chapter I am therefore going to develop the hypothesis
that impaired development of the right hemisphere plays an important
role in the problems of many developmental dyslexics. I shall
discuss:

1.   evidence that many dyslexics have disordered visuo-
      spatial function;

2.   The role of the right hemisphere in visuospatial and
      visuomotor functions;

3.   evidence that many developmental dyslexics have impaired
      development of the functions of the right hemisphere.

1.   Dyslexics' visuospatial function

My first important task is to make entirely clear the criteria
which we use to diagnose developmental dyslexia. Many studies
suffer from inadequate attention to this essential preliminary. If
reading ability were normally distributed with respect to I.Q. then
$2^1/_2\%$ of all children would be expected to read more than 1.96%
standard deviations behind the mean level for their age and I.Q.
(95% probability level); and equal numbers of males and females
would be affected. Instead up to 20% of boys, and 5% of girls
(Rutter & Yule, 1978), read below their expected standard, implying
that there is a significant excess of poor readers, especially among
males. This 'hump' on the distribution curve suggests in turn that
developmental dyslexics may be a separate population with
distinctive characteristics.

We therefore only call children 'dyslexic' if they meet this
simple operational criterion: their reading must be more than
2 S.D.s behind that expected from their scores on non verbal
subtests of the British Abilities Scales (BAS). The BAS
Similarities and Matrices tests have been shown not to penalise
children with specific reading difficulties (Thompson, 1982); and
therefore give a reliable guide to such children's fundamental
ability that is suitable for our purposes.

Some authorities suggest that, in addition to the reading
deficit, other common characteristics of dyslexics, such as
left/right confusions or sequencing problems, should be included in
the definition, and used to determine whether a child is 'truly'
dyslexic (Miles, 1983). However by excluding children who do not

have these symptoms, but whose reading is nevertheless significantly
backward, one is prejudging the basic issue of what causes any such
child to fail to learn to read. We therefore define as dyslexic any
child whose reading in the BAS single word reading test falls more
than 2 S.D.s behind their performance on the matrices or
similarities tests.

Dyslexics' unstable vision.

Many dyslexic children complain that they cannot see properly.
They say that letters and words seem to blur, change their
orientation and move around, so that they cannot tell what way round
or in what order they should be. Hence they confuse words, such as
'dog' with 'god' or 'was' with 'saw'. These symptoms are seldom the
result of any visual defect which can be detected by standard
clinical tests. In fact many children with very poor visual acuity
learn to read perfectly well. It appears that the problems of
dyslexics with visual symptoms are more complex. For some reason
they seem to be experiencing an unstable visual world.

Their frequent complaints of visual instability made me wonder
whether they might be suffering breakdown of the processes which
keep the visual world perceptually stable; these combat the stream
of images which smear across the retina each time we move our eyes.
This possibility occurred to me as a result of the research I had
been doing studying the mechanisms by which information provided by
the visual system is converted into motor signals capable of aiming
eye and limb movements accurately at a target (Stein, 1978). The
position of an image on the retina by itself provides incomplete
information about the real location of its parent object in space.
To determine accurately where it is in relation to the observer,
requires the association of its retinal locus with additional
signals about the direction in which the eyes are pointing when the
object is fixated.

Such association of ocularmotor and retinal signals enables the
maintenance of a representation of the true location of objects of
interest independently of eye position. The process of transforming
the retinal co-ordinates of an image into real space co-ordinates of
the object by making use of ocularmotor signals, is probably a
particular function of the right posterior parietal cortex as I
shall be discussing later.

Vergence control.

There are particularly intractable difficulties with
determining the direction and distance of objects when the eyes are
converged to look at near targets. Under these conditions the two
eyes are pointing in opposite directions with respect to the head;
i.e. in an arrowshead directed at the close object. Neither eye's
ocular motor signals alone can give unequivocal information about
the direction and distance of the object; these must be recovered

by triangulation from the angles of the two eyes with respect to the
frontal plane, and from their distance apart. This is a complex
calculation, and one which is very vulnerable to drugs and disease.

Imagine yourself inspecting the word 'dog'; but instead of
converging accurately on the letter 'o' your eyes are actually
converged on a plane behind the word. Then the 'd' is foveated by
the left eye and the 'g' by the right eye. But you have no
awareness of which eye is seeing what image. Furthermore, if your
eyes were suddenly to shift to converge on a plane in front of the
page, the right eye would change from fixating the 'g' to the 'd'
suggesting that the 'g' was now to the left of the 'd', and that the
word was 'god'. Such are the missequencing errors which are typical
of dyslexics.

What evidence is there that unstable convergence really does
explain some of the difficulties faced by dyslexics? In the
following pages I shall present evidence that many dyslexic children
suffer a disorder of visuomotor control which causes a vicious
circle. Poor visuomotor control leads to an impaired ability to
determine the location of objects reliably, which in turn hinders
the accurate aiming of eye movements towards them; i.e. an impaired
sense of visual direction worsens visuomotor control, and it can
lead to the visual reading problems outlined earlier.

The Dunlop Test.

It was Sue Fowler who started me thinking along these lines.
She had been using an orthoptic test introduced by Patricia Dunlop
(Dunlop, 1972) to study dyslexic children's visual problems. Her
test was derived from Ogle's original observations (Ogle, 1962) on
ocular dominance under vergence viewing conditions. He suggested
that stable dominance of one eye had to develop in order to be able
to determine the direction of objects reliably when the eyes are
converged. Hence he reasoned that its acquisition must be necessary
for developing an accurate sense of visual direction.

In the Dunlop Test the eyes are caused to diverge or converge
whilst inspecting small $(2^1/_2^0)$ fusion slides in a stereoscope with
moveable tubes – a synoptophore. The slides are identical, a house
with a central front door, apart from monocular 'controls': a large
post with a circle on top seen by the left eye is drawn on one side
of the front door, and a small post with an arrow on top is seen by
the right eye on the other side. These controls are introduced in
order to detect any monocular suppression (if the child fails to see
both the arrow and circle posts); and also to determine which eye
is the 'dominant' or 'reference' eye under these conditions. When
the eyes are made to converge or diverge in the test most people
experience, just before fusion breaks, a strong illusion that one of
the posts appears to move in relation to the door. Of course
neither post actually does move because post and door are on the
same slide. The eye which does not see its control post appear to

move in relation to the door is termed the 'reference eye'. In normal readers the post on one side always appears to remain stationary even when the test is repeated 10 times, as we do routinely. Such children are said to have a stable or 'fixed' reference eye; and this implies that they have acquired a reliable sense of visual direction. Sue Fowler and I found that up to two thirds of the dyslexic children we saw did not consistently see the post on the same side remain stationary. They had 'unfixed' or 'unstable reference' (Stein & Fowler, 1982). We believe that unstable Dunlop Test responses indicate that a child has failed to make reliable retinal/ocularmotor associations, hence he has an impaired sense of visual direction.

This finding has been repeated by us in several different ways (Stein et al., 1987), and by several other groups (Bishop et al., 1979, Bigelow & McKenzie, 1985, Masters, 1988). The differences between normals and dyslexics remain significant, even when the groups compared are matched on the basis of reading rather than chronological age (Stein et al., 1987). This kind of comparison is important because it rules out the possibility that the development of a stable reference eye in Patricia Dunlop's test may simply be the result of reading practice, the dyslexics failing to develop stability because they are such poor readers. However in our reading age match study, most of the younger normal readers, reading at the same level as the dyslexics, had stable reference, whereas the dyslexics did not. This argues that it is the development of stable reference which helps children to read rather than vice versa. The dyslexics cannot be charged with having had less reading experience than the normal controls because both groups had reached the same low reading level.

What does unstable reference in the Dunlop Test imply about the visuospatial abilities of dyslexic children? Nobody suggests that such large vergence changes as those which are called for in the Dunlop Test are required during normal reading. However vergence adjustments ($< \pm 0.5^{\circ}$) are required when reading a flat page; and we (Bracewell et al., 1987), and others (Collewijn et al., 1988), have found that vergence errors much larger than this ($< \pm 5^{\circ}$), are regularly made, then corrected, by normal subjects when shifting their gaze to a new lateral position in the same frontal plane. These corrections require each eye to refoveate the target independently, i.e. that the ocularmotor control system for each eye has available the retinal signals which that eye is providing together with eye position signals about the direction in which it is pointing. We argue that development of stable reference in the Dunlop Test indicates that these signals are available and reliably associated for each eye. In contrast unstable reference implies that the retinal and ocularmotor signals relating to each eye are mixed up; hence they are not available to direct each eye accurately, and, if necessary, independently of the other, for vergence control.

Vergence eye movement control.

We have confirmed these ideas by recording vergence eye
movements in normal and dyslexic children. The stimulus for undertaking these was partly theoretical, and partly the practical
problems which have arisen from attempting to use the Dunlop Test
clinically. It is highly subjective; and it is often difficult for
the child to understand what he is meant to be doing. It requires a
highly experienced tester to interpret the child's responses.
Therefore in order to obtain more objective records of dyslexics'
visuomotor control we began measuring children's vergence eye
movements during the Dunlop Test (Stein et al., 1988). It speedily
became apparent that, as we had suspected, children with unstable
Dunlop Test responses were unable to make accurate vergence
movements in the Test. Normal children are able to make smooth
symmetrical convergence responses when performing the Dunlop Test.
But many dyslexic children with the same reading age as normal
controls were unable to make convergence responses at all under
these conditions. Instead they tend to make inappropriate conjugate
movements so that after a very short while they begin to see double.

This pattern of impaired vergence eye movement control in the
Dunlop Test has proved to correlate well with subjective Dunlop Test
perceptual responses. Among 300 reading retarded children, Dunlop
Test perceptual and vergence responses were the same in 235 (73.5%);
and in 110 normal children the concordance was nearly 90%. As we
have reported several times for the Dunlop Test, approximately two
thirds (69%) of identified dyslexics proved to have poor vergence
eye movements, compared with only 2% of normal readers.

We then compared dyslexics' vergence eye movements with much
younger normal controls matched for reading rather than
chronological age (Stein et al., 1987), in order, as explained
earlier, to exclude the possibility that their ocularmotor control
was inferior simply because they had so much less reading experience
than age matched normal readers. We confirmed that the dyslexics
had even worse vergence control than these much younger normal
readers. Their poor ocularmotor control could not have been the
result of their lack of reading experience because the younger
controls had had the same limited amount, yet had good vergence
control. This result strongly implies that good vergence control is
a prerequisite for satisfactory reading progress.

The most common disagreement between Dunlop Test results and
vergence eye movement records was that in about 20% of dyslexics
(but only 5% of normals) the Dunlop Test indicated a stable
reference eye but the eye movement recordings still showed poor
vergence control. This and other evidence suggests that a stable
reference eye in the Dunlop Test often develops before accurate
vergence control is achieved. This is not unexpected if development
of stable reference is associated with acquisition of the good
visual direction sense which is required for accurately directing

vergence eye movements.

The remaining anomalous group – those whose vergence eye movements were good but whose Dunlop Test results indicated unstable reference eye, was the smallest (c.5%). We have found that many of these children exhibit unstable fixation; their eyes dart around, seemingly uncontrollably, even when they are asked to fixate the stationary calibration symbols. Such eye movements are normally conjugate however. We have not yet studied them in any great detail; but we believe that they may constitute a separate group of children with unstable fixation, not caused by impaired vergence control, but by some other factor.

Treatment of poor vergence control.

Our eye movement recording results have in general confirmed our hypothesis that many children's reading difficulties are a consequence of impaired visual direction sense associated with poor vergence control. This conclusion led us to attempt to improve these children's binocular control in the hope of helping their reading. Also we hoped that successful treatment would provide further evidence in favour of our hypothesis that impaired visuomotor control is a potent cause of children's reading failure.

Our first attempts were encouraging (Stein & Fowler, 1982). We gave 15 children with unstable Dunlop Test results a pair of spectacles with one lens occluded with opaque tape to wear only while reading. Our rationale was that these children's two eyes often fail to point accurately at the same letter; hence retinal and ocularmotor signals provide confusing cues about where the letter is situated. Consequently occluding one eye might help the children to sort out the confusion. The 15 children who wore the occluding spectacles became fixed on the Dunlop Test within a few months, and then improved their reading age by an average of over 12 months during the 6 months we followed them up; whereas 15 children with unstable reference whom we did not treat, remained unstable on the Dunlop Test and improved their reading by less than 6 months in the 6 months they were observed, i.e. their reading regressed relative to their age over the 6 months.

We have since confirmed these results in a double blind study designed to control for any placebo effect of the treatment (Stein & Fowler, 1985). Monocular occlusion was effective in improving vergence control in about half of dyslexic children with unstable visual direction sense as assessed by the Dunlop Test. The reading age of children whose vergence control improved increased by 12 months during the 6 months follow-up, whereas those whose vergence did not improve did not improve their reading.

Unfortunately we have found that monocular occlusion is not particularly effective for older children (over $8^1/_2$). We have been more successful with vergence exercises in older children however

(Stein et al., 1987). We teach them to maintain stable convergent
fixation on a close pencil tip by observing and holding still the
double images of a distant object. When vergence control is
improved by these exercises, the child's reading often improves
thereafter.

Stereoacuity.

Another consequence of impaired vergence control that we might
expect is reduced stereoacuity, since accurate determination of
binocular disparity requires very stable binocular fixation. So we
have been measuring stereoacuity in all the children we see, using
the 'Randot' test (Stein et al., 1987). As expected, stereoacuity
is indeed reduced in children with unstable vergence control
compared with normals. Moreover when we manage to improve
children's binocular control their stereoacuity improves also.

Dot localisation.

It follows from our hypothesis that impaired vergence control
is associated with poor visual direction sense, that dyslexic
children's visuospatial perception should be impaired not only for
letters, but when attempting to locate any small target accurately.
Larger targets are easier to locate simply because they are larger,
and because outside the macular area the problems of determining
which eye is seeing what are less severe.

It was therefore important to confirm that children with poor
vergence control also had impaired ability to localise small non
linguistic targets. Patricia Riddell therefore tested them in a dot
localisation task (Fowler et al., 1988). A small (10') conditioning
spot was displayed on a VDU for 2 seconds i.e. long enough for the
eyes to wander if the child had unstable fixation. 200 mS later a
test spot was flashed to the right or left of it and the child was
asked to indicate by pointing which way the spot had appeared to
move. The task difficulty was adjusted to give c.25% errors. 25%
was chosen as halfway between making the task too easy (0% errors)
and too difficult, in which case their responses would have been
random (50% errors in this two alternative forced choice paradigm).
The results were clear. As expected, children whose vergence
control was impaired made significantly more errors in the task than
children who had good binocular control.

We also measured the eye movements of some of the children
whilst they were performing the localisation task. As expected
those with poor vergence control made significantly more
inappropriate eye movements when they were meant to be fixating the
targets steadily than children with good binocular control; also
the amplitude of these was larger. These unintended eye movements
led them to make more errors than normal controls, as predicted by
our hypothesis.

Summary.

We have been able to show that many dyslexic children have poor visuomotor control associated with impaired ability to locate small targets accurately (impaired visual direction sense) which can explain many of their symptoms. Normal readers do not show these abnormalities. Treatment, either by means of monocular occlusion in younger children (under $8^1/_2$ years old), or vergence exercises, can help these dyslexics to improve their vergence control; and if this happens their reading often improves greatly. These observations support the hypothesis that impaired visuomotor control and visuospatial sense may cause many of dyslexics' difficulties. I should emphasise here, however, that we do not claim that all dyslexics' problems are visuospatial, merely that some are. It is clear that many dyslexics have the phonemic segmentation problems which were discussed earlier, in addition to or instead of, the visuospatial impairments described in this section.

2.   Visuospatial functions of the right hemisphere

The oversimple concept of left hemisphere dominance (which even led some commentators to wonder why we have a right hemisphere at all!) has given ground to Hughlings Jackson's alternative idea of complimentary specialisation (Hughling Jackson, 1898). According to the modern version of this idea, where the left hemisphere is specialised for the temporal sequencing required for speech production and comprehension, the right is essential for spatial sequencing, visuospatial perception and the spatial direction of attention and eye and limb movements. Evidence for these special functions of the right hemisphere comes from many quarters, including comparing perceptual abilities on the two sides of the body (divided field studies), imaging of cerebral activity using EEG and cerebral blood flow techniques, neuroanatomical studies, recording from single neurones (mainly in animals) and the results of lesions in man and animals.

Hemifield perceptual studies.

The rationale for comparing subjects' perceptual abilities on the two sides of the body is that the primary sensory pathways bring information to the contralateral hemisphere first. Any access of that hemisphere to ipsilateral signals requires transfer from the opposite side via the corpus callosum. Hence left sided superiority implies right hemispheric specialisation for the task under study, and vice versa. However equal abilities on the two sides do not necessarily imply a lack of hemispheric specialisation for the task; this outcome could result from transfer of the necessary ipsilateral information across the corpus callosum being very efficient.

A broad range of visuospatial functions have been shown to be better performed in the left hemifield (Young, 1983), suggesting that the right hemisphere provides superior facilities for the processing demands of the tasks. These include simple visual discriminations, such as intensity and colour differences, dot detection, dot localisation, line rotation and orientation judgements. Left hemifield superiority has also been found for stereoacuity, global stereopsis and distance judgements, the rotation and recognition of complex forms and for recognising faces.

In the somaesthetic domain similar left sided advantages have been found. The left hand is better at detecting raised dots, appreciating the orientation of unseen rods, bisecting them accurately, stereognosis of complex shapes, constructing with unseen blocks, even for the detection of letters in Braille, though not for decoding their meaning. In the auditory domain left ear advantages have been found for non linguistic sound analysis - e.g. the perception of tone, pitch and intonation and recognising the emotional connotations of music.

Sensorimotor association.

In a recent survey of the extensive literature on divided field studies Young (1983) pointed out that the largest differences between the two sides have usually been found for the most 'complex' tasks such as the recognition of faces, stereognosis and block construction. One important common feature of these complex tasks, is their requirement for accurate sensorimotor control; for example precise retinal/ocularmotor associations are required to determine the position of important features during the many fixations made when inspecting a face; and accurate somatomotor associations are essential to interpret the sensory reafference occurring during the many movements made by the fingers when palpating a complex object for stereognosis.

I have therefore speculated that the fundamental pressure for hemispheric specialisation came not from the requirements of perception, but from the need for accurate sensorimotor control (Stein, 1988); operations in space being organised by the right hemisphere, those in time by the left hemisphere. This argument is supported not only by the evidence of specialisation of the right hemisphere for visuospatial performance, and of the left for linguistic functions, but also by evolutionary and phylogenetic considerations.

Saccadic accuracy.

In the case of visuospatial functions the 'sensorimotor' theory of hemispheric specialisation predicts that large differences between the hemispheres appear, not because the tasks are very 'complicated', but because they demand accurate sensorimotor control. A simple example of such control is the integration of retinal and ocularmotor signals which is required, as described earlier, to transform the evanescent retinal co-ordinates of images fleetingly fixated, into a stable representation of the location of objects in real space. Therefore I predicted that aiming accurately at small targets ought to be a special function of the right hemisphere. To test this hypothesis, Martin Bracewell and I (1987) measured the accuracy with which subjects could aim saccadic eye movements at small targets, in azimuth (requiring conjugate, version, eye movements) and in depth (requiring accurate dysconjugate, vergence control).

Right handed subjects were asked to look at a central fixation spot for 1 second. This was then extinguished and 200 msec later a target spot flashed for 200mS to the left or right of it. The subjects were told to make a saccade as accurately as possible to where the target had appeared. Because it had by then disappeared they were not able to enlist the help of visual feedback to increase the accuracy of their saccades. Almost all subjects were significantly more accurate when making these version saccades into the left hemifield; the mean difference in azimuth accuracy between the two fields (c.25%) was as large as those seen in more complex tasks such as form or face recognition. The differences in vergence accuracy between the hemifields were even greater as the figure shows. I have been emphasising this theme and will continue to do so: accurate vergence control is most difficult to achieve, and is most vulnerable to drugs and disease; it is probably particularly dependent on proper functioning of the right hemisphere.

Hemispheric specialisation.

What do left sided superiorities in sensorimotor processing tell us about the mechanisms of hemispheric specialisation? Two alternative hypotheses are: (1) 'Strong' specialisation. The two hemispheres are absolutely specialised and the left hemisphere cannot perform spatial functions at all. Hence if visual material is projected to the left hemisphere it must be handed over the corpus callosum to the right cortex for visuomotor processing. This transfer takes time and degrades the signals; hence performance is inferior in the left hemifield.

An alternative hypothesis (2) is 'weak' specialisation. According to this idea both hemispheres participate in all kinds of processing but the right is better than the left for some tasks, and vice versa for others. Thus the left hemisphere gets involved in spatial processing but is simply worse at these operations than the right. No callosal transfer is necessary therefore; but left sided advantages follow from the right hemisphere's superior spatial abilities.

It has not yet proved possible to decide unequivocally which of these alternatives is correct. Divided field studies cannot provide the answer because callosal transfer of signals cannot be avoided. Measures of cerebral activity have repeatedly suggested that not only primary sensory areas, but also the association areas of both

right and left hemispheres are involved in most of the tasks
studied, whether linguistic or visuospatial, i.e. they favour the
'weak' hypothesis. On the other hand studies of split brain
subjects and patients with lesions tend to favour the 'strong'
hypothesis. Speech is unequivocally located in the left hemisphere
and visuospatial abilities in the right in most subjects, according
to these results.

Right posterior parietal cortex.

Measuring the relative size of homologous cortical areas in the
two hemispheres, recording regional cerebral ability and careful
assessment of the effects of lesions has enabled us to determine
which parts of each cerebral hemisphere are responsible for the
processing functions underlying hemispheric specialisation. In the
case of visuospatial function the association cortex in the
posterior part of the parietal lobe has turned out to be crucial.
In humans and higher primates this area is larger on the right side
than on the left (Geschwind & Galaburda, 1987);   during visuomotor
tasks it is more highly active than corresponding regions on the
left; and following lesions patients suffer the converse of all the
left sided advantages enumerated earlier, i.e. they are poor at
visual discriminations, face and form recognition; they misaim and
have particular problems with reading, judging distances etc.
(Benton, 1979).

The most common symptom of a right posterior parietal lesion is
left sided inattention or neglect, i.e. failure to notice stimuli in
the left side. Significantly left hemisphere lesions do not often
lead to right sided neglect; this requires bilateral damage, which
implies that the right hemisphere contributes to visuospatial
orientation even in the right hemifield. Many of the results of
parietal damage can be reproduced in animals by appropriately placed
lesions, although signs of particular specialisation of the right
posterior parietal cortex have not yet been found. By cooling the
posterior parietal cortex in monkeys trained to reach for lights in
either their right or left hemifields I was able to show that
parietal inactivation caused them to misaim (Stein, 1978b). Their
perception of the location of visual targets appeared to have become
distorted.

The success of such animal models means that a large body of
single unit recording data obtained by Hyvarinen (1982) and
Mountcastle (1975) and his colleagues who have studied the functions
of the posterior parietal cortex in primates, can be applied to the
problems of hemispheric specialisation. The essential findings, for
our purposes, are that discharge of posterior parietal neurones
normally precedes shifts of attention or eye or arm movements aimed
towards visual targets. They seem to encode both the retinal
location of the target and the position of the eyes at the time
(Andersen, 1985). Thus they are ideal candidates for performing the
retinal/ocular-motor associations described earlier, which are

necessary for converting the retinal co-ordinates of an image into a representation of its position in real space; this process has been alluded to repeatedly in this chapter. Another theme I have emphasised is the importance and particular difficulty of distance judgements and control of corresponding vergence eye movements. So it is not unexpected to find that posterior parietal neurones seem to encode not only version, but also vergence eye movements (Sakata, 1985).

One can summarise the function of the right posterior parietal cortex as to maintain a representation of the real position of objects around us, using retinal and ocularmotor cues. It seems that this representation is not a 'map' in the true sense of the word; there is no suggestion of a topo-graphical arrangement of cortical neurones representing adjacent areas of space. Rather there seems to be a distributed 'look up table' denoting the direction in which the 'mind's eye' (attention), the eyes or the limbs must point in order to aim at each object, i.e. the representation seems to be in terms of motor vectors in 'motor space'.

'Cognitive spaces'.

There are a number of psychological 'spaces' with which we think and work. Personal space is that occupied by our own body, its orientation with respect to gravity and in the world, the disposition of our limbs etc. To maintain 'morphosynthesis', as this perceptual process is called, requires the association of motor signals with proprioceptive and cutaneous signals provided by the limbs. This is analogous to the retinal/ocularmotor associations discussed earlier. This seems to be a special function of the region of posterior parietal cortex in front of area 7 known as area 5. Lesions here cause amorphosynthesis, and recordings show that neurones in area 5 carry both cutaneous, proprioceptive and motor signals (Mountcastle et al., 1978).

Peripersonal space is equivalent to the motor space alluded to earlier. It is the space immediately surrounding us within which we can touch objects. In it an accurate representation not only of the positions of the limbs and body, but also of near objects is maintained. Operating in it therefore requires, in addition to the functions attributed above to area 5, the retinal/ocularmotor associations which are known to take place in area 7 for locating targets visually. Extrapersonal space is the space beyond peripersonal, where we have less accurate information (visual and auditory only) about the position of objects.

Personal, peripersonal and extrapersonal space are all 'egocentric'. That is locations within them are of specified with respect to a co-ordinate system centred somewhere near the bridge of the nose. Conceptual space on the other hand is 'allocentric'. It uses an abstract set of co-ordinates which remain unchanged from wherever they are inspected. Thus, West and East are allocentric terms, specified absolutely, as on a map; whereas left and right are egocentric, since their direction in real space depends upon which way round you, the observer, happen to be looking at them. In conceptual, allocentric, space objects are located in relation to each other and a set of standard geographical co-ordinates, without reference to the observer.

Interestingly it seems probable that long term memorised items in conceptual space are not stored in the parietal cortex, but are retrieved when required by that region in order to generate the parietal sensorimotor representations currently in use. Bisiach and his colleagues (1978) found that patients with right posterior parietal cortex lesions omitted the buildings on the left side when describing the cathedral square in Milan as if entering from the cathedral end; but they could describe these buildings perfectly well when asked to imagine the square as though they were entering from the other end. Seen from this end they now omitted the side they had already described (now on the left side of their conceptual space). This suggests that all the required information was still retained in memory after the cortical lesion, but only the right sided motor map could be created for consciousness. In fact it seems likely that the basic allocentric storage may take place in the hippocampus.

Summary: The right posterior parietal cortex appears to be specialised to generate a representation of the direction and amplitude required of conscious shifts of attention towards objects in the environment, or of voluntary eye or limb movements aimed towards them. For eye movement control this requires precise association of retinal and ocularmotor signals. This is a particularly difficult operation for vergence eye movements, since the signals from each eye are different, but must be reliably compared to specify azimuth and distance accurately. Thus vergence eye movement control, and direction and distance judgements during vergence, are particularly vulnerable to right posterior cortical damage.

3. Right Hemisphere Function in Developmental Dyslexics

In this, unfortunately the shortest section, I wish to draw together the threads from the two preceding ones; to show that there is prima facie evidence supporting the hypothesis that the poor vergence control and inaccurate sense of visual direction which we have found in many developmental dyslexics may be the result of disordered development of the visuospatial processing functions of their right hemispheres. Again it is necessary to emphasise that we do not believe that this is dyslexics' only problem.

Acquired Dyslexia.

It is often alleged that acquired dyslexia only occurs after left hemisphere damage. However dyslexia alone, without aphasia, is rare after left sided damage (Vignolo, 1988); whilst dyslexia without dysgraphia is rarer still. The latter is a very important condition theoretically, because its existence implies that visual perceptual input to the reading system can be eliminated without damaging graphemic output. Dyslexia without dysgraphia requires a lesion involving not only the left angular gyrus, but also, very significantly, the posterior part of the corpus callosum or the right angular gyrus (posterior parietal cortex). This implies that to obtain isolated dyslexia, visuospatial signals provided by the right posterior parietal cortex need to be disconnected from left sided speech areas.

In fact, contrary to some claims, right posterior damage usually does lead to reading difficulties. Such patients are not often labelled 'dyslexic', because this problem is so obviously a consequence of their visuospatial disorder; it is merely one aspect of their left sided neglect. Nevertheless poorly aimed eye movements and missing out the left side of the page or the left side of words decimates reading, as was clearly recognised in the 19th century by Hughlings Jackson, by Gordon Holmes after the first world war and, more recently, by Hecaen (1978) who coined the term spatial dyslexia to describe the condition.

Left sided Neglect.

A common clinical test for neglect is to ask the patient to attempt to draw a clock. We ask all children referred to us to draw a clock. Many show clear evidence of left sided neglect. A neurologist might conclude that children who draw clocks in this way are suffering a right posterior cortical lesion. Yet nearly 60% of children with reading difficulties display significant impairment at drawing clocks, particularly on their left side. This figure is strikingly similar to the proportion of children we see with poor vergence control and impaired visual direction sense. We are currently investigating this aspect of their condition in greater detail, using a battery of neuropsychological tests for neglect. But clearly these preliminary observations are suggestive that the children have right posterior cortical damage of some kind.

Another result pointing to the same conclusion came when we analysed our dot localisation data (Fowler et al., 1988) with respect to the hemifield in which the dyslexic children made most errors. The children had inspected a target spot and then had been asked in which direction it had appeared to move when the test spot had flashed subsequently to the right or left of it. So we could compare the average numbers of errors they made in left and right visual fields. There was a very clear difference between the normal controls and the children with poor vergence control and impaired

visual direction sense. As expected the normals made slightly more
errors when the test spot flashed in the right visual field; but
the impaired children made their great excess of errors in the left
visual field. Even though they were almost as good as the normals
at detecting the test spot in the right field they were far, far
worse in the left visual field. Clearly, this difference supports
the hypothesis that impaired development of the specialised
visuospatial functions of the right hemisphere may underlie their
reading problems.

        Finally in this context I should re-emphasise the findings of
Brain electrical activity mapping and local cerebral blood flow
measurement (Mazziotta et al., 1982). Even linguistic activities
such as listening to speech and speaking, which were thought to be
exclusively left hemisphere functions have been found to be attended
by significant right hemisphere activity; whilst during reading the
right hemisphere is seen to be even more active. Interestingly in
Frank Duffy's comparisons between normal and dyslexic children's
cerebral activity during reading, one of the areas which showed the
greatest differences from normal was the right posterior parietal
cortex.

Summary and Conclusions

        In this chapter I have presented evidence that many dyslexics
have impaired visuomotor control which gives rise to an inaccurate
and unreliable sense of visual direction; this may be one cause of
their reading difficulties. Their visuomotor instability
particularly affects vergence eye movements; hence their distance
and direction judgements are especially poor when the eyes are
converged, as when reading. These problems do not affect normal
readers even when these are matched with dyslexics on the basis of
their reading ability rather than their chronological age, in order
to ensure that the dyslexics have had the same amount of reading
experience as the controls. The results of the reading eye match
confirm that dyslexics' visuomotor problems are probably a cause
rather than a consequence of their reading impairment.

        This conclusion is supported by the results we obtained from
attempting to treat these children's visuomotor deficit by means of
monocular occlusion or vergence exercises. When this was successful
in improving vergence control the accuracy of children's direction
sense improved, as did their reading.

        Accurate visuomotor control and visual direction sense depend
upon proper development of the specialised visuospatial functions of
the right hemisphere. The right posterior parietal cortex appears
to maintain a representation of the motor vectors required to direct
the mind's eye (attention), the ocularmotor system, and limb
movements accurately towards visual targets. Lesions of the right
posterior parietal cortex lead to neglect of the left side of space,
the misaiming of eye and limb movements and to impaired vergence

control; hence reaching and judgements of distance are especially
disturbed.

These facts make it natural to speculate that dyslexics' visual
problems may be a consequence of disordered development of the
specialised functions of the right hemisphere. I presented some
evidence that this is indeed the case. Right posterior cortical
damage does give rise to reading problems. Dyslexic children show
evidence of left sided neglect analogous to that found in patients
with right hemisphere lesions, and they make errors of visual
localisation especially in the left hemifield, again like patients
with right hemisphere damage.

Thus my over-all conclusion is that many dyslexic children have
impaired visuomotor control and visuospatial perception, as a result
of disordered development of the specialised functions of the right
hemisphere. These visuomotor abnormalities can often be alleviated,
in which case the children's reading difficulties may improve also.
But in ending I must again emphasise that the disordered right
hemisphere functions discussed in this chapter are seldom found in
isolation. Unfortunately many dyslexic children also have
linguistic problems, perhaps due to maldevelopment of the
specialised functions of the left hemisphere, which may continue to
impede their reading even after their visuospatial problems have
been conquered. It seems quite likely that both left and right
hemisphere disorders have a common genetic/developmental/endocrine
aetiology (Geschwind & Galaburda, 1987); but it remains to be
discovered precisely what this is.

References

Andersen, R.A., Essick, G.E. & Siegel, R.M. (1985). Encoding
    spatial location by posterior parietal neurones. Science,
    230, 456-458.
Benton, A.L. (1979). Visuospatial Disorders. In Clinical
    Neurophysiology, (ed. K.M. Heilman and Valenstein). Oxford
    University Press.
Bigelow, E.R. & McKenzie, B.E. (1985). Unstable ocular dominance
    and reading ability. Perception, 14, 329-335.
Bishop, D.V.M., Jancey, C. & Steel, A.McP. (1979). Orthoptic status
    and reading disability. Cortex, 15, 659-666.
Bisiach, E. & Luzzati, C. (1978). Unilateral neglect of
    representational space. Cortex, 14, 129-133.
Bracewell, M., Husain, M. & Stein, J.F. (1988). Differences in the
    accuracy of saccades in left and right visual fields.
    J.Physiol., 382, 98P.
Bradley, L. & Bryant, P. (1983). Categorising sounds and learning
    to read - a causal connection. Nature, 301, 419-421.
Code, C. (1987). Language, Aphasia and the Right Hemisphere.
    J. Wiley, Chichester.

Collewijn, H., Erkelens, C.J. & Steinman, R.M. (1988). Binocular
    coordination of human horizontal saccades. J.Physiol., <u>404</u>,
    157–182.
Dunlop, P. (1972). Dyslexia; the orthoptic approach. Australian
    J. Orthopt., <u>12</u>, 16–20.
Fowler, M.S., Riddell, P. & Stein, J.F. (1988). Binocular fixation
    and visual direction sense in backward readers. Physiological
    Society Meeting, Paris.
Geschwind, N. & Galaburda, A.M. (1987). <u>Cerebral Lateralization:</u>
    <u>Biological Mechanisms, Associations and Pathology.</u> The MIT
    Press, Cambridge, Mass. and London, England.
Hecaen, H. & Albert, M. (1974). Human Neurophysiology, Wiley, New
    York.
Hyvarinen, J. (1982). The Parietal Lobe of Primates. In <u>Studies</u>
    <u>in Brain Function 8.</u> Springer.
Hughlings–Jackson, J. (1898). <u>Selected Writings.</u> (ed. J.Taylor
    (1931). Hodder & Stoughton, London.
Larsen, B., Skinho, E. & Larsen, N.A. (1978). Regional cortical
    blood flow in right and left hemisphere during automatic
    speech. Brain, <u>101</u>, 193–211.
Lieberman, A.M., Cooper, F.S., Shankweiler, D.P. & Studdert Kennedy,
    M. (1967). A motor theory of speech perception. Psychol.Rev.,
    <u>74</u>, 431.
Masters, M.C. (1988). Orthoptic management of visual dyslexia.
    Brit.Orthoptic J., <u>45</u>, 40–48.
Mazziota, J.C., Phelps, M.E., Carson, R.E. & Kuhl, D.E. (1982).
    Ternographic mapping of human cerebral metabolism: auditory
    stimulation. Neurol., <u>32</u>, 921–937.
Miles, T.R. (1983). <u>Dyslexia: The Pattern of Difficulties.</u>
    Collins, London.
Mountcastle, V., Lynch, J., Georgopoulos, A., Sakata, H. & Acuna,
    C. (1975). Posterior parietal associating cortex – Command
    functions for operations within extra personal space.
    J.Neurophysiol., <u>38</u>, 871–908.
Ogle, K. (1962). The Optical Space Sense. In: Davson, H. <u>The</u>
    <u>Eye, Vol.IV.</u> Academic Press, New York and London.
Rutter, M. & Yule, W. (1975). The concept of specific reading
    retardation. J.Child Psychiatry, <u>16</u>, 181–197.
Sakata, H. (1985). Neural mechanisms of space vision in posterior
    parietal cortex of the monkey. Vis.Res., <u>25</u>, 453–463.
Stein, J.F. (1978a). Long Loop Motor Control in Monkeys. In:
    <u>Cerebral Motor Control in Man: Long Loop Mechanisms.</u> (ed.
    J. Desmedt). pp.107–123, Vol.4, Prog. in Clin.Neurophysiol.
    Karger, Basel.
Stein, J.F. (1978b). Effect of Cooling Parietal Lobe Areas 5 and 7
    on Visual and Tactile Performance of Trained Monkeys. In:
    <u>Active Touch.</u> (ed. G.Gordon). Pergamon Press, Oxford.
Stein, J.F. & Fowler, M.S. (1981). Visual dyslexia. Trends in
    Neurosciences, <u>4</u>, 77–80.
Stein, J.F. & Fowler, M.S. (1982). Diagnosis of dyslexia by means
    of a new indicator of eye dominance. Brit.J.Ophthalmol., <u>66</u>,
    332–336.

Stein, J.F. & Fowler, M.S. (1985). Effect of monocular occlusion on visuomotor perception and reading in dyslexic children. The Lancet, 13 July, 69–73.

Stein, J.F. & Fowler, M.S. (1988). Disordered vergence eye movement control in dyslexic children. Brit.J.Ophthalmol., 72, 162–166.

Stein, J.F., Riddell, P. & Fowler, M.S. (1987). Fine binocular control in dyslexic children. Eye, 1, 433–438.

Stein, J.F. (1988). Physiological Differences between the Hemispheres. In Aphasia. (ed. Clifford Rose). Whurr Wyke, London.

Vellutino, F.R. (1978). Psychological factors in specific reading disability. In Dyslexia. (ed. A.L. Benton). Oxford University Press, New York.

Vignolo, L.A. (1988). The Anatomical and Pathological Basis of Aphasia. In Aphasia. (ed. F.C. Rose). Whurr Wyke, London.

Young, A.W. (1983). Functions of the Right Hemisphere. Academic Press, London.

11
Motor Control in Man: Complex Movements Using One or Both Hands

J. C. Rothwell

INTRODUCTION

There have been many studies of simple, self-paced, self-terminated movements at a single joint (e.g. Angel, 1974; Hallett, Shahani & Young, 1975; Hallett & Marsden, 1979). Such movements, executed as rapidly as possible, have been termed "ballistic", and are produced by a triphasic pattern of electromyographic (EMG) activity in agonist and antagonist muscles. The duration, latency and size of these bursts varies with the velocity and extent of movement (see Wierzbicka, Wiegner & Shahani, 1986 for references) and is relatively constant from subject to subject. Because of its simplicity, this type of movement has been examined in a multitude of different diseases. Deficits have been found in the timing and duration of the EMG bursts as well as in the kinematics of the movement, which in some instances are relatively specific to certain disease states (see Hallett, 1983).

Motor behaviour in daily life is more complex than this. It can be envisaged as a continuous series of movements, some being executed at the same instant and others in a sequence. In order to mimic this increased complexity we have studied movements made up of two simple actions: elbow flexion and isometric power grip ("squeeze"). These movements were performed either simultaneously or sequentially ("squeeze then flex") with one or both arms. The question arises as to how the brain combines such simple actions into a single more complex movement. Are two separate motor programs concatenated, or is a new, more complicated program devised which has overall control of all aspects of the task? The data suggest that at least for these particular tasks, each separate action remains under the control of a separate program. The two programs are then run simultaneously or sequentially according to the instruction given to the subject. The study of patients with Parkinson's disease provides some insight into how the process of combining motor programs may be affected in disease states in man. The work described here was performed with Drs R.Benecke, B.L.Day,

J.P.R.Dick and C.D.Marsden.

METHODS

   The methods have been described in detail in two papers by
Benecke et al. (1986a,b;1987). Briefly, subjects were seated com-
fortably with the shoulder abducted to 90°, and the semipronated
forearm strapped to a lightweight manipulandum. The elbow joint
was coaxial with the pivot of the manipulandum, which was connected
to a potentiometer measuring elbow angle. The hand grasped a U-
shaped bar of aluminium that recorded the force of the hand squeeze
via a strain gauge mounted on one of the vertical arms of the U.
Subjects were asked to perform a 15° elbow flexion or a 30N squeeze,
both of which he could monitor on an oscilloscope screen before
him. The tasks were: i) elbow flexion alone, ii) squeeze alone,
iii) flex and squeeze at the same time (simultaneous task) or
iv) squeeze first and then flex (sequential task). Tasks (iii) and
(iv) were performed either using one arm for both movements, or
using one arm to flex and the other to squeeze. All movements were
self-paced with the instruction to move as rapidly as possible.
Accuracy of movement was not stressed. Four to five practice trials
were allowed before recordings began.

   Results from normal subjects were compared with those from a
group of ten patients with Parkinson's disease, seven of which were
studied 12hrs or more after stopping their normal drug therapy.

RESULTS

Simultaneous movements

   Normal subjects had no difficulty in executing simultaneous
movements of flex and squeeze using either one or both arms. The
combined movement appeared to be the sum of the two separate movements, both in terms of the underlying EMG pattern and the trajectory of the movement (Fig.1). Thus, the time taken to perform the
flex and squeeze components of the simultaneous movement was the
same as when each movement was performed on its own. (Mean $\pm$ 1 s.e.
data from 10 subjects using one arm: flex alone, 229 ± 14 ms;
squeeze alone, 156 ± 8 ms. In the simultaneous task, the movement
times were: flex, 244 ± 12 ms; squeeze, 150 ± 8 ms).

   The question arises as to whether the simultaneous movement
was, as it appeared to be, the sum of two separate movements, or
whether performance of a simultaneous movement required the preparation and execution of a novel, more complex motor program.

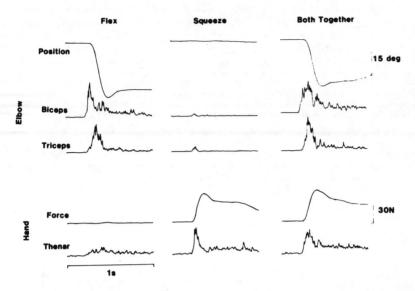

Fig. 1.   Typical average (of 10 trials each) records of simple
and simultaneous movements in a normal subject. The left column
shows data from a flex; the middle column for a squeeze; the right
column for a combined flex and squeeze executed at the same time.
Records are, from the top down, elbow angle, biceps EMG, triceps
EMG, squeeze force and thenar EMG. The combined task appears to be
the sum of the two single movements.

In order to distinguish these possibilities, we analysed the co-
variation of movement times between flex and squeeze in the simultaneous task. In some complex movements, such as handwriting
(Denier van der Gon & Thuring, 1965), typewriting (Terzudo &
Viviani, 1980) or speech articulation (Tuller et al. 1982), changes
in the timing of one part of the movement always are accompanied
by changes in timing of the other parts. For example, in writing
a letter "a", there is always a constant relation between the
speed at which the circular and straight parts are executed: if
one is slow, the other is equally slow. In the present simultaneous
flex and squeeze movement this was not the case. Although the
duration of the flex and squeeze components varied in any one subject from trial to trial there was no constant relation between
the two. The correlation coefficient relating movement times of
flex and squeeze ranged from −0.4 to +0.6 in ten subjects (mean,
0.16). On this basis it seems that a simultaneous flex and squeeze
is produced by the simultaneous execution of two separate motor
programs.

Examination of the bereitschaftspotential (BP) preceding such
movements suggests that the simultaneous execution of two separate
movements is organised differently to the execution of each movement separately. In nine normal subjects, the BP was larger and
began earlier prior to movement onset with a simultaneous flex and
squeeze compared with the BP prior to each movement on its own
(see Benecke et al., 1985). An example of this behaviour is shown
in fig.2. It may be that this extra activity reflects the increased
complexity of the simultaneous movement. This fits well with the
data of Roland et al. (1980a,b) who measured greater cerebral
blood flow over the supplementary motor area (SMA) during complex
finger movements as compared with simple finger flexions. Thus,
an increase in activity of the SMA may contribute to the changes
in the BP seen in the present experiments.

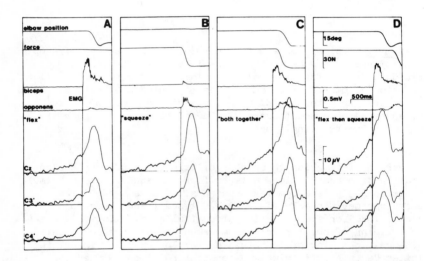

Fig.2. Increased bereitschaftspotential prior to simultaneous
and sequential motor acts as compared to simple movements. Averages
of 64 trials for each of the 4 tasks. The tasks (A-D) were performed self-paced in a cyclic order. A: simple goal-directed
elbow flexion over 15° (flex). B: simple goal-directed squeezing
of a strain gauge (squeeze); a U-shaped bar of alumninium was
attached at the end of the arm manipulandum, which could be grasped
between the thumb and fingers; the strain gauge was mounted on one
of the vertical arms of the U. C: simultaneous execution of flex
and squeeze (both together). D: sequential execution of first

flex and then squeeze (flex then squeeze). All movements had to be
performed with the right arm as fast as possible. Traces from top
to bottom in A-D are elbow position, squeeze force, EMGs of biceps
brachii (biceps) and opponens pollicis (opponens), and EEGs recorded over C_z, C3 (left arm area) and C4 (right arm area).
Vertical lines in A-D indicate EMG onset of the prime mover (biceps
for tasks A, C and D; opponens for task B). Negativity at the
scalp electrodes is indicated by an upwards deflection. The horizontal lines in the EEG traces show the baseline defined as the
mean activity over the first 250 ms of the sweep. Calibrations in
D apply to all tasks. Note the increase of the bereitschaftspotential in C and D as compared with A and B. (From Benecke et al.
1985, with permission).

It is not possible to say precisely which aspect of a simultaneous movement constitutes the important increase in complexity
referred to above. Our hypothesis is that superimposition of two
motor programs represents an extra stage in the preparation of a
movement, and that the SMA may play an important role in this
process. The results from the patients with Parkinson's disease
discussed below also are compatible with this theory.

Sequential Movements

As with the simultaneous task, no normal subjects experienced
any difficulty in performing a rapid, sequential, squeeze then
flex movement. Since there was no correlation in 9 subjects between the time taken to execute the two components of the movement
(mean correlation coefficient between time taken for squeeze vs.
flex = 0.12; range -0.4 to +0.5), it appeared that both components
remained under the control of separate motor programs. The BP
prior to such sequential movements was larger than to each movement executed alone (see fig.2), again suggesting that sequences
are treated as more complex than single simple movements by the
CNS.

An unexpected limiting feature became apparent when we
analysed sequential movements of squeeze then flex. Even though
the subjects were instructed to flex their elbow as soon as the
squeeze had ended, there was a pause of about 85ms between the
end of squeeze and beginning of flex. Since the duration of the
squeeze was some 150ms, this gave rise to an interonset latency
between the movements of 230 ms. The reason for this unnecessarily
long interval became apparent when subjects were asked to decrease
the interonset interval to less than 200ms. Fig.3 illustrates
an example of what happened in one typical subject. When the
subject performed the sequence with a short interonset interval,
the speed of the second (flex) movement was slower than normal.
The shorter the interval, the slower the second movement. Subjects
were able to perform sequences with short interonset intervals,
but it seemed that they unconsciously chose the minimum interval

which allowed them to execute the second flexion, movement at maximum speed. In this particular task, that interval was about 230ms. Why there is this limitation in the performance of rapid sequential movements is unknown.

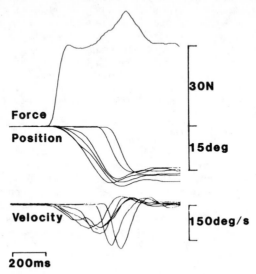

Fig.3.   Slower speed of the second movement at short inter-onset latencies. A normal subject was instructed to start the elbow flexion during the execution of squeeze. Traces are:force of squeeze (average of 6 trials, top upgoing trace), 6 superimposed position signals for flex (second downgoing traces), and 6 corresponding superimposed velocity signals for flex (both traces). Note the prolonged movement times with lower velocities at inter-onset intervals less than 200ms (from Benecke et al. 1986, with permission).

Patients with Parkinson's disease

It is well-known that movements about a single joint are executed more slowly than normal by patients with Parkinson's disease (Draper & Johns, 1964; Berardelli et al., 1985). Study of more complex simultaneous and sequential movements reveals further abnormalities which are consistent with the hypothesis that such movements involve an extra stage in motor control,   above those used in performance of each movement separately. Ten patients were studied on the simultaneous task. Their separate movements of "flex" and "squeeze" were performed, as expected, more slowly than normal (mean ± 1 s.e.   movement times: flex, 349 ± 25; squeeze, 221 ± 9 ms). However, when both movements were made simultaneously the speed of each component decreased further (movement times: flex, 557 ± 50; squeeze, 309 ± 25). Thus, the patients experienced additional difficulties in combining two separate movements over and above the problems seen where each single movement was made on its own. This extra difficulty might be explained by the following mechanism. One of the prime output targets of the basal ganglia is the SMA (see for example, Jurgens, 1984). If this area of the brain does have a role in combining two separate movements, then the abnormal basal ganglia input in Parkinson's disease may compromise its function, leading to the deficit described above.

A similar phenomenon may account for the performance of the same patients in sequential tasks. In the squeeze then flex task, the speed of the initial squeeze was the same as when executed alone (movement time for squeeze, 254 $\pm$ 12ms), but that for the flexion movement was markedly increased (445 $\pm$ 33ms). Additionally, the interonset interval between the two component acts was far longer than normal (normal, 224 $\pm$ 11; patients, 425 $\pm$ 14ms). The pause between the end of squeeze and start of flex was therefore some 170 ms, rather than 85 ms as in normals. As with simultaneous movements, the additional difficulty experienced by the patients may reflect the need for an extra stage in motor control necessary when two separate movements are combined in a sequence.

Finally, is it possible to say whether the same extra stage of processing is needed for both simultaneous and sequential combinations of flex and squeeze? In the experiments above, both simultaneous and sequential tasks appeared to be equally affected in the patients. Despite this similarity, there is one line of evidence that suggests that different processes may be involved in combining two simple movements in these different tasks. In the experiments described above, both component movements were performed with the same arm. However, if the squeeze was made with one arm and the flex with the other, the results were different. The patients' component movements were no longer very much slower in the complex tasks than they were when each was executed on its own. (Movement times in 5 patients: flex alone, 338 $\pm$ 20; squeeze alone, 190 $\pm$ 5; flex simultaneous, 363 $\pm$ 30; squeeze simultaneous, 212 $\pm$ 6; flex sequential, 356 $\pm$ 18; squeeze sequential, 216 $\pm$ 9ms). In contrast, the interonset interval in the sequential task still was very much longer than the normal 230ms (mean interval in 5 patients, 380 $\pm$ 17ms). The conclusion from these bilateral movements is that different processes are involved in controlling the timing and speed of complex tasks involving flex and squeeze.

CONCLUSIONS

When two simple tasks, flexion at the elbow and squeeze of the hand, are performed simultaneously or sequentially as fast as possible, both movements still appear to be controlled by separate motor programs. Running of two such programs together to form a complex movement is accompanied by changes in the bereitschafts-

potential which may reflect increased activation of the supplementary motor area in this type of task. In patients with
Parkinson's disease, such complex movements are affected more than
one would have predicted from examining the performance of each
component movement on its own. This suggests that an extra stage
in motor control is necessary when two simple movements are combined together and that this process is affected in Parkinson's
disease.

ACKNOWLEDGEMENTS

    This work would have been impossible without the guiding
hands of Mr H.C. Bertoya and Mr R. Bedlington in the construction
and maintenance of much of the equipment used in the experiments.
The work was funded by the Medical Research Council.

REFERENCES

Angel,R.W. (1974). Electromyography during voluntary movement: the
two burst pattern. Electroencephal. clin. Neurophysiol., 36, 493-
498.

Benecke,R., Dick,J.P.R., Rothwell,J.C., Day,B.L. & Marsden,C.D.
(1985). Increase of the Bereitschaftspotential in simultaneous and
sequential movements. Neurosci. Lett., 62, 347-352.

Benecke,R., Rothwell,J.C., Dick,J.P.R., Day,B.L. & Marsden,C.D.
(1986a). Performance of simultaneous movements in patients with
Parkinson's disease. Brain, 109, 739-757.

Benecke,R., Rothwell,J.C., Day,B.L., Dick,J.P.R. & Marsden,C.D.
(1986b). Motor strategies involved in the performance of sequential movements. Exp. Brain Res., 63, 585-595.

Benecke,R., Rothwell,J.C., Dick,J.P.R., Day,B.L. & Marsden,C.D.
(1987). Disturbance of sequential movements in patients with
Parkinson's disease. Brain, 110, 361-379.

Berardelli,A., Rothwell,J.C., Dick,J.P.R., Day,B.L. & Marsden,C.D.
(1985). Scaling of the size of the first agonist EMG burst during
rapid movements in patients with Parkinson's disease. J Neurol.
Neurosurg. Psychiat., 49, 1273-1279.

Denier van der Gon,J.J. & Thuring,J.P. (1965). The guiding of
human handwriting movements. Kybernetik, 2, 145-148.

Draper,I.T. & Johns,R.J. (1964). The disordered movement in
parkinsonism and the effect of drug treatment. Bull. Johns Hopkins
Hosp., 115, 465-480.

Hallett,M. (1983). Analysis of abnormal voluntary and involuntary movements with surface electromyography. Advances in Neurology, 39, 907-914.

Hallett,M. & Marsden,C.D. (1979). Ballistic flexion movements of the human thumb. J Physiol., 294, 33-50.

Hallett,M., Shahani,B.T. & Young,R.R. (1975). Analysis of stereotyped voluntary movements in man. J Neurol. Neurosurg. Psychiat., 38, 1154-1162.

Jurgens,U. (1984). The efferent and afferent connections of the supplementary motor area. Brain Res., 300, 63-81.

Roland,P.E., Larsen,B., Lassen,N.A. & Skinhoj,E. (1980a). Supplementary motor area and other cortical areas in organisation of voluntary movements in man. J Neurophysiol., 43, 118-136.

Roland,P.E., Skinhoj,E., Lassen,N.A. & Larsen,B. (1980b). Different cortical areas in man in organisation of voluntary movements in extrapersonal space. J Neurophysiol., 43, 137-150.

Terzuolo,C.A. & Viviani,P. (1980). Determinants and characteristic of motor patterns used for typing. Neuroscience, 5, 1085-1103.

Tuller,B., Kelso,J.A.S. & Harris,K.S. (1982). Interarticular phasing as an index of temporal regularity in speech. J Exp. Psychol. Human Percept. Perform., 8, 460-472.

Wierzbicka,M.M., Wiegner,A.W. & Shahani,B.T. (1986). Role of agonist and antagonist muscles in fast arm movements in man. Exp. Brain Res., 63, 331-340.

III
Phonetics and Phonology

12
The Speech Code

Gunnar Fant

THE CONCEPT OF THE SPEECH CODE

The notion of a code implies relations between message units and signal units. In speech communication, we are concerned with the relation of language units to units of the speech act. This is the speech code, also referred to as the phonetic code. How are units of spoken messages encoded in the acoustic signal that radiates from a speaker's mouth and reaches our ears to be heard and understood? We may extend this notion of the speech code to relations within a chain of successive encoding stages within the processes of speech production and speech perception. Our main reference for the speech signal is the speech wave as observed from oscillographic and spectrographic records. These have the potential advantage of preserving maximally complete specifications of the physical aspect of speech. Of course, such records lack information that the speakers conveys through facial expressions and other aspects of body language which possesses its own code of socially acknowledged patterns.

Studies of underlying articulatory processes cannot provide as complete and exact descriptions as the speech wave analysis. However, speech wave patterns are inherently complex and need to be interpreted by reference to possible underlying articulatory patterns and perceptual constraints. The encoding rules within the speech chain, e.g., relating articulatory movements and resonator configurations to speech wave patterns have become important constituents of the overall code (Fant, 1960; 1980). Articulatory interpretation of spectrograms is a key to the understanding of the speech code.

The speech chain model becomes more illusive when applied to brain functions. We loose insight in encoding mechanisms and signal structure. We are left with partial insights that can serve

as basis for speculations about general aspects of the code. The
same is true of hearing and speech perception. The close ties
observed between articulation and language units have influenced
theories of a coordinated speech production/speech perception brain
mechanism, e.g., the motor theory of speech perception developed by
Alvin Liberman (Liberman and Mattingly, 1985). However, we do
possess a substantial amount of general knowledge of auditory
mechanisms and speech perception, such as frequency selectivity of
the ear, critical bands of hearing, time constants, masking and
adaptation that enable us to perform auditory adapted speech wave
analysis (Carlson and Granström, 1982). Auditory constraints allow
a substantial data reduction of sampled speech wave patterns. In
addition, a general knowledge of phonetically relevant auditory
patterns contribute to the development of a less complex and more
precise specification of the code.

     When discussing the speech code, we are apparently faced with
two different communication situations. One employs a human listener. The other employs a human or a computer attempting to read
a spectrogram of an unknown text. The strategies we develop for
the latter tasks may only in part reflect the true speech code but
they are of great technical importance. The basic strategy, as
already mentioned, is to ask ourselves "How has this been produced?" and "How can this be perceived?". In both situations, the
listeners' or the spectrogram reading persons' expectancy becomes
an important part of the decoding process. We hear what we expect
to hear and sometimes nothing else. Lindblom (1987; 1988) has
pointed out the trading relations between distinctiveness and redundancy. Even so-called clear and careful speech often displays
omissions and substitutions on the phonological level as well as
far-going reductions in produced speech patterns. We encounter a
continuity of reductions from complete forms to a total extinction
of information-bearing elements of a phoneme. These are important
aspects of the speech code which we are usually not aware of.

     To the speech code also belong the specifics of individual
voice types and speaking and reading style as well as deviant
speech behavior. Any consistent regularities that can be subjected
to a descriptive analysis may be incorporated in the speech code.

APPLICATIONS

     By now, it is evident that the subject of the speech code
becomes more or less synonymous to general and experimental phonetics or general speech research. Fig. 1 symbolizes the many bran-
ches of speech research in communication engineering, acoustics,
linguistics, phonetics, psychology, physiology, medicine, rehabilitation, speech and language teaching etc. which are concerned with
aspects of the speech code.

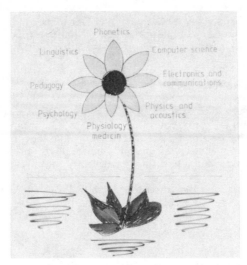

Fig. 1. Speech sciences.

Speech technology has supplied us with talking computers that are capable of converting any arbitrary text in ordinary spelling to a fairly intelligible synthetic speech. We may also program and train computers in a limited task of recognition of spoken words. I shall not go into details here but it may suffice to state that computers are good readers but bad listeners which is the reverse of general dyslexic behavior. The reading ability has found many applications in aids for the blind and in aids for speech handicapped persons. In these applications, the input to the synthesis is a string of alphanumerical signs, i.e., a digital representation of the text which is retrieved from a computer or from an optical character recognition system scanning a text for a blind user. The text-to-speech conversion unit in a prosthesis for a nonspeaking person receives its input string of characters from a computer keyboard tailored to suit the user's specific motoric capabilities.

Here in Sweden my colleagues Karoly Galyas and Irene Dahl have been engaged in successful applications of speech synthesis in teaching aids for children with reading and spelling difficulties (Dahl and Galyas, 1987). The technical development of such training aids and speech prosthesis now includes means of lexical prediction, i.e., letting the computer suggest a possible continuation given the first entries of a word. We are also in the process of including improved optional choices of speaker category, i.e., child versus adult voice, female versus male voice.

However, text-to-speech synthesis still lacks elements of naturalness and intelligibility which could be improved on. Speech synthesizers are often said to have a foreign accent. This is more or less pronounced and it can be tiring to listen to synthesizers, especially if they have not been programmed to stop now and then and to take a pause for breathing and afterthought. Anyhow, these shortcomings do generally not disturb a handicapped person who is dependent on his aid.

INVARIANCE AND VARIABILITY

The relative success of speech synthesis has created an illusion that we have a profound insight in the speech code. This illusion becomes especially apparent when we try to operate in the reverse direction, that is, given a record of the speech wave and attempting to decipher what was said.

Automatic speech recognition is still in a primitive stage of development, generally limited to single-word utterances and speaker-adapted functions which require an initial calibration and training to fit the specific voice.

Why is this so? Why could we not develop rules for identification of phonemes irrespective of talker and context to convert speech to writing? Or even better, why not attempt a decoding of speech in terms of the phonetic inventory of natural sound classes, e.g., the distinctive features of Jakobson, Fant, and Halle (1952)? A limited number of about ten features would suffice to describe most of the phonemic contrasts in the languages of the world. Could one not simply implement their acoustic attributes in a computer program as a simple recipe for speech recognition? This naive thought has been followed up and it has failed for obvious reasons.

Distinctive features are in the first place minimal units of a phonemic inventory. The information-bearing acoustic correlates, on the other hand, are highly sensitive to the particular context. An invariant, common denominator can be formulated but its descriptive power will be diluted and is found insufficient for recognition work. Still one can claim a relational invariance, and this is a main point of distinctive feature theory. Irrespective of context, two phonemes differing in one feature only will display a difference along a specific critical dimension. The contrast conveys a distinction. Feature theory thus implies a choice situation and a relational invariance within an inventory. The criterion for selection is otherness rather than identity.

IN QUEST OF THE SPEECH CODE

Let us go further into the nature of the speech code. There are often great differences between words pronounced in citation form under laboratory conditions and in real everyday speech. Unstressed forms may differ much from stressed forms. However, even a normal, clear reading of a text presents problems. The information-bearing elements are subject to considerable contextual variations, temporal spread, fusion, and overlay of other simultaneous features that complicate a rational description and analysis (Fant, 1962). Still there exist typical quantal effects (Stevens, 1972).

The phonological segments of the message level are discrete units while articulation is continuous. In the speech wave, i.e., in the domain of a time-frequency-intensity spectrogram, we find a mixture of continuous pattern variations and discrete breaks related to points in time when the vocal tract is opened from being closed, i.e., at the release of an obstruction, or vice versa, at the instant of complete closure being reached. Onsets and offsets of the voice source or of a noise source may also provide distinct boundaries. Even though a single phoneme occasionally may have its main physical counterpart in a single acoustic segment, this is usually not the case. In the speech wave, we may find more segments or less segments than in the phonological string and segmentation criteria may loose their precision or become ambiguous due to the continuity of the underlying articulatory gestures.

Thus, once a segmentation has been attempted, we find that one phoneme generally influences several successive acoustic segments and conversely, due to coarticulation, that a single physical segment is generally influenced by several successive phonemes. A typical instance of this temporal spread of information-bearing elements is that the patterns of formant transitions into or out of a physical segment become important cues to the identity of the phoneme conventionally ascribed to the segment. An example is the positive transition in all formants at the release of a labial closure and the systematically different patterns of dental/alveolar or velar/palatal release. A stylized version of the speech code along these lines was developed at Haskins Laboratories (Liberman, Ingemann, Lisker, Delattre, and Cooper, 1959). It was based on experiments with simplified synthetic speech stimuli. A similar attempt to structure patterns of real speech has been performed by Fant (1962; 1968).

However, in spite of accumulated acoustic-phonetic knowledge, we still lack an insight in the full code sufficient for speech recognition purposes. Even if we could develop a perfect talent of reading spectrograms of unknown texts, we would still have difficulties in transforming visual recognition strategies to schemes suitable for automatic computer analysis. Visual information-processing capacity and memory are by far superior. Still lacking well-defined visual strategies and invariance criteria, most people involved in speech recognition research have now turned to non-phonetic approaches employing statistical methods of pattern matching of larger units than single phonemes. An interesting new line of approach is to develop computer analogs of "neural network" that are trained to perform specific recognition tasks.

This is a real challenge.   Shall we give up our attempts to
force the speech code, or shall we rely on computers to acquire
recognition competence that is as inaccessible to objective analysis and understanding as our competence as listeners?

In my view, the phonetic approach should be followed up.   But
how shall we get access to the complete code?   The issue of invariance versus variability has been the subject of a whole conference, see Perkell and Klatt (1986).   Instead of worrying about the
lack of invariance, we should pay more attention to means of
structuring variability.   Our present projects of speech analysis
center around large data banks of stored speech from which we may
perform statistical analysis of any contextual and individual factors of interest (Carlson and Granström, 1986; Fant, Nord, and
Kruckenberg, 1986; Nord, 1988).   The data bank analysis thus provides a combination of reference data and rules for predicting
variations with respect to specific sequences of phonemes and to
underlying morphological and syntactic constructions and semanti-
denotations which manifest more directly in the prosodic frame of
intonation and stress patterns, emphasis, junctures, and pauses.
We apparently need to develop a more integrated view of the interactions between "inherent" features assigned to speech segments and
"prosodic" features which operate over larger units of time (Fant,
1987).

Spectrographic patterns of the same utterance produced by
different speakers may vary considerably in spite of relative small
differences in apparent qualities (Fant, Nord, and Kruckenberg,
1986). An example is shown in Fig. 2.   The three subjects have
produced the voiced stop /g/ in the Swedish word "legat" with
varying degree of articulatory closure, which is complete for
subject JS, incomplete for subject JJ, and even more reduced for

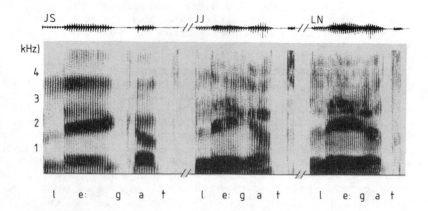

Fig. 2. Three degrees of articulatory contrast in a vowel-/g/-vowel
        sequence.   Oscillograms and broad-band spectra.

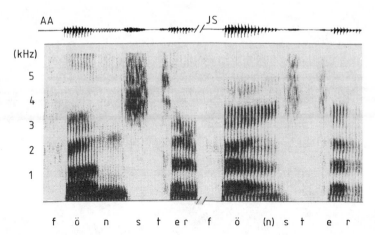

Fig. 3. Left pattern, speaker AA: normal appearance of a nasal
consonant /n/. Right, speaker JS: The nasal consonant is
produced with incomplete alveolar occlusion and thus mani-
fests through nasalization only.

subject LN. The weak gesture towards closure for subject LN is
sufficient to evoke the percept of a voiced stop but one may argue
that the "top-down" expectancy adds to the identification. Another
instance of incomplete articulatory closure is illustrated in Fig.
3. Here the subject AA at the left of the figure produces a well-
defined boundary between the vowel /ö/ and the following nasal
consonant /n/. The subject JS, on the other hand, does not produce
a complete oral closure during the /n/ which therefore becomes
realized as a nasalized vowel with no apparent boundary between the
/ö/ and the /n/. This is a quite common phenomenon in a sequence
of a vowel followed by a nasal and an obstruent.

Some phonemes are produced with a complex combination of
coordinated articulatory activity while a minimal phonetic distinction often involves a single selective modification which may
change several aspects of the spectrographic pattern. Such a case
is illustrated in Fig. 4. Here the contrastive nonsense words
/kaka:ka/, /gaga:ga/, /papa:pa/, /baba:ba/, /tata:ta/, /dada:da/
illustrate the pair wise relations between unvoiced and voiced
stops. The major articulatory correlate of this distinction is the
difference in the opening and closing gestures of the vocal cords.

This example could support motor theories of speech perception
(Liberman and Mattingly, 1985). But could not the complex of
auditory cues trigger the response more directly (Fant, 1967)? The
spectrograms in Fig. 4 were produced with so-called broad-band filtering which enhances the appearance of formants, i.e., vocal tract

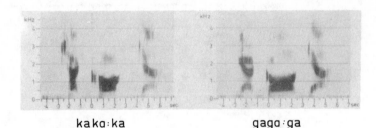

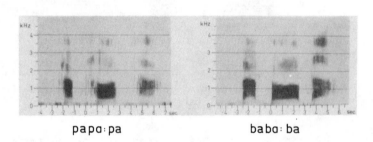

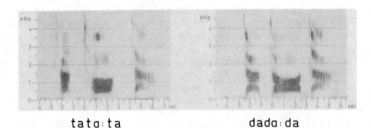

Fig. 4. Three-syllable nonsense words with the second vowel long
and stressed. A basic cue to the unvoiced feature is that
consonantal segments become prolonged and more intense
while a preceding or following vocalic segment is short-
ened. The voiced/voiceless distinction is highly reduced in
the final syllable.

resonances.   In Fig. 5, I have for comparison also included a
narrow-band filtering. The utterance is intimately related to our
symposium "Academia Rodinensis".   The narrow-band spectrogram displays a fine structure of harmonics within less evident formant
bands.   This feature is related to the longer time constant associated with the narrow filter.   I leave it to the reader to digest

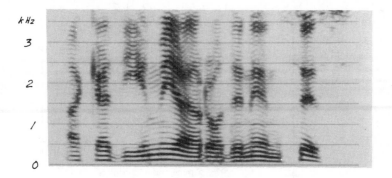

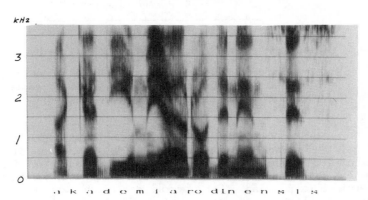

Fig. 5. Narrow-band above and broad-band spectrogram below of the
         text: "Academia Rodinensis".

details of the picture. I shall limit myself to comments on the
first few segments. The F2-F3 proximity at the end of the first
segment indicates the velar-palatal articulation of the /k/. If
the second vowel were to be identified out of context, it would
have been given a phonetic symbol /e/ rather than /a/. Here, in an
unstressed position, the coarticulation with the immediate consonantal frame becomes dominant.

SPEECH PROSODY

    Studies of the speech code have dealt more with inherent
features than with speech prosody. Although prosodics only in part
serves a distinctive function, the major importance is as a decoding facilitator. An incorrect prosody inhibits the listeners' perceptual and cognitive processes. This is an additional incitement
for improving prosody in speaking aids.

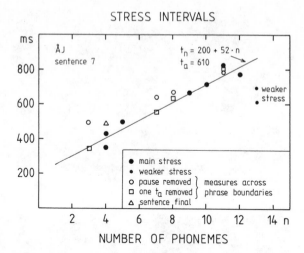

Fig. 6. Inter-stress interval durations versus number of phonemes.
Intervals spanning a phrase boundary with pause attain a
duration with an extra mean interval added.

Recent prosodic research at KTH (Fant, Nord, and Kruckenberg,
1986; 1987; Fant and Kruckenberg, 1988) has been directed to
studies of both objective and subjective measures of syllabic
stress and syntactic boundary markings. Segmental durations, final
terminal lengthening effects, and local pitch excursions and voice
source perturbations may be combined into objective measures. A
continuity of variations in the objective signal domain has its
correspondence in a more or less continuous perceptual scaling.

A special attention has been laid on the study of rhythmical
qualities in text reading. We have fresh evidence for a suggestion
of Lea (1980) that inter-stress intervals, defined by distances
from a stressed vowel to the next stressed vowel of the sequence
acts as synchronizing impulses for an internal clock which guides
the time we take in making pauses between phrases and sentences.

We have found that the average duration of inter-stress intervals not spanning a syntactic boundary sets the basic temporal
module of the internal clock. In rhythmical reading an inter-stress
interval spanning a phrase boundary with a pause tends towards the
sum of an inter-stress interval predicted from the number of phonemes contained plus one unit of the inner clock beat, i.e., an
average inter-stress interval is added. At sentence boundaries
with longer pauses, there is a tendency of one or two additional
clock units being added. In other words, noting that we always
have a terminal lengthening before and to some extent after pauses,
we may restate this finding as an expectancy that the sum of the

physical pause and terminal lengthening equals an integer multiple of the rhythmical time constant. This is illustrated in Fig. 6.

Durations of inter-stress intervals are thus largely imposed by language and do not appear to be adjusted to retain isochrony while the rhythmical demand becomes apparent in the planning of pauses. Even without such perfect synchrony, e.g., when a phrase boundary is realized without a pause, the final lengthening alone is capable of signalling the appearance of the boundary.

The constants of the regression line relating inter-stress intervals to number of phonemes appear to be a key to the analysis of components of individual reading and talking styles. These constants should also be of interest in contrastive language studies.

References

Carlson, R. and Granström, B. Eds. (1982). The Representation of Speech in the Peripheral Auditory System. Elsevier Biomedical Press, Amsterdam.

Carlson, R. and Granström, B. (1986). A Search for Durational Rules in a Real-speech Data Base. Phonetica, 43, 140-154.

Dahl, I. and Galyas, K. (1987). Experiences with the Use of Computer Programs with Speech Output in Teaching Reading and Writing. In European Conference on Speech Technology, Edinburgh, II. (eds. J. Laver and M.A. Jack). CEP Consultants, Edinburgh.

Fant, G. (1960). Acoustic Theory of Speech Production. Mouton, The Hague.

Fant, G. (1962). Descriptive Analysis of the Acoustic Aspects of Speech. Logos, 5, 3-17.

Fant, G. (1967). Auditory Patterns of Speech. In Symposium on Models for the Perception of Speech and Visual Form, 1964. (ed. W. Wathen-Dunn). The MIT-Press, Cambridge, MA.

Fant, G. (1968). Analysis and Synthesis of Speech Processes. In Manual of Phonetics. (ed. B. Malmberg). North-Holland, Amsterdam.

Fant, G. (1980). The Relation Between Area Functions and the Acoustical Signal. In Proc. IXth ICPhS, Copenhagen, III. (eds. E. Fischer-Jørgensen and N. Thorsen). University of Copenhagen.

Fant, G. (1987). Interactive Phenomena in Speech Production. In Proc. XIth ICPhS, Tallinn, Estonia, 3. Estonian Academy of Sciences.

Fant, G., Nord, L., and Kruckenberg, A. (1986). Individual Variations in Text Reading. A Data-bank Pilot Study. STL-QPSR (KTH,
Stockholm), No. 4, 1-17.

Fant, G., Nord, L., and Kruckenberg, A. (1987). Segmental and
Prosodic Variabilities in Connected Speech. An Applied Data-bank
Study. In Proc. XIth ICPhS, Tallinn, Estonia, 6, Estonian Academy
of Sciences.

Fant, G. and Kruckenberg, A. (1988). Some Durational Correlates of
Swedish Prosody. Paper presented at the Seventh FASE Symposium,
SPEECH 88, Edinburgh.

Jakobson, R., Fant, G., and Halle, M. (1952). Preliminaries to
Speech Analysis: The Distinctive Features and Their Correlates.
Acoustics Lab., MIT Tech. Rep. No. 13; also MIT-Press, VIIth print-
ing (1967).

Lea, W.A., ed. (1980). Trends in Speech Recognition, Prentice
Hall, London.

Liberman, A.M. and Mattingly, I.G. (1985). The Motor Theory of
Speech Perception Revised. Cognition, 21, 1-36.

Liberman, A.M., Ingemann, F., Lisker, L., Delattre, P., and Cooper,
F.S. (1959). Minimal Rules for Synthesizing Speech. J.Acoust.Soc.
Am., 31, 1490-1499.

Lindblom, B. (1987). Adaptive Variability and Absolute Constancy
in Speech Signals: Two Themes in the Quest for Phonetic Invariance. In Proc. XIth ICPhS, Tallinn, Estonia, 3, Estonian Academy
of Sciences.

Lindblom, B. (1988). The Status of Phonetic Gestures. Paper presented at the Conf. on Modularity and the Motor Theory organized in
June 1988 at Haskins Laboratories in honor of Alvin M. Liberman.

Nord, L. (1988). Acoustic Phonetic Studies in a Swedish Data Bank.
Paper presented at the Seventh FASE-meeting, SPEECH 1988, Edinburgh.

Perkell, J. and Klatt, D., eds. (1986). Invariance and Variability of Speech Processes. L. Erlbaum, New York.

Stevens, K.N. (1972). The Quantal Nature of Speech: Evidence from
Articulatory-acoustic Data. In Human Communication: A Unified
View. (eds. E.E. David and P.B. Denes). McGraw-Hill, New York.

13
Neuropsychological and Neuroanatomical Studies of Developmental Language/Reading Disorders: Recent Advances

P. Tallal and W. Katz

This chapter[1] summarizes some recent findings from the San Diego Longitudinal Study (Tallal and Curtiss, 1979-1988) and the San Diego Center for Neurological Studies (Tallal et al., 1985-1990) concerning cognitive, linguistic, and neurodevelopmental changes associated with developmental language and reading dysfunctions. These studies have been designed to further our understanding of the neuropsychological profiles which characterize language/reading-impaired children, and to develop theories pertaining to the biological bases for these disorders. A primary focus of this research has been to investigate the deficiencies which arise in language/reading-impaired populations confronted with tasks requiring the precise temporal manipulation of auditory, visual, or tactile stimuli. This work has been motivated by a large body of previous research suggesting that language/reading-impaired children, as a group, demonstrate difficulties in neurophysiological tasks which involve discrete timing components for perceptual, memory, and motor function.

In some of the first studies conducted by Tallal and colleagues examining phonetic processing in language-impaired children, Tallal and Piercy (1973a, 1973b, 1974) observed that a well-specified group of specifically language-impaired children (i.e., children who show no evidence of hearing loss, mental retardation, autism or frank neurological problems) were significantly impaired on tasks requiring the rapid processing and storing of nonverbal auditory or visual perceptual information. On the other hand, if this information was presented over a longer period of time, these deficits were no longer apparent. For example, whereas normally developing

---

[1]This research was funded by NINCDS #NS-92332 and grant #NS-22343 as part of the Multidisciplinary Research Center for the Study of the Neurological Bases of Learning, Language, and Behavior Disorders in Children.

children (ages 6-9) required 8 ms between two nonverbal tones to discriminate them at a 75% level of accuracy, language-impaired children required over 300 ms to respond at the same level of accuracy. A similar deficit was also noted in subjects' serial memory performance. While language-impaired children were unable to remember a series of even three successive tones of 75 ms duration, the same children could correctly remember a series of five successive tones when the duration of the tones was increased to 250 ms.

These striking perceptual defects led the investigators to explore whether there were matched deficits in the production systems of these subjects, that is, in nonverbal motor output. Tallal, Stark and Mellits (1985a) demonstrated that language-impaired children perform significantly more slowly than normal children in timed motor tasks, including rapid sequential movements of the hands and oral cavity. This type of finding has been reported by other researchers (e.g., Johnson and Weismer, 1983) who noted that, although language-impaired children did not differ from normal children on a task of mental rotation based on the number of accurate responses, they required consistently longer processing time as compared with normal children to respond correctly.

The next step in this research was to determine whether these nonverbal processing and production deficits indeed relate to the use of speech and language in language-impaired children. Tallal and colleagues addressed this issue by conducting a number of studies using synthesized speech as stimuli. The use of synthetic speech allowed for the concise manipulation of strictly temporal features (such as VOT and rate of formant transition), while leaving frequency parameters constant. Tallal and Piercy (1975) demonstrated that language-impaired children show difficulties in the discrimination of stop-CV syllables (e.g., /ba/ and /da/) when these stimuli are synthesized, having very brief (40 ms) formant transitions. On the other hand, there are no such difficulties when the duration of the formants are increased to 80 ms. Over the next few years, Tallal and colleagues conducted experiments using a number of synthetic stimuli, including fricative-vowel syllables, CVC syllables, consonant cluster, and synthetic syllable pairs which when blended could form words (e.g., /be/-/bi/, /ba/-/di/, etc.). Although there were variations as a function of stimulus type and of the exact parameters used in generating synthetic stimuli on different computers, a consistent finding was that language-impaired children evidence difficulties in processing stimuli whose acoustic cues are brief and are followed in rapid succession by other acoustic cues.

In more recent studies, Tallal, Stark and Mellits (1985b) have examined the predictive value of these basic perceptual/motor integration deficits with respect to the degree of language impairment in language-impaired children. This was done by assessing the receptive language abilities of a large group of well-defined language-impaired children and rank-ordering these children according to their degree of receptive language impairment (based on standardized language tests). The children were then rank-ordered based on their scores on a series of nonverbal and speech temporal processing tests.   Multiple correlations were conducted with these data in an attempt to determine the extent to which the nonverbal/speech data would predict the severity of receptive language impairment.   The results demonstrated a correlation of .85, significant at the .001 level.   Multiple regression data showed that 72% of the variance related to the level of receptive language dysfunction could be accounted for by the language-impaired children's ability to discriminate and sequence nonverbal acoustic tones and speech stimuli containing brief duration temporal cues.

Finally, it was asked to what extent could specific neuropsychological abilities, alone, discriminate or diagnose language-impaired from normal children.   More specifically, it was sought to determine whether there is a particular pattern of neuropsychological deficits that is characteristic of developmentally language-impaired children and, if so, to what extent could this pattern of deficits, alone, correctly classify children as normal or language-impaired.   To address these questions, a large neuropsychological battery of nonverbal and speech perception, motor, and memory tests was given to language-impaired and matched, control subjects.   This neuropsychological test battery incorporated auditory, visual, tactile, and cross-modal stimuli.   The perceptual test battery included the assessment of detection, association, temporal resolution, sequencing, rate-processing, and serial memory skills.   In addition, nonverbal and verbal motor tests evaluated rate of production and sequencing abilities.   A comprehensive neurological "soft sign" battery measured general motor control and coordination, balance and station, tactile sensation and perception, and laterality.   Demographic and case history variables were also documented.   In short, this experiment was designed to take into account not only neuropsychological variables, but also almost any other possible factors which might be involved in language impairment diagnoses.   A step-wise discriminant function analysis was then employed, examining the extent to which the independent variables correctly assign individuals to the defined outcome groups.

The results demonstrated that six variables, assessing basic perceptual and motor abilities, when combined, correctly classified 100% of the normal children as normal and 96% of the language-impaired children as language-impaired.   These variables were found to have in common the assessment of specific temporal capabilities, either in perception or production.   The six variables included rapid syllable production, two measures of two-point simultaneous tactile discrimination, discriminating between speech syllables characterized by brief formant transitions, cross-modal integration at rapid rates of presentation, and sequencing the letters "e" and "k" when presented rapidly in succession.   Importantly, the same tasks given at slower presentation rates did not enter the discriminate function equation.   Each of the variables entering the equation had in common the necessity to produce or perceive information either simultaneous or very rapidly in succession, regardless of whether the information was verbal or nonverbal.

Anticipatory labial coarticulation in language-impaired children

We have discussed the fact that language/reading-impaired children appear to have difficulties in the temporal control necessary for the production of certain speech segments. Similarly, developmental disorders involving a large degree of articulatory impairment (known as "developmental dyspraxia" or "developmental dyspraxia of speech") have been characterized by a deficit in programming the position and sequence of volitional speech movements (Rosenbek & Wertz, 1972). These disorders have been related to problems in the sequencing of sound elements and to reductions in the complexity of word shapes (Smartt et al., 1976; Marquardt et al., 1985). These data suggest that the speech production difficulties of language-impaired children might involve mistiming in the anticipation of coarticulatory (or sound sequencing) gestures. To explore this hypothesis further, we have designed experiments investigating anticipatory labial coarticulation in normal and language/reading-impaired children.

Anticipatory labial coarticulation refers to anticipation of labial rounding of a subsequent vowel during production of the consonantal portion of an utterance. For example, in the English word /su/, adult speakers generally begin lip-rounding for the rounded vowel /u/ even while producing the preceding fricative /s/, whereas no such rounding occurs for the /s/ of /si/. Recent investigations have shown that most normal adult speakers of American English reliably demonstrate anticipatory labialization in their read speech (Lubker & Gay, 1982; Soli, 1981). Also, recent findings indicate that anticipatory labialization difficulties may be involved in the speech production errors of anterior and posterior aphasic subjects (Katz, 1987; Katz et al., 1988; Ziegler and Von Cramon, 1985, 1986). These data suggest that segment transitionalizing abilities are fundamental to the speech production process, and are probably acquired early in language acquisition. Current data for children are somewhat controversial, but in general suggest that the ability to anticipate labial gestures is acquired early in the course of language development (Sereno et al., 1987). If language/reading-impaired children evidence coarticulatory impairments, this would provide an additional means for understanding the basis of their speech and language difficulties. If, on the other hand, these subjects do not show coarticulatory irregularities, this would suggest that segment-transitional (or syllabic) processing is relatively spared in children with specific language dysfunctions, and would suggest that, for these subjects, timing difficulties do not show up at the syllable or lexical levels of the phonology.

In a series of pilot investigations, we have videotaped and audiotaped five 8-year-old language/reading-impaired children and five age-matched controls while the subjects were speaking the sentences "I said /si/" and "I said /su/." The apparatus used is described in Figure 1. A video camera with a zoom lens was used to obtain high-quality images of lip position at 33 ms intervals. The audio track of the video-recorder was connected to an oscilloscope, registering an image of the speech waveform.

This image was simultaneously videotaped with a second camera, and a combined image of the mouth and speech waveform was generated using a

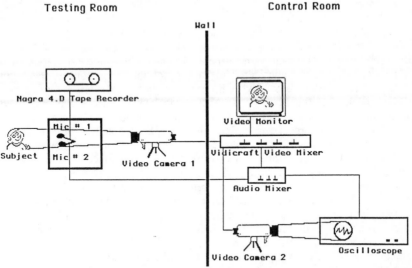

Figure 1. Apparatus used for visual tracking of anticipatory coarticulation.

mixer. The videotapes were then edited frame by frame, and hard copies were generated for three specific points in the speech production process: (1) after the first 33 ms of frication, (2) at an approximate midpoint of frication, and (3) at the midpoint of the steady-state vowel. Hardcopy images of the lips were then given to a group of independent raters, who were instructed to mark on a test sheet whether the picture represented production of the word "Sea" or "Sue."

Identification scores for productions made by each of the subject groups were found to be well above chance (83% for adults and 72% for children). As expected, scores for the vowel midpoint were significantly higher than for the fricative stimuli, and there was significantly greater identification for the fricative midpoint stimuli than for the initial 33 ms of frication. Interestingly, the scores for the normal children were found to differ significantly from those of the language/reading-impaired children, with the scores of the impaired children more resembling those of adults. These data suggest that in these 8-year-old language/reading-impaired subjects, anticipatory coarticulatory problems do not appear to be involved in speech production difficulties. Although it is premature to draw conclusions at this early stage of investigation, these pilot data show that the technique of having viewers rate videotaped images of speech is a viable means of analyzing coarticulation in the speech of children and adults. Having established this technique for measuring coarticulation in 8 year olds, we plan to correlate this data with acoustic, perceptual, and kinematic measures, and to then begin examining younger children. This should allow for a developmental investigation of the earliest stages of coarticulatory, speech motor-control abilities.

Phonological disorders in dyslexia

Early childhood language impairment is not the only developmental communication disorder considered to have a possible phonological basis. In recent years, developmental dyslexia has also been considered to possibly involve specific dysfunctions at the phonological level. Tallal has suggested that temporal processing disorders may constrain phonological processing. In particular, temporal processing deficiencies have been noted to be a potential underlying factor in dyslexic subjects' speech production difficulties (Di Lollo et al., 1983; Zurif and Carson, 1972). Tallal and colleagues (Tallal, 1980a, 1980b; Tallal and Stark, 1982) have conducted a series of studies with dyslexic children examining the temporal processing abilities of these subjects. The results demonstrated that within the dyslexic population there are two subgroups. The larger subgroup demonstrated temporal processing deficits similar to those reported for language-impaired children, whereas the smaller subgroup did not. The larger subgroup also demonstrated deficits on standardized speech and language tests, whereas the smaller subgroup responded within normal limits. In addition, the larger subgroup demonstrated considerable deficits with phonetic encoding tests, whereas the other subgroup of dyslexic children did not. A further analysis demonstrated that there was a highly significant correlation between the degree of nonverbal acoustic temporal processing deficits and decoding deficits in the children. Thus, the basis of phonological decoding deficits in some dyslexic children may be an inability to process temporal acoustic cues which are necessary for the fine-grained phonological analysis which underlies decoding skills.

A second method of examining the similarities between childhood language impairment and dyslexia is to follow language-impaired children from an early age, in order to determine what the outcomes are in terms of their academic achievement. This data is currently being analyzed as part of the San Diego Longitudinal Study of Specific Language Impairment (P. Tallal and S. Curtiss). Since 1979, the development of 89 language-impaired children and 60 matched controls have been traced longitudinally from ages 4 to 8 years. Currently under investigation are the outcomes of preschool language impairment on subsequent linguistic development, academic achievement, and social and emotional development. Preliminary results of this study have shown that by age 6, over 75% of the children who were originally identified at age 4 as seriously language-impaired could be correctly discriminated from matched control children, based solely on their spelling scores. These percentages increased to approximately 80% correct identification by age 8. In addition, over 85% of the 6-year-old children could be correctly identified from controls based solely on their reading vocabulary and reading comprehension scores. This longitudinal study demonstrates the co-occurrence of developmental language disorder and developmental reading disorder in the same child, only at different ages. Furthermore, the data implicate a similar underlying temporal processing deficit in both developmental dyslexia and developmental dysphasia, at least for some subtypes.

Thus, some developmentally language-impaired and developmentally reading-impaired children may not represent two distinct diagnostic groups. Rather, a single developmental disability affecting specific processing constraints on particular aspects of the language learning system may occur at different ages. It is possible that a similar underlying neural mechanism may interfere with phonological analysis, resulting in speech and language disorders in young preschool-age children, and subsequently reading development in older school-age children.

Brain imaging studies of developmental language disorders

Having carefully isolated the behavioral phenotype associated with language and reading impairment in children, Tallal and colleagues have begun studies aimed at describing the neuroanatomical deficits associated with these impairments. Because, by definition, specific language and reading disorders do not involve neurobehavioral disorders associated with frank neurological damage, little has been known about the neuroanatomical bases for these disorders. There have been few actual anatomical or physiological studies of developmental language or reading disorders reported in the literature. Only one child with a specific developmental language disorder has ever come to autopsy (Goldstein et al., 1958). This autopsy was of a 9-year-old child who had acquired some expressive language but had considerable difficulty processing speech when it was spoken at a normal rate. His autopsy revealed old, bilateral infarctions of the Sylvian region and severe retrograde degeneration of both medial geniculate nuclei. Galaburda and Kemper (1979) have reported the results of autopsy studies on the brains of adults with a life-long history of language and reading disorders. At autopsy, these brains showed signs of neurological abnormalities, all confined to the left hemisphere. There was no evidence of left hemisphere neuron loss or gliosis; however, there was a marked area of polymicrogyria with adjacent molecular layers of the gyri fused, no cortical lamination, and no cell-free layer. These abnormalities were confined to the posterior parts of Hechel's gyrus into the left planum temporale (an area roughly corresponding to Wernicke's Area). Galaburda and Kemper speculated that these abnormalities may be involved in the language impairments of these patients.

In light of the scarcity of direct autopsy data, the advent of Magnetic Resonance Imaging (MRI) has offered a unique opportunity to explore issues of brain morphology in childhood language and reading disorders. Recently, Jernigan, Hesselink and Tallal (1987) reported preliminary results from MRI studies of language- and reading-impaired children. Based upon the work of Galaburda and Kemper, and upon the theories of Geschwind and colleagues (Geschwind, 1979; Geschwind and Behan, 1984), it was hypothesized that dyslexic and dysphasic children will show abnormal patterns of lateralization in the peri-Sylvian language zones[*]. To date, ten language-impaired children between the ages of 8 and 10, five (age- and IQ-matched) normal children, and 9 IQ-matched (13- to 20-year-old) children with global mental retardation have been examined. For each subject, a total of 49 MRI sections were obtained, and the images were analyzed by a method designed to image grey matter, white matter, and cerebrospinal fluid. This analysis method involves image preprocessing by means of an interactive computer program. Using this program, an operator views a pseudo-colored, signal-strength image of the brain, and designates the center of each isolated brain region. An iterative algorithm then checks for contiguous pixels that are within a predicted range. Artifacts are removed by high-pass filtering, and the final data are then used to display estimates of grey matter, white matter, and cerebrospinal fluid in each of 4 brain quadrants (Figure 2).

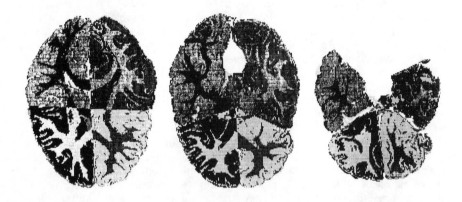

Figure 2.   Coronal sections from the MRI imaging
techniques of Jernigan et al., showing
grey matter, white matter, and cerebrospinal fluid in each of four brain
quadrants.

Of primary interest is the morphology of the cerebrum inferior to the Sylvian vessels (i.e., the level separating temporal from parietal lobes). The results showed that, whereas all 5 of the control children scanned had a larger left than right posterior region of the brain, 6 of the 10 language-impaired children had a larger right than left posterior region. These 6 children also had a decrease in grey matter and increase in fluid in these

---

* see also Sherman, Rosen, and Galaburda in this Volume (Eds' comm.)

regions. This was not, however, the case for the children with global mental retardation. Although 8 of the 9 mentally retarded children showed reversed asymmetries, this was not associated with a decrease in grey matter or increase in fluid in these specific brain regions. Rather, the retarded children showed less overall cerebral volume, which was uniform across both hemispheres. Thus, these results suggest that specific language and reading disorders (and not mental retardation, per se) may be correlated with differences in posterior brain asymmetry.

A second series of neuroanatomical studies in progress are using Positron Emission Tomography (PET) imaging techniques to investigate metabolic abnormalities associated with language and reading disorders. This work, done in collaboration with M. Buchsbaum and F. Wood, is designed to elucidate cortical areas associated with auditory and visual processing of rapid stimuli in normal and language-impaired subjects. In the first series of experiments, normal adults and adults with a history of language and reading impairment are given radioactively labelled glucose, and are then asked to detect sequentially presented stimuli by pressing a button when a target appears. For the visual stimuli, degraded numbers were used, and for the acoustic stimuli, synthetic CV stimuli (/ba-da-ga-pa-ta-ka/) masked with white noise were employed. During these tasks, event related potentials were also recorded in order to estimate the brain electrical activity associated with stimulus recognition and detection. Immediately after task completion, a topographic scan of cortical glucose uptake was obtained. In this manner, both electrical and metabolic estimates of processing were registered. To date, eight adult dysphasic subjects with a history of childhood developmental aphasia have been tested. Interestingly, several of these subjects have shown difficulties in recognizing place of articulation distinctions in the synthetic speech stimuli. If these techniques prove to be reliable, it is planned to next examine stimuli containing rapid vs non-rapid formant transitions, in an effort to further examine the physiological correlates of processing rapid temporal stimuli in normal and language/reading-impaired subjects.

Genetic factors in developmental language and reading disorders

Although some researchers have postulated a possible genetic etiology for childhood language disorders, there has been little systematic investigation of these issues. There have been a number of case histories reported (e.g., McReady, 1926; Arnold, 1961; Borges-Osorio & Salzano, 1985) in which families had several members showing language disorders. A number of group studies have also been completed (Ingram, 1959; Bishop and Edmundson, 1986; Robinson, 1987) which suggest the presence of familial aggregation for specific language impairment. However, these studies are somewhat difficult to interpret due either to lack of clear diagnoses of language impairment (Ingram), lack of sufficient discussion of familial data (Bishop and Edmundson), or the failure to include non-language-impaired control subjects in the probands (Robinson).

Tallal, Ross, and Curtiss (in press) have recently completed a series of studies investigating familial aggregation and sex-ratios in families of language/learning-impaired children. These studies are based upon extensive questionnaires completed by the parents and family of the children participating in the San Diego Longitudinal Study of Specific Language Impairment. In the study of familial aggregation, 89 well-defined, four-year-old, language-impaired children and 60 controls (matched on age, IQ, and SES) were selected over a two-year period. The biological parents of these children were each requested to fill out a separate questionnaire relating to family history of language, reading, writing, and academic achievement. The results showed that families of impaired children reported higher rates of affected first-degree relatives than did families of matched controls. Significantly higher incidence of maternal and paternal childhood language/learning disabilities, as well as sibling disability rates, were reported.

Tallal and colleagues next sought to investigate the extent to which this familial aggregation reflects genetic or environmental influences. This study examined whether the pattern of family history data for this population would lend support to any known modes of sex-linked genetic transmission. One of the more commonly known facts about the prevalence of developmental language disorders in children is that there are reportedly higher ratios of boys than girls (2-3:1) affected. This finding was replicated in the present study. However, the most interesting results of the present investigation are that the increase in sex-ratio of boys to girls only occurred in families that had an affected mother (Figure 3). That is, whereas non-affected parents and affected fathers had approximately equal male and female offspring ratios, affected mothers had a 3:1 male:female offspring ratio and a 5:1 ratio of affected offspring. These results fail to support the sex-linkage hypothesis, but instead, support an autosomal dominant mode of transmission, with greater penetrance through mothers than fathers. In autosomal dominant disorders, only one gene is necessary to express the disorder, and these disorders are also characterized by a high rate of spontaneous mutation and variable penetrance.

These data are particularly interesting in light of recent theories concerning fetal testosterone levels, secondary sex-ratio, and brain development. In studies investigating factors affecting the secondary sex-ratio in humans, increased male births have been highly associated with maternal stress and abnormal levels of gonadal hormones, especially testosterone (James, 1986). Both the effects of stress on hormonal secretion, and the effects of hormones on brain development, have been implicated in neurodevelopmental language and learning disorders. In one prominent theory, Geschwind and Behan (1982) have suggested that developmental learning disorders may be linked to both left-handedness and immune disorders through the action of testosterone on brain development. These authors propose that abnormal testosterone levels, or unusual sensitivity to testosterone in utero, can alter brain anatomy such that normal cerebral asymmetry fails to develop.   Although other studies are needed to independently confirm and extend the present questionnaire-based data, the results lend support to theories proposing hormone-mediated brain development deficits, because elevated testosterone levels (or testosterone sensitivity thresholds) during fetal life might also explain the unusual secondary sex-ratios observed.

        In summary, we have briefly presented some of the theories and recent research results of Tallal and colleagues at the San Diego Center for Neurological Studies. By investigating the behavioral, neuroanatomical, and neurophysiological attributes of language deficiencies in children, it will hopefully be possible to obtain a broader perspective from which to better understand these disorders.

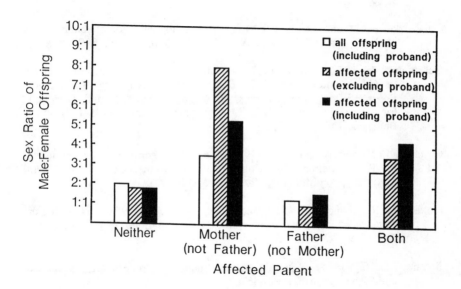

Figure 3.   Sex-ratio of offspring by number and sex of affected parents of dyslexic children

REFERENCES

Arnold, G.E. (1961). The genetic background of developmental language disorders. Folia Phoniatr. **13**, 246-254.

Bishop, D.V.M., Edmundson, A. (1986). Is otitis media a major cause of developmental language disorders. Br. J. Disord. Comm. **1**, 321-328.

Borges-Osorio, M.R., and Salzano, F.M. (1985). Language disabilities in 3 twin pairs and their relatives. Acta Genet. Med. Gemoll. (Roma) **34** (1-2), 95-100.

Di Lollo, V., Hanson, D. and McIntyre, J. (1983). Initial stages of visual information processing in dyslexia. J. Exp. Psych., Hum. Perc. Perf. **9**, 923-935.

Galaburda, A.M. and Kemper, T.M. (1979). Cytoarchitectonic abnormalities in developmental dyslexia: A case study. Ann. Neurol. **6**, 94-100.

Geschwind, N. (1979). Anatomical foundations of language and dominance. In C.L. Ludlow and M.E. Doran-Quine (Eds.), The Neurological Bases of Language Disorders in Children: Methods and Directions for Research, in NINCDS Monograph Series, 145-153. NIH: Bethesda, Md.

Geschwind, N. and Behan, P.O. (1984). Laterality, hormones and immunity. In R. Guillemin, M. Cohn, and T. Melnechuk (Eds.), Neural Modulation of Immunity. Raven Press, New York.

Goldstein, R., Landau, W.H., and Kleffner, F.R. (1958). Neurological assessment of some deaf and aphasic children. Trans. Am. Otol. Soc., Vol. 46, 122-136.

Ingram, T.T.S (1959). Specific developmental disorders of speech in childhood. Brain **82**, 450-467.

James, W.H. (1986). Hormonal control of sex ratio. J. Theor. Biol. **118**, 427-441.

Jernigan, T.L., Hesselink, J., and Tallal, P. (1987). Cerebral morphology on magnetic resonance imaging in developmental aphasia. Soc. Neurosci. Abstr. **13**(1), 651.

Johnson, J., and Weismer, S. (1983). Mental rotation abilities in language disordered children. J. Sp. Hear. Res. **26**, 397-403.

Katz, W. (1987). Anticipatory labial and lingual coarticulation in aphasia. In J. Ryalls (Ed.), Phonetic Approaches to Speech Production in Aphasia and Related Disorders. College-Hill Press, San Diego.

Katz, W., Schoenle, P., Machetanz, J., Hohne, J., Wenig, P., Veldscholten, H. (1988). A kinematic analysis of anticipatory coarticulation in an anterior aphasic subject using electromagnetic articulography. Presentation at 1988 Academy of Aphasia, Montreal, Canada.

Lubker, J.M, and Gay, T. (1982). Anticipatory labial coarticulation: Experimental, biological, and linguistic variables. J. Ac. Soc. Am. 17 (2), 437-447.

Marquardt, T.P., Dunn, C., and Davis, B. (1985). Apraxia of speech in children. In J.K. Darby (Ed.), Speech and Language Evaluation in Neurology: Childhood Disorders. Grune & Stratton, Orlando.

McReady, E.B. (1926). Deficits in the zone of language (word-deafness and word-blindness) and their influence in education and behavior. Am. J. Psychiatr. 6, 267.

Robinson, R.J. (1987). The causes of language disorder. Proceedings of the First International Symposium on Specific Speech and Language Disorders in Children. Reading, England.

Rosenbek, J. and Wertz, R. (1972). A review of 50 cases of developmental apraxia of speech. Language, Speech and Hearing Services in Schools 3, 23-33.

Sereno, J.A., Baum, S.R., Marean, G.C., and Lieberman, P. (1987). Acoustic analyses and perceptual data on anticipatory labial coarticulation in adults and children. J. Acoust. Soc. Am. 81, 512-519.

Smartt, J., LaLance, L., Gray, J., and Hibbert, P. (1976). Developmental apraxia of speech: A Tennessee Speech and Hearing Association subcommittee report. J. Tenn. Sp. Hear. Assoc. 20, 21-39.

Soli, S. (1981). Second formants in fricatives: Acoustic consequences of fricative-vowel coarticulation. J. Acoust. Soc. Am. 70, 976-984.

Tallal, P. and Piercy, M. (1973a). Defects of non-verbal auditory perception in children with developmental aphasia. Nature 241, 468-469.

Tallal, P. and Piercy, M. (1973b). Developmental aphasia: Impaired rate of non-verbal processing as a function of sensory modality. Neuropsychologia 11, 389-398.

Tallal, .P and Piercy, M. (1974) Developmental aphasia: Rate of auditory processing and selective impairment of consonant perception. Neuropsychologia 12, 83-93.

Tallal, P. and Piercy, M. (1975). Developmental aphasia: The perception of brief vowels and extended stop consonants. Neuropsychologia 13, 69-74.

Tallal, P. (1980a). Auditory temporal perception, phonics, and reading disabilities in children. Brain and Language 9, 182-198.

Tallal, P. (1980b). Language and reading: Some perceptual prerequisites. Bulletin of the Orton Society, Vol. 30, 170-178.

Tallal, P. and Stark, R.E. (1982). Perceptual/motor profiles of reading impaired children with or without concomitant oral language deficits. Ann. of Dyslexia 32, 163-176.

Tallal, P., Stark, M., and Mellitts, D. (1985a). Identification of language-impaired children on the basis of rapid perception and production skills. Brain and Language 25, 314-322.

Tallal, P., Stark, M., and Mellitts, D. (1985b). The relationship between auditory temporal analysis and receptive language development: Evidence from studies of developmental language disorder. Neuropsychologia 23, 527-534.

Tallal, P., Ross, R., and Curtiss, S. Familial aggregation in specific language impairment. J. Sp. Hearing Disorders, in press.

Tallal, P., Ross, R., and Curtiss, S. Unexpected sex-ratios in families of language/learning-impaired children. Psychoneuroendocrinology, in press.

Zurif, E. and Carson, G. (1970). Dyslexia in relation to cerebral dominance and temporal analysis. Neuropsychologia 8, 351-361.

14
Reading is Hard just because Listening is Easy

Alvin M. Liberman

In their work on reading and the difficulties that attend it, investigators have commonly omitted to ask the questions that are, in my view, prior to all others: why is it easier to perceive speech than to read, and why is it easier to speak a word than to spell it? My aim is to repair these omissions. To that end, I divide my talk into two parts. First, I say why we should consider that the greater ease of perceiving and producing speech is paradoxical, by which I mean to suggest that the reasons are not to be found among surface appearances. Then I propose how, by going beneath the surface, we can find the reasons, and so resolve the paradox.

THE PARADOX

Before developing the paradox, I should first remind you that perceiving and producing speech <u>are</u> easier than reading or writing, for this is the point from which I depart and to which I will, at the end, return. The relevant facts include the following. (1) All communities of human beings have a fully developed spoken language; in contrast, only a minority of these languages has a written form, and not all of these are in common use. (2) Speech is first in the history of the race, as it is in the child; reading and writing are later. (3) For the proper development of speech, a neurologically normal child need only be placed in an environment where language is used; reading and writing typically require formal tuition. And, (4), most people master speech well enough to find it useful; many fail utterly, or nearly so, to read or write.

Consider, now, in how far this is a paradox. It is paradoxical, first, because the eye, not the ear, is the better organ. By any standard one can think of, the eye is a broader

197

channel than the ear, capable of transmitting more information
about the environment and at a far higher rate. One supposes,
indeed, that few human engineers would ever have tried to put so
rapid a flow of information as language requires through so narrow
a bottleneck as the ear affords. Which is, we might suppose,
another demonstration of the validity of the observation by
Francois Jacob that nature is not so much an engineer as she is a
tinker.

Another aspect of the paradox is that, by comparison with the
sounds of speech, the letters of print are by far the cleaner
signal. Think of the precise edges that set letters apart from
their backgrounds, and contrast this with the fuzzy patterns one
sees in a spectrogram of speech, where information that is most
important for linguistic purposes is often among the least
prominent parts of the signal.

A further contribution to the paradox is that, unlike human
beings, machines find it much easier to 'read' print than to
'perceive' speech. Thus, 'reading' machines (optical character
readers, so called) can, without too much difficulty, be made to
work according to the phonologic (hence, the alphabetic)
principle. That is, given a machine designed to recognize the /d/
in 'hid', it will, without further ado, recognize the /d/ in 'do'.
Not so for machines that are supposed to perceive speech. Not
only do they have trouble generalizing from one occurrence of /d/
to another, but they also cannot readily discover about the word
'hid' that it has three phonological segments, while 'do' has only
two. Though all words are combinations and permutations of a
small set of such segments, they cannot readily be made to appear
so to an automatic speech recognizer.

We come, then, to a fact that is, at once, the crux of the
paradox and the key to its resolution: the relation between
signal and language is relatively simple for an alphabetic
representation but inordinately complex for speech. Because this
is the key fact, I will develop it in greater detail as we go
along. For now, it will suffice to say that it is true. An
alphabetic orthography is, with occasional exceptions, a
relatively straightforward reflection of the phonological or
morphophonological structure of some language. Speech conveys the
same structure, but in a far less straightforward way.

RESOLVING THE PARADOX

Taking into account that speech and writing systems must
communicate words, we should first remind ourselves that all words
are combinations and permutations of the specifically linguistic
elements we know as consonants and vowels. These are governed, of
course, by phonology, the component of every language that forms
all its words--past, present, and future--by a systematically

constrained application of the combinatorial principle. Thus, as
several members of the symposium have said (I. Y. Liberman, 1988;
Lindblom, 1988), the critically important function of phonology is
to allow the inventory of words--i. e., of phonological
structures--to be vastly larger and more flexible than it could be
if, as in all nonlinguistic forms of natural communication, the
signal for each meaningful element were holistically different
from the signals for all others. It need not matter, not in
principle at least, whether the phonological structures are
conveyed acoustically, optically, or, for that matter, chemically.
What does matter is that these structures should exist, however
abstractly, and so provide the basis for a large lexicon. Thus,
the unique characteristic of words, as opposed to all
nonlinguistic vehicles of communication, is that their meanings
are given, not by a direct link to the physical signals (sounds,
sights, smells, etc.), but, indirectly, via the phonological
structures these signals convey. We should suppose, therefore,
that every word, whether spoken or written, refers to such a
structure. If the language system is to find the meaning of a
word, it must, perforce, know which word--i. e., which
phonological structure--it is to find the meaning of.

It is, of course, nonetheless true that, just as nonhuman
animals can respond more or less appropriately to some spoken
words, treating them nonphonologically as if they were so many
sounds, so, too, can would-be readers respond to printed words as
if they were pictures or optical shapes of some nondescript sort.
But such responses do not engage the language system; hence they
stand apart from the kind of communication that language alone
makes possible.

Granting, then, that words are systematic phonological
structures, let us imagine a circumstance in which reading and
writing would be, at worst, no harder than listening and speaking,
and then see why, under that circumstance, language as we know it
could not have developed. For that purpose, consider how the
phonological structures might have been realized by the speaker as
articulatory gestures and sounds. Perhaps the most
reasonable-seeming possibility is that, since nature had elected
to transmit the phonological structures acoustically, she would
have defined its elements in acoustic terms. In that case, there
would have been, for each consonant or vowel, a discrete and
invariant sound, providing an acoustic 'alphabet' entirely
analogous to one of the optical alphabets used for reading and
writing. Speaking a word would then have been exactly equivalent
to spelling it--that is, to setting out the sequence of consonants
and vowels it comprised. Listening to such an explicitly
segmented sound would, of course, have made its phonological
spelling equally plain. To convert, then, from this acoustic
alphabet to one conveyed optically, by letters, would have been
trivially straightforward and trivially easy; anyone who could

produce and perceive speech would have had only to learn a few perfectly transparent associations. Consequently, reading and writing would have been at least as easy as speaking and listening. But there would have been no language worth trying to read or write, for producing and perceiving an acoustic alphabet would have been so tedious and time-consuming as to have precluded the use of those larger syntactic structures that take advantage of essential groundwork by phonology to give language its truly productive character.

What makes speech, as we know it, possible is that the consonants and vowels are defined ultimately, not as sounds, but as gestures or, more properly, as the remote and abstract structures that control them (Liberman and Mattingly, 1985; cf. Browman and Goldstein, 1985; Fowler, 1986). The important consequence is that the elements of these controlling phonetic structures can be variously overlapped and merged--that is, coarticulated--and so produced at rates many times faster than is possible with an acoustic alphabet. Such coarticulation is carried out--presumably, it can only be carried out--by a biologically coherent module adapted specifically to this function. This module is special on at least two counts: its constituent gestures are a distinct set, used for producing phonetic structures and for nothing else; and their coarticulation is so coordinated as to gain high rates of transmission--about ten consonants and vowels per second, on average--and yet retain information about their underlying structure (Mattingly and Liberman, in press, a). But what is relevant to our concern is that, like all such specialized modules, this one operates at a precognitive level, below the threshold of awareness. As a result, speaking a word does not require knowing how it is spelled, or even that it has a spelling. Given that the speaker has thought of the word, the phonetic module takes care of the rest, automatically selecting and regulating the string of consonants and vowels the word comprises.

Coarticulation also speeds the perception of speech, since it folds into a single piece of sound information about several successive elements of the phonetic structure (Liberman et al., 1967). But this considerable gain in efficiency comes at a cost: there is now a complex and specifically linguistic relation between the sound and the phonetic structure it conveys. The nature of the complexity has often been described (see, for example, Liberman and Mattingly, 1985; Fant, 1962). I would speak only of the one aspect that is most relevant to our concern: the acoustic segments do not correspond directly to the segmentation of the phonological structure; accordingly, they correspond no better to the segments of the alphabetic representation. Thus, to take the example offered to this symposium by Isabelle Liberman (1988), the word 'bag' has three phonological segments, but only one segment of sound. Any attempt to divide the sound into the linguistic segments that underlie it will produce three syllables, 'buh ah guh', which are not, on their face, recognizable as the word 'bag'.

How, then, do listeners cope? The answer my colleagues and I have offered is that they rely on a phonetic module, specifically adapted for processing the speech signal so as to recover the coarticulated gestures that produced it (Liberman and Mattingly, 1985; Mattingly and Liberman, in press, a), Mattingly and Liberman, in press, b). This module is, of course, merely the other face of the one that governs the processes of coarticulation. Thus, there is but a single module with two complementary and specifically linguistic processes, one for producing phonetic gestures, the other for perceiving them. I will return to this property of the phonetic specialization later, for it is central to understanding why speech, but not reading or writing, could have evolved in the race, and why speech, but not reading or writing, can develop without formal instruction in the child. But, for the moment, the important point is that, just like the processes that underlie the production of phonetic structures, those that manage their perception take place below the level of awareness. Thus, the phonetic module automatically recovers the 'spelling', which it uses, just as automatically, to find the word in the listener's lexicon. So, to perceive a word, one need only listen to the sound. There is no need to puzzle out the underlying linguistic structure, or even to know that it exists; the phonetic module does all the hard, analytic work.

Of course, recovering the phonetic structure is not quite enough, for, as is well known, the invariant form of the word--that is, its phonological and morphophonological structure--undergoes systematic changes on its way to the phonetic surface. This occurs, both within and across word boundaries, as a function of context, stress, rate, and dialect. Thus, the voiceless fricative of 'bats' becomes the voiced fricative of 'balls'; the voiceless alveolar stop of 'bat' becomes (in American English) the voiced flap of 'batter' (as if 'batter' were the comparative form of 'bad'); all the vowels of 'telegraph' change in 'telegraphy'; and the initial semivowel of 'you', though reasonably preserved in 'Will you...?', usually becomes a voiced affricate in 'Did you...?' Surely, reading and writing would be even harder than they are if the orthography rendered words in all their myriad phonetic forms, which is presumably why all alphabetic systems, excluding only those used for technical linguistic purposes, are pitched at a reasonably abstract phonological level.

To speculate about how the speaker-listener manages the interconversion of phonetic and phonological structures, and about how much of it is attributable to the constraints of articulation and coarticulation, would take us far beyond the purpose of this essay. What is relevant for now is simply that the interconverting processes are, for the most part, just about as automatic as those of the phonetic module.

As for readers, the point is that the orthographic spelling is, by and large, closer to the invariant phonological form of the word than any of its phonetic realizations is likely to be. Therefore, readers are well advised to identify the word directly from the information about its internal structure that the orthography offers. Indeed, there is little else they can do, for orthographies, whether broadly phonological or narrowly phonetic, do not specify how words (or pseudowords) are to be pronounced -- that is, how the movements of the speech organs are to be governed. There is, then, no way that readers can get to a word via an articulatory or acoustic route, either explicitly or implicitly. The order must rather be the reverse: readers first apprehend the word; that done, they have the articulatory representation automatically available to them, ready to be used in working memory for coping with the syntax (Shankweiler and Crain, 1986; I. Y. Liberman, 1988; cf. Gathercole and Baddeley, 1988; Kean, 1988), and also for pronouncing the word should circumstances call for reading aloud.

So it is that a specialized, precognitive module, part of the larger specialization for language, automatically interconverts between spoken words and their internal structure. Consider, now, how this pertains to the four points I made at the outset about what it means to say that reading is hard and speech is easy.

(1) Speech is universal because, being managed by a module specifically adapted for the purpose, it evolved with our species. Writing systems are artifacts, hence comparatively rare.

(2) Speech could evolve, and thus come first in the history of the race, while reading and writing could not, because of the very different ways they meet a requirement that is imposed on all communication systems: what counts as structure for the sender must count for the receiver; otherwise, communication does not occur. Though rarely taken into account by theories about the processes of spoken and written language, this requirement, which Mattingly and I have called the requirement for parity, is real (Mattingly and Liberman, in press, b). To say how it is met in the development of the system is to test any theory of the biology and psychology of language or, indeed of any natural communication system. To tie it to our immediate concern is to go to the core of the difference between spoken and written language.

In this connection, consider again that there is, in speech, a phonetic module, specialized to conduct the producing and perceiving aspects of its business in a common coin of

specifically   linguistic   gestures.   This   provides   a   built-in
guarantee that, at every stage of   evolutionary   development,   the
perceptions   of   the   listener   will   be in the same domain as the
intentions of the speaker, a domain that is, for both,   inherently
and singularly linguistic: message sent and message received will
always be made of the same stuff.   Thus, parity   is   at   the   very
heart   of   the   phonetic   module.   No   conventions,   no cognitive
interventions from outside the phonological system, no translation
across   domains   were required in order to link, to each other and
to   language,   what   must   otherwise   have   been   wholly   separate
modalities of perception and action.   There was but one modality,
and it was essentially   linguistic;   hence,   speech   was   free   to
evolve.

Obviously,   the   alphabet   did   not   enjoy   this   biological
advantage.   It   had no module adapted to its linguistic purposes,
so its use had, necessarily, to rest on modalities of   action   and
perception   that   evolved   entirely   apart   from   language.   As a
consequence,   parity   could   only   have   been   established   by
arbitrarily   associating these modalities to each other and to the
linguistic structures they were required, somewhat unnaturally, to
convey.   Accordingly,   a   writing system was a triumph of applied
linguistics,   half   discovery,   half   invention.   The
discovery--surely   one   of   the most important ever made--was that
the words people had been speaking for so many thousands of   years
did   not   differ   from   each   other holistically, but rather by an
internal structure made of a small number of   phonological   units.
The   invention   that exploited this discovery was the notion that,
if these units were to be represented by arbitrary optical shapes,
then   reading   and   writing would be possible for all who knew the
language, provided they   could   become   reasonably   aware   of   its
phonological   structure, and so appreciate what the optical shapes
were all about.   Thus, an alphabet, though based   on   one   of   the
naturally   evolved structures of language, can only have developed
in cultural evolution, out of conscious, cognitive effort.

(3) For exactly the same reason that speech could   evolve   in
the   race--viz.,   that   parity is intrinsic to the system--it can,
and does, develop without formal   tuition   in   the   child.   Thus,
there   is not in the child, any more than there was in the race, a
need for cognitive intervention   to   establish   the   link   between
phonological   structures   and   the   sounds   of   speech.   In   the
acquisition of speech, it is the phonetic   module   that   'learns',
automatically   adjusting   its   internal   precognitive   processes
according to the stage of its development and   the   conditions   of
the   linguistic environment (Mattingly and Liberman, in press, b).
Reading and writing cannot develop in this epigenetic way for   the
same   reason that they did not evolve in the race: parity must be
imposed, and,   typically,   that   requires   special   experience   or
instruction to   lead   the   child to the same discovery about words
that had earlier been made by those who   developed   the   alphabet.

Only after parity is established can the child properly apply the alphabetic principle, and only by practice can he then make such application automatic.

(4) To explain why fewer children fail at speech than at reading and writing, I need only say what has been the point of the whole talk: reading and writing present a cognitive hurdle that speaking and listening do not. Because of the phonetic module, there is nothing in the child's normal experience with spoken language that necessarily acquaints him with the fact that words have an internal structure. Indeed, the automaticity of the module tends rather to make this fact obscure. Yet it is precisely this fact that must be understood if the alphabet is to make sense, and if its advantages are to be properly exploited. (Elbro, 1988; I. Y. Liberman, 1988; Lundberg, 1988; Olson, 1988).

References

Browman, C.P. and Goldstein, L.M. (1985). Dynamic Modeling of Phonetic Structure. (ed. V. Fromkin). In Phonetic Linguistics. Academic Press, New York.

Elbro, C. (1988). Morphemic Awareness Among Dyslexics. Paper presented at the Seventh Inernational Symposium on Developmental Dyslexia and Dysphasia. Academia Rodinensis Pro Remediatone, Wenner-Gren Center, Stockholm.

Fant, C.G.M. (1962). Descriptive Analysis of the Acoustic Aspects of Speech. Logos, 5, 3–17.

Fowler, C.A. (1986). An Event Approach to the Study of Speech Perception From a Direct Realist Perspective. J. of Phon., 14, 3–28.

Gathercole, S.E. and Baddeley, A.D. (1988). The Role of Phonological Memory in Normal and Disordered Language Development. Paper presented at the Seventh Inernational Symposium on Developmental Dyslexia and Dysphasia. Academia Rodinensis Pro Remediatone, Wenner-Gren Center, Stockholm.

Kean, M-L. (1988). Grammatical Capacity in Developmental Dyslexia: Issues for Research. Paper presented at the Seventh Inernational Symposium on Developmental Dyslexia and Dysphasia. Academia Rodinensis Pro Remediatone, Wenner-Gren Center, Stockholm.

Liberman, A.M., Cooper, F.S., Shankweiler, D.P., and Studdert-Kennedy, M. (1967). Perception of the Speech Code. Psychol. Rev., 74, 431–461.

Liberman, A.M. and Mattingly, I.G. (1985). The Motor Theory of Speech Perception Revised. Cogn., 21, 1-36.

Liberman, I.Y. (1988). Phonology and Beginning Reading Revisited. Paper presented at the Seventh Inernational Symposium on Developmental Dyslexia and Dysphasia. Academia Rodinensis Pro Remediatone, Wenner-Gren Center, Stockholm.

Lindblom, B. (1988). On the Evolution of Spoken Language: Some Remarks on the Origin of the 'Phonetic Code'. Paper presented at the Seventh Inernational Symposium on Developmental Dyslexia and Dysphasia. Academia Rodinensis Pro Remediatone, Wenner-Gren Center, Stockholm.

Lundberg, I. (1988). Lack of Phonological Awareness--a Critical Factor in Developmental Dyslexia. Paper presented at the Seventh Inernational Symposium on Developmental Dyslexia and Dysphasia. Academia Rodinensis Pro Remediatone, Wenner-Gren Center, Stockholm.

Olson, R.K. (1988). Defects in Disabled Readers' Phonological and Orthographic Coding: Etiology and Remediation. Paper presented at the Seventh Inernational Symposium on Developmental Dyslexia and Dysphasia. Academia Rodinensis Pro Remediatone, Wenner-Gren Center, Stockholm.

Mattingly, I.G. and Liberman, A.M. (in press, a). Specialized Perceiving Systems for Speech and Other Biologically Significant Sounds. In Functions of the Auditory System. (eds. G.M. Edelman,, W.E. Gall, and W.M. Cowan). Wiley, New York.

Mattingly, I.G. and Liberman, A.M. (in press, b). Speech and Other Auditory Modules. In Signal and Sense: Local and Global Order in Perceptual Maps. (eds. G.M. Edelman, W.E. Gall, and W.M. Cowan). Wiley, New York.

Shankweiler, D. and Crain, S. (1986). Language Mechanisms and Reading Disorder: A Modular Approach. Cognition, 24, 139-168.

Acknowledgments. Preparation of this paper was aided by a grant to Haskins Laboratories (NIH-NICHD-HD-01994). The notions offered here are adapted from the contributions of the many colleagues, at Haskins Laboratories and elswhere, who have been concerned with the role of phonological structures in reading.

15
Phonology and Beginning Reading Revisited

Isabelle Y. Liberman

The research of my colleagues and me has, for many years, been guided by the assumption that most problems in learning to read and write stem from deficits in the language faculty, not from deficiencies of a more generally cognitive or perceptual sort. A paper by Alvin Liberman (1988) says in detail how and why we were initially led to that assumption. My aim here is rather to describe the assumption itself, offer data in support, and finally to develop the implications for the teacher and clinician.

A CONTRAST BETWEEN LISTENING AND READING

But first, I should offer some background (Liberman, 1987). To that end, I will consider a few facts about words: how they are produced and perceived, and how differently they are processed in spoken and written language. All words are, of course, formed of combinations and permutations of phonological elements called consonants and vowels. The obvious advantage of forming words in this way is that by using no more than two or three dozen different elements, we can and do produce a large and vastly expandable vocabulary numbering tens of thousands of words. If, on the other hand, each word had to be uniquely and holistically different from every other word, the number we could produce would be limited to the number of different individual signals--sounds, if you will--that a person can efficiently make and perceive; that number is, of course, exceedingly small.

An alphabetic writing system--the one we're concerned with--represents the same string of phonological segments--consonants and vowels--that we use in speaking, the string that distinguishes one word from all others. Then why should it be so hard for many beginning readers to grasp the alphabetic principle? Why can they not quickly begin to read and

write as well and as easily as they can already speak and listen?
The exact nature of the difficulty has been developed in greater
detail elsewhere (A. M. Liberman, 1982, 1988; A. M. Liberman,
Cooper,   Shankweiler,   &   Studdert-Kennedy,   1967).   I should
nevertheless summarize the argument here.

     Consider how you and I produce a word like "bag", or more to
the point, how we do not produce it. We do not say B A G; we say
"bag".   That is, we fold three phonological segments--two
consonants and one vowel--into a single segment of sound. This we
do by a process called "coarticulation". In the case of "bag", we
overlap the lip movement appropriate for the initial consonant B
with the tongue movement appropriate for the medial vowel A, and
then smoothly merge that with the tongue movement appropriate for
the final consonant G.   Such coarticulation, it should   be
emphasized, is not careless speech. It is the very essence of
speech, the only basis on which phonological structures can be
produced at the rapid rates that make words, phrases, and
sentences feasible.

     Consider now the consequences for perception.   When one
examines a schematic spectrogram sufficient to produce the word
"bag" (A.M. Liberman, 1970), one sees that the three phonologic
segments are thoroughly merged in the sound stream. The vowel is
not limited to a medial position, but covers the entire length of
the syllable.   Information about the initial consonant continues
well beyond the middle of the signal.   Moreover, the center
portion of the acoustic signal is providing information not just
about the vowel, but about all three perceptual segments at once.

     Now we must ask how a listener knows that the word is "bag"
and not "tag" or "big" or "bat". The answer is that all this is
managed by a biologically coherent system, specifically adapted to
the production and perception of phonetic structures.   In
production, the specialization automatically converts   the
phonological representation of the word into the coarticulated
movements that convey it.   In perception, this specialization
effectively runs the process in reverse: it automatically parses
the sound so as to recover the coarticulated gestures--that is,
the segmented phonetic structure--that caused it.

     But notice that all of this is automatic, carried out below
the level of conscious awareness. Thus, to say "bag", speakers
need not know how it is spelled--that is, what sequence of
consonants and vowels it comprises. They have only to think of
the word. The phonetic specialization in effect spells it for
them.   Matters are correspondingly automatic for listeners: on
hearing the sound "bag", they need not consciously analyze it into
its three constituent elements.   For, again, the phonetic
specialization does it all, recovering the segments and matching
them to the word stored in the lexicon; the listeners are none the

wiser about the very complex process that has been carried out on their behalf.

The relation of all this to reading and writing has long seemed to us quite obvious (Liberman, 1971). For if readers and writers are to use the alphabetic principle productively--that is, if they are to deal with words they have never seen in print--they must be quite consciously aware of the phonological structure the letters represent. But nothing in their normal linguistic experience has prepared them for this. Never have the processes by which they normally speak and listen revealed to them that words have internal phonologic structures, and never before have they been in a situation which required them to know that such structures do, in fact, exist.

What then are beginners to make of the three letters that form the word bag? If we tell them the letters represent sounds, then we are misleading them, because they know, and we should know, that there are three letters but really only one sound. If we tell them the letters represent abstract and specifically phonologic gestures, then we are conveying the true state of affairs, but, as a practical matter, that explanation is not likely to help them read.

These considerations led us to several hypotheses. The first was that awareness of phonological structure might be a problem for preliterate children. The second was that individual differences in this ability might be related to success in reading. A third hypothesis was that training in phonological awareness would have a positive effect on reading achievement. The fourth hypothesis was that the weakness in phonological awareness displayed by beginners who have difficulties in learning to read might reflect a more general deficiency in the biological specialization that processes phonological structure in speech. Now I turn to the relevant data.

AWARENESS OF PHONOLOGICAL STRUCTURE IN PRELITERATES

What data do we have about awareness? Some 15 years ago we began to examine developmental trends in phonological awareness by testing the ability of young children to segment words into their constituent elements (Liberman, Shankweiler, Fischer & Carter, 1974). We found that normal preschool children performed rather poorly. We learned further that of the two types of sublexical units--the syllable and the phoneme--the phoneme, which happens to be the unit represented by our alphabet, presented the greater difficulty by far. About half the four- and five-year-olds could segment by syllable, but none of the four-year-olds and only 17% of the five-year-olds could manage segmentation by phoneme.   Even at six there was a difference--10% failed on the syllables but 30% failed on the phonemes.

The answer to our first hypothesis is clear from these results and those of studies by many other investigators (see Stanovich, 1982 for a review): Awareness of the phonemic segment, the basic unit of the alphabetic writing system, is indeed hard to achieve, harder than awareness of syllables, and it develops later, if at all. It was also apparent that, like any cognitive achievement, it develops to varying degrees at varying rates in different children. Moreover, a large number of children have not attained awareness of either level of linguistic structure--syllable or phoneme--even at the end of a full year in school. If linguistic awareness does indeed provide entry into the alphabetic system, as we think it does, then these children are the ones we need to worry about.

AWARENESS OF PHONOLOGICAL STRUCTURE AND LITERACY

Much evidence is now available to support our second hypothesis, namely, that awareness of the phonological constituents of words is important for the acquisition of reading. The evidence comes from numerous studies here and abroad. These have all shown that phonological awareness is significantly related to reading success in young children. In English, there are , to name only a few, studies by Liberman (1973); Goldstein (1976); Fox & Routh (1980); Treiman & Baron (1981); Blachman (1984); Bradley & Bryant (1983); Mann & Liberman (1984) and Olson (1988). All these findings have been supported and indeed extended in Swedish by the carefully controlled, pioneering studies of the correlates of reading disability carried out by Lundberg and his associates in Umeå (1980, 1988) and also by the recent studies by Magnusson and Naucler in Lund (1987). In Spanish we cite work by de Manrique and Gramigna (1984), in French by Bertelson's Belgian laboratory (Bertelson, 1988; Morias, Cluytens, and Alegria, 1984),and in Italian by Cossu and associates (Cossu, Shankweiler, Liberman, Tola & Katz, 1988).

THE EFFECT OF TRAINING IN PHONOLOGICAL AWARENESS

Thus there is now a great deal of evidence to support the hypothesis that deficiency in phonological awareness is related to success in reading. The evidence comes, as we have seen, from studies covering a wide range of ages, many language communities, and a variety of cultural and economic backgrounds, ranging from inner city and rural poor to suburban affluent.

It is of special interest, then, to find that phonological awareness can be taught even in preschool (Ball & Blachman, in press; Content, Morais, Alegria, & Bertelson, 1982; Lundberg, 1988; Lundberg, Frost, & Petersen, 1988; Oloffson & Lundberg, 1983; Vellutino & Scanlon, 1987). Early evidence for the value of such training cames from a landmark study by Bradley & Bryant (1983). In the first of a pair of experiments, they found high correlations between preschoolers' phonological awareness as measured by rhyming tasks and the children's reading and spelling scores several years later. In the second experiment, they found that children with initially low levels of phonological awareness who were trained in the phonological classification of words were later superior in reading and spelling to groups who had had semantic classification training or no training at all. Those trained, in addition, to associate letters with the phonemes were even more successful. New evidence for the positive effects of phonological training on reading achievement has recently been reported by Lundberg (1988) and by Vellutino (Vellutino and Scanlon, 1987).

THE SOURCE OF INDIVIDUAL DIFFERENCES IN AWARENESS

What the research data have shown thus far can be summarized by four major points. The first is that despite adequate speech, preliterate children and adults are not necessarily aware that words have an internal phonological structure. Since the alphabet represents that structure, they are therefore not in a position to use the alphabetic principle. The second is that there are individual differences in the ease with which children become aware of phonological structure. Third, these differences correlate with success in learning to read. And finally, explicit training in the analysis of phonological structure produces not only better speech analysers but also better readers.

Now we should ask whence comes the abnormally great difficulty that some children have in developing the awareness? There are two possibilities: the problem could reflect difficulty with any cognitive tasks that require analytic ability or, alternatively, it could point to a deficiency in the phonological processor that causes it to set up phonological structures weakly. In the latter case, the difficulty in awareness would be only one of many symptoms of the deficiency. We will consider the phonological alternative.

Most of the research I have mentioned thus far has concentrated on deficiencies in phonological awareness. Now, I will consider evidence that the deficiency in awareness may be symptomatic of a more general deficiency or weakness in the neurobiological device that carries out all phonological processes. In speech, phonologic structures are thus set up more weakly.

The evidence comes from comparisons of good and poor readers in their performances on tasks of short-term memory, speech perception, speech production, and naming.

Because verbal short-term memory depends on the ability to use phonological structures to hold linguistic information in memory (Conrad, 1964; Liberman, Mattingly, & Turvey, 1972), we would expect people with phonological deficiencies to have difficulties with short-term memory tasks. In many studies poor readers have, in fact, been found to have such difficulties. Typically, poor readers recall fewer items than age-matched good readers (Gathercole & Baddeley, 1988; Shankweiler, Liberman, Mark, Fowler, & Fischer, 1979; Wagner & Torgesen, 1987), but their memory difficulties occur mainly when the items require verbal rendering. If the test materials do not lend themselves to verbal description, as in the memory for nonsense shapes or photographs of unfamiliar faces, the poor readers are not at a disadvantage (Katz, Shankweiler, & Liberman, 1981; Liberman, Mann, Shankweiler, & Werfelman, 1982).

A deficiency in the phonological processor is suggested also by the research of Brady and associates (Brady, Shankweiler, & Mann, 1983) on the speech perception of poor readers. They found that poor readers need a higher quality of signal than good readers for error-free performance in the perception of speech but not of non-speech, environmental sounds. Underlying deficits in phonological processing have also been posited by Hugh Catts (1986) to explain his finding that reading disabled students made signficantly more errors than matched normals on three different tasks in which their speech production was stressed.

A similar conclusion was reached by Robert Katz (1986) in regard to the naming problems of poor readers in the second grade. The fact that poor readers tend to misname things could lead us to infer that their problem is semantic. But Katz's research with the Boston Naming Test suggests that this may be a wrong inference. The poor readers' incorrect responses to the pictured objects were sometimes nonwords closely but imperfectly resembling the target word in its phonological components ("gloav" for glove). Here the phonological problem is easily seen. In another kind of error, the phonological difficulty is less obvious. For example, a frequent response to the picture of a volcano was the word "tornado" which is so different in meaning that a semantic source of the error would seem likely. However, it is noted that the incorrect response has structural characteristics in common with the target word; for example, volcano has the same number of syllables, an identical stress pattern, and similar vowel constituents as tornado. More critically, it was clear that the children often actually knew the correct meaning of the word, since in subsequent questioning about the pictured object, they produced a description of a volcano, not a tornado.

Further evidence that phonological and not semantic weakness was the basis for many of the poor readers' naming errors was provided in a test of identification. Each item previously misnamed was afterwards tested for recognition by having the child select from a set of eight the one picture that best depicted the meaning of the word. In many cases, the correct object was now selected. Thus, it was possible that the poor readers had acquired internal lexical representations of many of the objects whose·names they had not been able to produce accurately.

SOME IMPLICATIONS FOR INSTRUCTION

Given all that we know about the important relations between phonological ability and reading acquisition, what can we say about instructional procedures? We surely must deplore a currently popular instructional procedure, dubbed by its creators the "psycholinguistic guessing game" (Goodman, 1976). In this widely used procedure and its offshoot, the so-called "whole language" method, teachers are directed not to trouble beginners with details about how the internal phonological structure of words is represented by the letters. Instead, children are encouraged to read words however they can--for example, by recognizing their overall visual shapes--then, using their so-called normal and natural language processes, to guess the rest of the message from the context.

The "whole language" proponents seem not to have considered that before one can get to the true meaning of a sentence, one but must first get to its actual constituent words--approximations will not be enough. And to get to those actual words properly, whether one is a beginner or a skilled reader, one cannot rely on visual shape but must apply the alphabetic principle. This does not mean, incidentally, that one must necessarily sound out the words letter by letter. As we have often said elsewhere (See Liberman, Shankweiler, Liberman, Fowler & Fischer, 1977), every reader must group the letters so as to put together just those strings of consonants and vowels that are, in the normal process of speech production, collapsed into a single pronounceable unit. There is no simple rule by which a reader can do this. Acquiring the ability to combine the letters of a new word into the appropriate pronounceable units efficiently and automatically, is an aspect of reading skill that separates the fluent reader from the beginner who has barely discovered what an alphabetic orthography is all about.

Fortunately, many children--the lucky 75% or so--do discover the alphabetic principle on their own and begin to apply it. They begin to discover for themselves the commonalities between similarly spoken and written words. When tested in kindergarten as preliterates, these children turn out to be the ones with strengths in the phonological domain. Unfortunately, for the many children with phonological deficiencies--children who do not understand that the spoken word has segments and who have not discovered on their own that there is a correspondence between

those segments and the letters of the printed word, the current
vogue for the so-called (and from my point of view, misnamed)
"whole language" and "language experience" approaches are likely
to be disastrous. Children with deficiencies in the phonological
domain who are taught in that way are likely to join the ranks of
the millions of functional illiterates who stumble along, guessing
at the printed message from their little store of memorized words,
unable to decipher a new word they have never seen before.

For those beginners who do not discover the alphabetic
principle on their own, an introductory method that provides them
with direct instruction in what they need to know is critical
(Liberman, 1985; Liberman & Shankweiler, 1979).

Direct instruction, as I see it, would begin with language
analysis activities, which are incorporated into the daily reading
lesson. These activities can take many forms, limited in number
and variety only by the ingenuity of the teacher. Adaptations of
three exercises that my colleagues and I advocated about ten years
ago (Liberman, Shankweiler, Blachman, Camp & Werfelman 1980) have
been shown by Blachman (1987) to be successful even in inner city
schools with a history of reading failure. They are outlined in
Figure 1. Borrowing a procedure originally devised by the Soviet
psychologist, Elkonin (1973), Blachman presented the child with a
simple line drawing representing the word to be analyzed. A
rectangle under the drawing is divided into squares equal to the
number of phonemes in the pictured word. The children are taught
to say the word slowly, placing a counter in the appropriate
square of the diagram as each phoneme is articulated. Later, as
the child progresses, the counter can be color coded--one for
vowels, another for consonants, and the letter symbols for the
vowels can be added one by one. The procedure has many virtues:
First, the line drawing, in effect, keeps the word in front of the
children throughout the process of analysis so that they do not
need to rely on short-term memory to retain the word being
studied. Second, the diagram provides the children with a linear
visual-spatial structure to which they can relate the
auditory-temporal sequence of the spoken word, thus reinforcing
the key idea of the successive segmentation of the phonemic
components of the word. Third, the sections of the diagram call
the children's attention to the actual number of segments in the
word, so that they need not resort to uninformed guessing.
Fourth, the combination of drawing, diagram, and counters provides
concrete materials that help to objectify the very abstract ideas
being represented. Fifth, the procedure affords the children an
active part to play throughout. Finally, the color coding of the
counters leads the children to appreciate the difference between
vowels and consonants early in their schooling. The subsequent
addition of letters to the counters can reinforce other kinds of
grapheme study.

ELKONIN (1973)

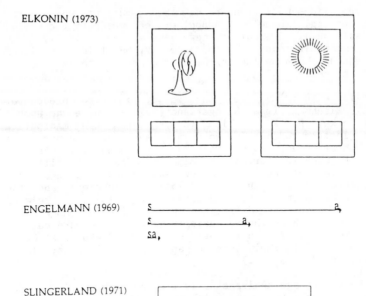

ENGELMANN (1969)

SLINGERLAND (1971)

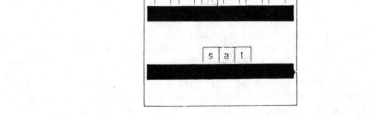

Figure 1. Language analysis activities (after Blachman, 1987 and Liberman, Shankweiler,

Blachman, Camp, and Werfelman, 1980)

In a second activity, this one adapted from Englemann (1969), Blachman taught the children how to read the combination of a consonant followed by a vowel as a single unit. For this purpose, the initial consonant selected to be written on the blackboard by the teacher and read by the children is the continuant "s". It is chosen because, unlike the stop consonants (ptk and bdg), it can be pronounced in isolation and held over time. It is held until the teacher writes the second letter, the vowel, which is then read (as "ă"). The length of time between the initial consonant and the final vowel (as well as the line drawn between them) is then reduced step by step until the two phonemes are, in effect produced as a single sound--"să". By adding stop consonants in the final position and pronouncing the resultant words, the children can begin to collect a pool of real words (for example, sad, sap, sag, sat). Thereafter, new vowels and, finally, new consonants can be introduced in the same way, built into new words which subsequently can be incorporated into stories to be read and written by the child.

A similar effect can be produced by a third procedure, adapted by Blachman from Slingerland (1971). There she uses a small desk pocket-chart on which the children can manipulate individual letters to form new words and learn new phonemes. The words thus constructed, along with a few nonphonetic "sight" words, can be used in stories and poems to be read and written by the child. Note that the child is now reading and writing words the structure of which is no longer a mystery and the understanding of which can be used productively to form related words. (Note also how different this is from a common basal reader approach in which the readability level of the word cat is rated at Grade 1.0-2.0 but that of the word cap is at Grade 3.1-4.1 (Cheek, 1974) simply because cap happens to appear later in many basal reader series.)

All these language analysis activities and others like them can be played as games in which the introduction of each new element not only informs but delights. The beginning reader with adequate phonological ability will require only a relatively brief exposure to such activities. For such readers, these can be followed, or even accompanied by practice with interesting reading materials from other sources, and the further enhancement of vocabulary and knowledge that comes with expanded reading and life experience. But the beginners with weakness in phonological skills, as identified by the language analysis games, who may include as many as 20-25% of the children, will learn to read only if the method includes more intensive, direct, and systematic instruction about phonological structure. Research support for this view has been presented many times for at least 20 years (see Chall, 1983 or Pflaum, Walberg, Karegianes, & Rasher, 1980). It is surely time to put the research into practice.

REFERENCES

Ball, E. W. and Blachman, B. A. (1987). Phoneme Segmentation Training: Effect on Reading Readiness. Paper presented to the Annual Conference of the Orton Dyslexia Society, San Francisco.

Bertelson, P. (1987). The Onset of Literacy: Cognitive Processes in Reading Acquisition. MIT Press, Cambridge, MA.

Blachman, B. (1984). Relationship of Rapid Naming Ability and Language Analysis Skills to Kindergarten and First-grade Achievement. J. Ed. Psych., 76, 610-622.

Blachman, B. (1987). An alternative classroom reading program for learning disabled and other low-achieving children. In Intimacy with Language: A Forgotten Basic in Teacher Education. (ed. W. Ellis).Orton Dyslexia Society, Baltimore.

Bradley, L. and Bryant, P. E. (1983). Categorizing Sounds and Learning to Read -- A Causal Connection. Nature, 30 419-421.

Brady, S. A., Shankweiler, D., and Mann, V. A. (1983). Speech Perception and Memory Coding in Relation to Reading Ability. J. Exper. Child Psych., 35, 345-367.

Catts, H. W. (1986). Speech Production/Phonological Deficits in Reading Disordered Children. J. Learn. Dis., 19(8), 504-508.

Chall, J. (1983). Learning to Read: The Great Debate (updated edition). McGraw Hill Book Company, New York.

Conrad, R. (1979). The Deaf Child. Harper & Row, London.

Cheek, E. H. Jr. (1974). Cheek Master Word List. Educational Achievement Corporation, Waco, Texas.

Content, A., Morais, J., Alegria, J., and Bertelson, P. (1982). Accelerating the Development of Phonetic Segmentation Skills in Kindergartners. Cahiers de Psych., 2, 259-269.

Cossu, G., Shankweiler, D., Liberman, I. Y., Tola, G., and Katz, L. (1988). Awareness of phonological segments and reading ability in Italian children. Appl. Psych., 9. 1-16.

Elkonin, D. B. (1973). U. S. S. R. In Comparative Reading. (ed. J. Downing). MacMillan, New York.

Engelmann, S. (1969). Preventing Failure in the Primary Grades. Science Research Associates, Chicago.

Fox, B. and Routh, D. K. (1980). Phonetic Analysis and Severe Reading Disability in Children. J. Psycholing. Res., 9, 115-119.

Gathercole, S. E. and Baddeley, A. D. (1988). The role of phonological memory in normal and disordered language development. Paper presented at the Seventh International Symposium on Developmental Dyslexia and Dysphasia. Academia Rodinensis Pro Remediatone, Wenner-Gren Center, Stockholm.

Goldstein, D. M. (1976). Cognitive-Linguistic Functioning and Learning to Read in Preschoolers. J. Exper. Psych., 68, 680-688.

Goodman, K. S. (1976). Reading: A Psycholinguistic Guessing Game. Theoretical Models and Processes of Reading (eds. H. Singer and R. B. Ruddell) International Reading Association, Newark, DE.

Helfgott, J. (1976). Phoneme Segmentation and Blending Skills of Kindergarten Children: Implications for Beginning Reading Acquisition. Contemp. Ed. Psych., 1, 157-169.

Katz, R. B. (1986). Phonological Deficiencies in Children With Reading Disability: Evidence from an Object-Naming Task. Cogn., 22, 225-257.

Liberman, A. M. (1970). The Grammars of Speech and Language. Cogn. Psych., 1/4, 301-323.

Liberman, A. M. (1982). On Finding that Speech is Special. Am. Psychol. 37(1), 148-167.

Liberman, A. M. (1988). Reading is Hard Just Because Listening is Easy. Paper presented at the Seventh International Symposium on Developmental Dyslexia and Dysphasia. Academia Rodinensis Pro Remediatone, Wenner-Gren Center, Stockholm.

Liberman, A. M., Cooper, F. S., Shankweiler, D. P., and Studdert-Kennedy, M. (1967). Perception of the Speech Code. Psych. Rev., 74, 431-461.

Liberman, A. M., Mattingly, I. G., and Turvey, M. (1972). Language Codes and Memory Codes. In Coding Processes and Human Memory. (eds. A. W. Melton and E. Martin), New York.

Liberman, I. Y. (1971). Basic Research in Speech and Lateralization of Language: Some Implications for Reading Disability. Bull. Orton Soc., 21, 71-87.

Liberman, I. Y. (1973). Segmentation of the Spoken Word and Reading Acquisition. Bull. Orton Soc.,23, 65-77.

Liberman, I. Y. (1985). Should So-called Modality Preferences Determine the Nature of Instruction for Children with Learning Disabilities? In Dyslexia: A Neuroscientific Approach to Clinical Evaluation. (eds. F. H. Duffy and N. Geschwind). Little, Brown, Boston.

Liberman, I. Y. (1987). Language and Literacy: The Obligation of the Schools of Education. In Intimacy with Language: A Forgotten Basic in Teacher Education. (ed. W. Ellis). The Orton Dyslexia Society, Baltimore.

Liberman, I. Y., Mann, V., Shankweiler, D., and Werfelman, M. (1982). Children's Memory for Recurring Linguistic and Nonlinguistic Material in Relation to Reading Ability. Cortex, 18, 367-375.

Liberman, I. Y. and Shankweiler, D. (1979). Speech, the Alphabet and Teaching to Read. In Theory and Practice of Early Reading. (eds. L. B. Resnik and P. A. Weaver). Erlbaum, Hillsdale, NJ.

Liberman, I. Y. and Shankweiler, D. (1985). Phonology and the Problems of Learning to Read and Write. Remed. Spec. Ed., 6, 8-17.

Liberman, I. Y., Shankweiler, D., Blachman, B., Camp, L., and Werfelman, M. (1980). Steps Toward Literacy. In Auditory Processing and Language: Clinical and Research Perspectives. (eds. P. Levinson and C. Sloan). Grune and Stratton, New York.

Liberman, I. Y., Shankweiler, D., Fischer, F. W., and Carter, B. (1974). Explicit Syllable and Phoneme Segmentation in the Young Child. J. Exper. Child Psych., 18, 201-212.

Lundberg, I. (1988). Lack of Phonological Awareness--a Critical Factor in Developmental Dyslexia. Paper presented at the Seventh International Symposium on Developmental Dyslexia and Dysphasia. Academia Rodinensis Pro Remediatione, Wenner-Gren Center, Stockholm.

Lundberg, I., Frost, J., and Petersen, O.-P. (1988). Effects of an Extensive Program for Stimulating Phonological Awareness in Preschool Children. Read. Res. Quart., 23/3, 263-284.

Lundberg, I., Olofsson, A., and Wall, S. (1980). Reading and Spelling Skills in the First School Years, Predicted from Phonemic Awareness Skills in Kindergarten. Scand. J. Psych., 21, 159-173.

Magnusson, E. and Naucler, K. (1987). Language Disordered and Normally Speaking Children's Development of Spoken and Written Language: Preliminary Results from a Longitudinal Study. Report Uppsala Univ. Ling. Dept., 16, 35-63.

Mann, V. and Liberman, I. Y. (1984). Phonological Awareness and Verbal Short-term Memory. J. Learn. Dis., 17, 592-598.

de Manrique, A. M. B. and Gramigna, S. (1984). La Segmentacion Fonologica y Silabica en Ninos de Preescolar y Primer Grado. Lect. y Vida, 5, 4-13.

Morais, J., Cluytens, M., and Alegria, J. (1984). Segmentation Abilities of Dyslexics and Normal Readers. Percep. Motor Skills, 58, 221-222.

Olofsson, A. and Lundberg, I. (1983). Can Phonemic Awareness be Trained in Kindergarten? Scand. J. Psych., 24, 35-44.

Olson, R., Wise, B., Conners, F., and Rack, J. (1988). Deficits in Disabled Readers' Phonological and Orthographic Coding: Etiology and Remediation. Paper presented at the Seventh International Symposium on Developmental Dyslexia and Dysphasia. Academia Rodinensis Pro Remediatone, Wenner-Gren Center, Stockholm.

Pflaum, S. W., Walberg, H. J., Karegianes, M. L., and Rasher, S. P. (1980). Reading Instruction: A Quantitative Analysis. Ed. Res., 9, 12-18.

Read, C. and Ruyter, L. (1985). Reading and Spelling Skills in Adults of Low Literacy. Remed. Spec. Ed., 6, 43-52.

Shankweiler, D., Liberman, I. Y., Mark, L. S., Fowler, C. A., and Fischer, F. W. (1979). The Speech Code and Learning to Read. J. Exper. Psych.: Human Learn. Mem., 5, 531-545.

Slingerland, B. H. (1971). A Multisensory Approach to Language Arts for Specific Language Disability Children: A Guide for Primary Teachers. Educators Publishing Service, Cambridge, MA.

Stanovich, K. E. (1982). Individual Differences in the Cognitive Processes of Reading: I. Word Coding. J. Learn. Dis., 15, 449-572.

Treiman, R. A. and Baron, J. (1981). Segmental Analysis Ability: Development and Relation to Reading Ability. In Reading Research: Advances in Theory and Practice, 3. (eds. G. E. MacKinnon and T. G. Walker). Academic Press, New York.

Vellutino, F. R. and Scanlon, D. (1987). Phonological Coding and Phonological Awareness and Reading Ability: Evidence from a Longitudinal and Experimental Study. Merrill-Palmer Quart., 33/3, 321-363.

Acknowledgments. Preparation of this paper was aided by grants to Haskins Laboratories (NIH-NICHD-HD-01994) and to Yale University/Haskins Laboratories (NIH-21888-01A1).

16
Lack of Phonological Awareness—A Critical Factor in Dyslexia

Ingvar Lundberg

INTRODUCTION

One basic assumption concerning developmental dyslexia is that the underlying deficit is <u>specific</u> to the reading task. Thus, one would expect to find reading disabled children with perfectly normal intellectual functions and linguistic abilities. Their only problem would specifically be related to the very act of reading and spelling. However, when reading disabled and normal children are compared all sorts of cognitive differences have been found indicating that dyslexic children actually suffer from quite general cognitive deficits. This is in fact a serious undermining of the assumption of specificity (Stanovich, 1986).

Numerous studies have demonstrated inferior performance among dyslexic children in a large number of linguistic and cognitive tasks including naming speed, syntax, vocabulary, and comprehension. Working memory deficits have also often been observed (Cohen. 1982; Baddeley, 1984). The reading disabled child has been characterized as an inactive learner who does not apply cognitive strategies within her/his capabilities (Torgesen. 1982). Taube (1988) has demonstrated the intricate interplay between reading disability, metacognition and self concept. Thus, the link between reading disability and global processes like the ones mentioned does not support the specificity hypotheses. However, the key to understanding reading disability may still not be found among those generalized linguistic and cognitive functions. It could even be the case that the observed general deficits are the <u>results</u> of reading disability rather than its cause. If so, it could be more profitable to look at an early stage of development where specificity might be more characteristic.

There is an emerging consensus in cognitively oriented research that the primary difficulty experienced by dyslexic children occurs at the word level rather than the text level. A beginning reader must discover that units of print map on to units of sound. This principle must be acquired if a child is to progress successfully in reading. The reason why dyslexics cannot read well is thus their poor decoding ability (see Gough & Tunmer, 1986; Snowling, 1980). Pushing the question one step further and asking why decoding is difficult leads us to phonological awareness. Let us assume that children with dyslexic disposition start school with a clearly delayed development of phonological awareness as their characteristic problem. This lack of ability entails problems in segmentation of the speech stream into units of phoneme size which prevents the child from understanding the alphabetic principle. This specific problem might then develop into more generalized deficits. Thus, the initial reading failure, based on a rather specific deficit, may be the entrance into an evil cycle of escalating learning problems of increased generality (see also Stanovich, 1986 and Taube, 1988).

The ultimate reason for lack of phonological awareness may well be biological. Richard Olson's paper at this conference indicates a genetic linkage for phonologically based word recognition problems, whereas evidence of cerebral abnormalities, or rather differences, in early fetal development has been presented by Albert Galaburda and coworkers. Here I am going to stay at the behavioral or psychological level and take a closer look at the relationship between phonological awareness and early reading acquisition to see if the hypothesis of early specificity can get empirical support. The implications of positive findings may be extremely important as far as preventive and remedial actions are concerned.

Why is segmentation of the speech stream into smaller units such a difficult task for some children? In speech, phonemic segments are merged in the sound stream through complicated rules of coarticulation (Liberman, Cooper, Shankweiler & Studdert-Kennedy, 1967). The acoustic characteristics of a phoneme are modified by the other phonemes in a word or syllable, and the cues for recognizing the phonemes in a word occur simultaneously as well as sequentially. Thus, there are no separable packets of information in the acoustic stream like the sequence of separate letters in printed words. Usually there are not even discernable pauses between successive words in speech. Phonemic cues are also altered by more global features like speech rate, stress contour, fundamental frequency, and dialectal variation (Repp & Liberman, 1984). All users of spoken language are, by a long evolution, provided with neurological mechanisms that normally function automatically to cope with the complicated processing of the phonological structure of speech. Explicit awareness of the phonemic segments, however, is a rather different thing. It is a question of abstraction and reflection which apparently does not come easy and naturally to many children.

I will here briefly review a series of investigations from our laboratory which, taken together, may clarify the relationship between phonological awareness and reading such that our conception of reading disability might be more precise and educational implications can be drawn.

Comparison of disabled and normal readers

With few exceptions the relationship between phonological awareness and reading has been studied with unselected groups of children. In one of our studies (Lundberg, 1982), however, poor readers and age- and sex-matched normal readers of equal intelligence level were compared on a metaphonological task. The poor readers were referred to clinics for reading remediation by their ordinary class-room teachers. The task was a deletion task which required explicit segmental analysis and active manipulation of the segmental representation. Thus, the child was asked to tell what was left when part of a word was subtracted (e.g. /lo/ from "melody" or /s/ from "school"). The difficulty of the task is well illustrated in the following case: An eight-year dyslexic boy reacted violently, when he was told that /dile/ had been deleted from the word "crocodile". Instead of trying to analyze the word, he answered with resentment: "You have cut off his tail!". Apparently he was not able to shift his attention from content to linguistic form. No wonder he had serious trouble learning to read.

From each of the grades 2, 3, 4, 5, and 6 we selected 10 disabled and 10 normal readers. In grade 2, the normal readers gave correct responses to 71 per cent of the items, whereas the disabled readers only solved 20 per cent correctly. In grade 3, the performance of the normal readers increased to 78 per cent. The poor readers, however, showed a dramatic improvement from grade 2 to grade 3. Now, they scored 62 per cent correct. From grade 3 on, there was a steady increase for both categories, although the difference between normal and disabled reader was significant in all grades.

Although the results are apparently suggestive, the correlational nature of the study is obvious. As we all know, correlation does not prove causality. We cannot rule out the possibility that segmentation skill is the result of reading skill rather than being a prerequisite for reading acquisition. Thus, we need to approach the relationship between phonological awareness and reading with different designs of the investigations.

Early prediction of reading disability

If it turns out that children with low phonological awareness at a prereading stage are likely to become poor readers later in school, we have come a bit closer to a causal interpretation of the relationship between phonological awareness and reading. What develops later in time can hardly be the cause of something preceding it. However, even a longitudinal study may entail problems and be open to alternative interpretations. Some unknown factor outside our control might be the common underlying cause of the observed relationship between phonological awareness and reading ability. Thus, we have to attempt to rule out the influence of such factors by including measures of, for example. general intellectual abilities and the general decentration ability to shift attention from content to form in non-linguistic tasks. Without such controls we cannot rule out the possibility that the observed correlation is spurious and reflects nothing but a common factor of cognitive maturity. Our specificity hypothesis is then, of course, impossible to test.

In our first longitudinal study (Lundberg, Olofsson & Wall, 1980) 200 children were followed from kindergarten to grade 2. A broad set of metalinguistic tests were given in kindergarten. The testing program also included non-linguistic decentration tests (visual analysis) and Raven (a non-verbal test of general cognitive ability). Reading and spelling was assessed with several measurements in grade 1 and 2. A causal model was set up and tested with path-analytic methods. Without going into details we can here report that more than half the variance (54%) of reading and spelling ability in grade 2 could be accounted for by phonological awareness in preschool, which also means that poor reading and spelling can be accurately predicted on the basis of preschool measures of phonological awareness. Thus, we have identified a specific precursor of reading disability, indicating support for the specificity hypothesis.

Related studies from our laboratory (Tornéus, 1984; Lundberg, 1985; Olofsson, 1985) have clearly demonstrated the uniqueness or specificity of the metaphonological factor. It has a low correlation to general cognitive ability and stands out as a pure factor when the various tests on phonological awareness together with a large number of other assessments are entered a factor analysis. It also meets the requirements of an underlying causal factor in reading acquisition when it is part of more comprehensive. causally formulated, LISREL-models (Tornéus, 1984; Olofsson, 1985).

The effect of training

Not even a well controlled longitudinal study can guarantee that there is no unknown factor at work which can invalidate a causal interpretation of the observed relationship between phonological awareness and reading. Testing the validity of the causal hypothesis requires an experimental approach, where phonological awareness is treated as an independent variable under active manipulation. A proper training study is thus a crucial step in our inquiry.

There are several requirements that should be met in a training study. First, adequate control groups should be included to check for general effects which have nothing to do with the hypothesis per se, such as increased motivation or confidence due to the extra attention given to a treatment group. Secondly, there should be a sharp separation between the independent variable (phonological awareness) and the dependent variable (progress in reading), i.e. the metaphonological training program should not include elements of reading instruction. If phonemic awareness is taught while the children are learning to read, it would be difficult to determine the effectiveness of the phonological awareness training. Thirdly, the outcome measure should be a measure of reading and spelling and not something related to it such as nonsense word reading. Fourthly, a check of specificity should be included in the design. Does the training affect general linguistic and cognitive abilities or is it specifically related to reading and spelling? To answer this question measures of such general abilities as well as a different school subject like mathematics should be included in the set of outcome measures.

Taken together, two of our training studies meet all the requirements mentioned. In the first study (Olofsson & Lundberg, 1983, 1985), 95 preschool children were divided into three experimental groups and two control groups. Phonological awareness was assessed at the start of the investigation. Then followed an 8-week training period for the experiment children with daily excercices and games designed to stimulate phonological awareness (puns, rhyming, comparing words, initial sound deletion, syllable segmentation, phoneme counting etc.). The three experimental groups differed in terms of the degree of structure or systematicity with wich the training program was run. To meet our first methodological requirement, one control group had a training program which was equivalent to the main program except for the fact that it only included non-linguistic sounds.

It was shown that the development of phonological awareness among nonreaders could be stimulated by systematic training. On the average, the experiment group with the most systematically implemented program outperformed all other groups on a posttest assessment of phonological awareness. We could conclude that preoccupation with letters was not of critical importance to get conscious access to the phonemic level of language. However, the long term effects of the training on later reading and spelling acquisition in school were difficult to evaluate. Great variance, ceiling effects and group heterogeneity prevented far reaching conclusions.

In our next training study to be considered here (Lundberg, Frost & Petersen, 1988) a larger number of children were included (235 in the experiment group and 155 children in the control group). The assessment program was also much broader and included functional linguistic abilities and Raven and mathematics at the school level. Furthermore, the training program in the experimental group was considerably more extensive, including daily excercices for eight months during the preschool period. Only very few children demonstrated any ability to read. Even their letter knowledge was rudimentary.

Once again we could convincingly demonstrate that phonological awareness could be successfully trained among nonreaders outside the context of formal reading instruction and without the help of letters. We could also demonstrate that the training effect was specific to the metaphonological domain. Within that domain we made distinctions among three basic factors: rhyming, syllable-word manipulation, and a phonemic factor. This model was strongly supported in a confirmatory factor analysis. The main training effect could now be localized to the phonemic factor.

Now, the long-term effects on reading and spelling in school was confirmed. The children who had enjoyed the benefit of metaphonological training in kindergarten significantly outperformed the non-trained children in reading as well as in spelling in both grade 1 and grade 2. (See Table 1).

Table 1. Reading and spelling performance for the experimental group and the control group in grade 1 and grade 2.

		Experimental group	Control group
Reading	grade 1	55.7	47.9
	grade 2	124.7	104.4
Spelling	grade 1	10.6	5.8
	grade 2	15.5	11.7

As pointed out by Bryant & Bradley (1985) it is not enough to assess literacy skills in school when evaluating the effects of a metaphonological training program. The theory concerns a specific connection between phoneme segmentation in kindergarten and later reading and spelling. Then we should not expect a relationship with other educational skills like mathematics. Thus, a mathematics test was given in school. Now, the control group actually outperformed the experimental group. This result justifies the conclusion that the pre-school training of phonological awareness is specifically related to reading and spelling.

The longitudinal design permitted a replication of the earlier prediction study. The set of predictors now included, except for a large number of metaphonological tests, tests of language comprehension, vocabulary, letter knowledge, prereading ability, Raven. A multiple regression analysis was performed with performance in grade 2 as criterion. As far as reading was concerned only two independent variables entered the equation. At the first step phonemic skills (which not included rhyming and word-syllable manipulation) yielded an R = .58. The second step included language comprehension and now R increased to .60. For spelling in grade 2 only phonemic skills entered the equation (R = .61). All remaining independent variables were insignificant. Thus, the single most powerful preschool predictor of literacy skills in school is phonemic awareness.

Phonemic awareness among dyslexic children

By now, we have obtained answers to many questions. The well established finding of a strong relationship between phonological awareness and progress in learning to read and spell has, in the light of our longitudinal studies and training studies, been interpreted as a causal relationship. We have demonstrated that phonological awareness can be developed among illiterate children without confronting them with written language. Especially vulnerable to instructional impacts are skills requiring the handling of phonemic segments. Thus, we seem to know what is learned during metalinguistic games and excercices in preschool. We have also found that the training facilitates the acquisition of reading and spelling in school. This effect is not just a general facilitation of cognitive skills but is restricted to the domain of literacy tasks. The general instructional implications of our findings are rather obvious.

However, in spite of our suggestive evidence, there are reasons to be cautious in assigning phonemic awareness a central role in dyslexia. Most of our studies of the relationship between phonological awareness and reading have not specifically investigated children who have been diagnosed as dyslexic, as distinct from generally poor readers. Thus, while difficulty with

phonemic segmentation may contribute to poor reading, it is not fully clear
that it is a causal factor in dyslexia. To strengthen the evidence on this issue
more direct data from dyslexic children should be obtained.

In the training study just reviewed (Lundberg et al., 1988), data from
219 children were available as a basis for the selection of a dyslexic subgroup
according to a conventional criterion of underachievement. The selection
variables were Raven-scores, number of correctly read words over a period of
15 minutes in grade 1 and grade 2, the number of correctly spelled words on
a word dictation test in grade 1 and in grade 2. In Lundberg (1985) a
regression technique was used to define dyslexia, where the main statistical
problems (regression effects) were avoided by repeating the whole testing
program after 6 months. The population on which the selection of dyslexics
was based was constituted of more than 700 children. Here a somewhat
simpler procedure was used, but yet with a criterion of stability. Children
were defined as dyslexics if they met the following criteria: (1) Raven-scores
within the normal range, i.e. more than one third of the children scored
lower on the test. (2) Reading scores both in grade 1 and in grade 2 below
the 20th percentile. (3) Spelling scores both in grade 1 and in grade 2 below
the 20th percentile. Out of the 219 cases, 13 children or about 6 per cent
met all these criteria. This proportion is pretty close to what was found in
Lundberg (1985).

Table 2. Phonemic awareness skills in kindergarten among 13 cases of
dyslexia.

Case	Sex	Pre-phon	Post-phon
1	boy	0	6
2	boy	0	4
3	boy	0	9
4	boy	0	12
5	boy	0	4
6	girl	0	10
7	girl	0	8
8	boy	0	0
9	girl	2	8
10	boy	0	1
11	boy	0	5
12	boy	3	3
13	boy	0	10

Let us now take a retrospective look at these 13 cases of well defined dyslexia and see what level of phonologcial awareness they had reached during the preschool year. Table 2 presents the cases with their performance on the tasks requiring phoneme manipulation (deletion of initial phoneme, phoneme segmentation, phoneme blending) in the beginning of the preschool year (Pre-phon) and at the end of the year (Post-phon).

Only 3 of the 13 cases were girls, which is in agreement with earlier findings, for example Lundberg (1985) where 8 out of 46 dyslexic children were girls. The maximum performance on the tests was 24 points. At the pretest level no dyslexic case showed any sign of being able to handle linguistic units of phoneme size. In he population the mean performance was also low and amounted only to about 2 points. The post-phon measurement was done after eight months of systematic training. Now the population mean was 10 points. Three of the dyslexic cases (case 4, 6 and 13) had reached that level, whereas the majority still had marked difficulties in handling the phonemes (in particular case 2, 5, 8, 10, 11, and 12). Thus, none of our dyslexic children demonstrated phonemic awareness at the start of the preschool year when they were about six years old. A few of them, however, seemed to benefit from the training program and started school with an average level of phonemic awareness. But still they failed in learning to read and spell. In these cases it seems difficult to hold the view that lack of phonemic awareness is the underlying cause of their dyslexia.

Our cases do not seem to suffer from any functional language problems. With the exception of case 9 all scores fell within the normal range. What we have, then, is a group of children with general cognitive functions (according to Raven) within the normal range, normal language ability but with serious problems in learning to read and spell during their first school years. Most of the children in this group had also a slow development of phonological awareness during the preschool period despite rather intense and systematic stimulation. Our earlier investigations indicated that phonological awareness is an important prerequisite for reading and spelling acquisition. A not too far fetched inference then is that lack of phonemic awareness is a critical factor in many cases of dyslexia. Thus, some tentative support for the specificity hypothesis has been presented in this paper.

REFERENCES

Baddeley, A. (1981). The concept of working memory: A view of its current state and probable future development. Cognition. **10**, 17-23.

Bradley, L. & Bryant, P. (1985). **Children's reading problems.** Basil Blackwell, Oxford.

Cohen, R.L. (1982). Individual differences in short-term memory. In **International Review of Research in Mental Retardation, vol 11.** (ed. N. Ellis). Academic Press, New York.

Gough, P. & Tunmer. W.E. (1986). Decoding, reading, and reading disability. Remedial and Special Education. **7**, Issue 1. 6-10.

Liberman, A.M., Cooper. F.S.. Shankweiler. D.. & Studdert-Kennedy. M. (1967). Perception of the speech code. Psychological Review. **74**, 431-461.

Lundberg, I. (1982).Linguistic awareness as related to dyslexia. In **Dyslexia: Neuronal, cognitive and linguistic aspects.** (ed. Y Zotterman). Pergamon Press, Oxford.

Lundberg, I. (1985). Longitudinal studies of reading and reading difficulties in Sweden. In **Reading research: Advances in theory and practice, vol 4.** (eds. G.E. MacKinnon and T.G. Waller). Academic Press, New York.

Lundberg, I., Frost, J.. & Petersen. O.-P. (1988). Effects of an extensive program for stimulating phonological awareness in preschool children. Reading Research Quarterly. **23**, (in press).

Lundberg, I., Olofsson. Å.. & Wall. S. (1980). Reading and spelling skills in the first school years predicted from phonemic awareness skills in kindergarten. Scandinavian Journal of Psychology.**21**, 159-173.

Olofsson. Å. (1985). **Phonemic awareness and learning to read. A longitudinal and quasi-experimental study.** University of Umeå. Umeå.

Olofsson, Å. & Lundberg, I. (1983). Can phonemic awareness be trained in kindergarten? Scandinavian Journal of Psychology. **24**, 35-44.

Olofsson, Å. & Lundberg, I. (1985). Evaluation of long-term effects of phonemic awareness training in kindergarten: Illustrations of some methodological problems in evaluation research. Scandinavian Journal of Psychology, **26**, 21-34.

Repp. B.H. & Liberman. A.M. (1984). Phonetic categories are flexible. Haskins Laboratories: Status Report on Speech Research. SR-77/78.

Snowling. M. J. (1981). Phonemic deficits in developmental dyslexia. Psychological Research. **43**, 219-234.

Stanovich. K.E. (1986). Matthew effects in reading: Some consequences of individual differences in the acquisition of literacy. Reading Research Quarterly. **21**, 360-407.

Taube. K. (1988). **Reading acquisition and self-concept.** University of Umeå. Umeå.

Torgesen. J.K. (1982). The learning-disabled child as an inactive learner: Educational implications. Topics in Learning and Learning Disabilities. **2**, 45-52.

Tornéus. M. (1984). Phonological awareness and reading: A chicken and egg problem? Journal of Educational Psychology. **76**, 1346-1358.

17
Deficits in Disabled Readers' Phonological and Orthographic Coding: Etiology and Remediation

Richard Olson, Barbara Wise, Frances Conners and John Rack

Theories about the processes involved in word recognition in reading have typically recognized two component skills. A phonological component is required when a new word must be "sounded out" by phonological rules or by analogy to known words. The essential characteristic of phonological coding is the mapping of sub-word orthographic units to phonology. A second component coding process is often invoked for the rapid recognition of familiar words. This process has commonly been referred to as reading words by "sight". In our theory, this second coding process in word recognition involves representing specific orthographic sequences of letters for familiar whole words. An orthographic representation is at least necessary for readers to distinguish common homophones in English (e.g., bear bare), and many theorists have argued that orthographic coding is the dominant process in skilled reading of familiar words. For our purposes, the important distinction between the two word coding processes is that orthographic coding involves a link to phonology and meaning at the whole-word-lexical level, whereas phonological coding involves a mapping between sub-word letter patterns and phonology.

We have been studying phonological and orthographic coding, along with a variety of other component reading and language processes, in disabled and normal readers. Many of our subjects have been identical and fraternal twins for behavior-genetic analyses of reading and language disorders. In this paper we will focus on the phonological and orthographic components of word recognition where some of the most interesting results have been found. We will begin with a discussion of the relations between phonological coding, orthographic coding, and word recognition. It will be shown that there is a unique deficit in phonological coding for most disabled readers that retards their progress. Then we will shift to our main focus, which is the relative influence of genetic and environmental factors on disabled readers' component reading and language skills.

*Supported by NIH grants HD 11681, HD 22223, and HD 2S07RR07013-22.

Phonological coding has been a long-time favorite of researchers looking for specific deficits in disabled readers. It was measured in the present study by having subjects read 45 one syllable and 40 two syllable nonwords aloud. Sample stimuli are presented in Table 1. The Phonological Coding variable was the first principal component of percent correct, oral latency for correct responses, and phonological accuracy ratings for errors.

Table 1

SAMPLE NONWORD STIMULI FOR THE PHONOLOGICAL CODING TASKS

45 ONE SYLLABLE NONWORDS			40 TWO SYLLABLE NONWORDS		
TER	CALCH	DOUN	TEGWOP	STALDER	FRAMBLE
ITE	SHUM	SED	POSKET	BLIDAY	SHIMPOLK
LUT	STRALE	HOAM	VOGGER	GRIBBET	VLINDERS

The second component process in word recognition, Orthographic Coding, was measured by having subjects designate the word in 80 word-pseudohomophone pairs such as the ones shown in Table 2. Note that the phonological codes for the pairs are identical, so the subjects must use their orthographic knowledge of the word to make a correct response, just as they must often do to discriminate the proper meaning for common homophones in English. The Orthographic Coding variable was based on the first principal component of percent correct and response time.

Table 2

SAMPLE WORD AND PSEUDOHOMOPHONE PAIRS FROM THE ORTHOGRAPHIC TASK
(PRESS BUTTON ON SIDE FOR WORD)

40 EASY WORDS: (ROOM RUME)   (RAIN RANE)   (SLEEP SLEAP)

40 DIFFICULT WORDS: (SAMMON SALMON)   (EXPLANE EXPLAIN)

There were several indications that Phonological Coding and Orthographic Coding are at least partially independent processes in the development of disabled readers' word recognition. The first evidence is the separate contributions of Phonological Coding and Orthographic Coding to variance in a sample of 172 disabled readers. Table 3 shows the correlations between Phonological Coding, Orthographic Coding, and performance on a Timed Word Recognition test. (This test required subjects to initiate an oral response within two seconds to be scored correct). After adjusting for age, Phonological and Orthographic Coding were both strongly correlated with Timed Word Recognition, but their correlation with each other was rather low. Hierarchical regression analyses indicated that both Phonological Coding and Orthographic Coding accounted for substantial independent variance in Timed Word Recognition.

Table 3

CORRELATIONS FOR AGE-ADJUSTED TIMED WORD RECOGNITION AND
COMPONENT WORD CODING SKILLS FOR 172 DISABLED READERS
(INDEPENDENT VARIANCE FROM HIERARCHICAL ANALYSES IN PARENTHESES)

	PHONOLOGICAL CODING	ORTHOGRAPHIC CODING
TIMED WORD RECOGNITION	.68 (30%)	.57 (18%)
PHONOLOGICAL CODING		.25

A second perspective on Phonological and Orthographic Coding showed that Phonological Coding was uniquely deficient in most disabled readers. This perspective was based on a comparison of disabled and normal readers' Coding profiles in a reading-level-match design (see Table 4). The disabled sample used for matching included nearly all of a group of disabled twins and affected siblings in the older age range. Likewise, the matched normals included nearly all the twins and siblings in their younger age range. Thus, we avoided the problem of unrepresentative samples that Jackson and Butterfield (1988) have warned us about in reading-level-match studies. The inclusion of a second word recognition measure, on which subjects were not matched, allowed us to address their concern about potential regression artifacts due to error variance in the selection measure.

Table 4

DISABLED DEVIATIONS FROM YOUNGER NORMAL SUBJECTS FOR 172 PAIRS
MATCHED ON PIAT WORD RECOGNITION

	NORMAL	DISABLED
MEAN AGE (RANGE)	10.3 (7.7-13.8)	15.6 (10.8-22.9)
PIAT GRADE/AGE GRADE	1.33 (min 1.0)	.65 (max .85)
PIAT WORD REC. GL.	6.5	6.5
TIMED WORD REC.	.0	+.10 ($p > .05$)
PHONOLOGICAL CODING	.0	-.78 ($p < .001$)
ORTHOGRAPHIC CODING	.0	+.38 ($p < .001$)

For the present analyses, reading level is a ratio defined by
the subjects' word-recognition grade-level on the PIAT national
norms, relative to their expected grade-level by age (see the second
line in Table 4). This ratio is a convenient way of expressing
reading level in samples with a wide age range. Normal subjects
selected for the reading-level-match scored at least 1.0 on the
PIAT-grade/age-grade ratio and their average was 1.33. The mean
score for all children referred from the schools for our normal
sample was 1.19 (including some children who actually met our
criteria for reading disability when they were tested in the
laboratory). This mean for the referred normal sample was very
close to the average for all children in our sampling area on a
variety of nationally normed reading tests. The disabled sample
mean was substantially lower at .65, with a maximum cut-off of .85.

Table 4 shows that having been matched on PIAT Word
Recognition, the disabled readers were not significantly different
from normal subjects on the unmatched Timed Word Recognition task.
However, the disabled readers were significantly lower in
Phonological Coding, and significantly higher in Orthographic
Coding. This pattern replicates the results of our earlier study
with groups of 50 older disabled and 47 younger normal subjects
matched on mean word recognition (Olson, 1985). The results provide
some of the strongest evidence for a Phonological Coding deficit in
most disabled readers since Maggie Snowling's initial report in
1980. It should be emphasized that there was a wide range of
Phonological Coding within our disabled sample. Some disabled
readers could read nonwords as well or even slightly better than
younger normal children at the same reading level. These subjects
would best fit the developmental lag view, but a substantial
majority of our disabled readers displayed a Phonological Coding
deficit.

The Orthographic Coding advantage for most disabled readers is
consistent with John Rack's (1985, 1986) studies showing that
disabled readers may compensate for their poor Phonological Coding
by relying more on Orthographic Coding.

Bryant and Goswami (1986) have suggested that the deficit in
Phonological Coding and related language skills implies a causal
role in reading disability. Backman, Mamen, and Ferguson (1984)
suggested the additional implication of a constitutional basis for
the phonological deficit. Of course there could be environmental
factors such as poor phonics instruction or early language
experience that caused both the deficit and associated reading
problems. Behavioral-genetic analyses can be used to address this
issue. Genetic etiology was assessed by contrasting the
similarities of identical or monozygotic (MZ) twins with those of
same-sex fraternal or dizygotic (DZ) twins. Both types of twins
share similar environments, but monozygotic twins have the same
genes while dizygotic twins share only half their genes.

The normal twins described in Table 5 must have both members of each pair reading in the normal range. Of course the disabled pairs must have at least one member who meets our criteria for reading disability. The most severely reading disabled twin is called the proband. The better twin, who may or may not be reading disabled, is called the cotwin.

Table 5

THE TWIN SAMPLE (MZ AND DZ COMBINED)

| VARIABLE | NORMAL TWINS (104 PAIRS) | DISABLED TWINS | |
| | | PROBANDS | COTWINS |
		(117 PAIRS)	
MEAN AGE (RANGE)	12.8 (7.7–20.4)	13.5 (8.4–20.2)	13.5
PIAT GRADE / AGE GRADE	1.19 (MIN .9)	.68 (MAX .9)	.87
AGE ADJUSTED PIAT REC.	.0 sd	–2.27 sd	–1.32 sd
WISC–R FULL SCALE IQ	112	99	101
WISC–R PERFORMANCE IQ	112	103	104
WISC–R VERBAL IQ	111	95	98

The third line in Table 5 presents the disabled probands' and cotwins' average reading deficit in standard deviation units from the normal twins. You can see that the cotwins of the disabled probands have regressed substantially toward the reading level of the normal twins. A comparison of identical and fraternal cotwin regression is the basis for evaluating genetic etiology.

There were significant differences in I.Q. between the normal and reading disabled twins. However, when the variables in the heritability analyses were controlled for their relation to I.Q., there was little change in the significance levels or in the heritability estimates.

Table 6 shows the mean standard–deviation scores, relative to the normal twin mean, for the identical and fraternal twin probands and cotwins. Both word recognition tests show significantly greater regression toward the normal mean for the fraternal cotwins. Under the assumption that identical and fraternal twins have an equal degree of shared environment, the smaller amount of regression toward the normal mean for the identical cotwins is presumed to be due to their identical genes.

We used a convenient regression model developed by DeFries and Fulker (1985) to analyze the statistical significance of MZ and DZ cotwin differences and to obtain heritability estimates (see

DeFries, Fulker & LaBuda, 1987, for a recent application). The
average heritabilities for the two tests of word recognition suggest
that about half of the variance in the disabled probands'
word-recognition deficits is due to genetic factors and about half
is due to environmental factors. (Remember that in these analyses
we have identified the proband as the twin with the lowest score on
the PIAT Word Recognition test. Therefore, the heritability
estimates for variables other than PIAT Word Recognition, including
the Timed Word Recognition test, are essentially estimates of the
degree to which the correlations between those variables and PIAT
Word Recognition are due to heritable influences).

Table 6

DISABLED TWINS' DEVIATIONS FROM NORMAL MEANS AND HERITABILITIES

VARIABLE	IDENTICAL MZ (64 PAIRS)		FRATERNAL DZ (53 PAIRS)		HERITABILITY
	PROBAND	COTWIN	PROBAND	COTWIN	(95% CONF.)
PIAT REC.	−2.27	−1.53	−2.26	−1.07	.40 $\pm$ .21
TIMED REC.	−1.90	−1.56	−1.86	−0.99	.61 $\pm$ .26
PHONOLOGICAL	−1.90	−1.53	−1.91	−0.65	.93 $\pm$ .39
ORTHOGRAPHIC	−1.54	−0.95	−1.34	−0.96	−.16 $\pm$ .51

    The heritability estimates for the two component coding
variables are significantly different. The very high heritability
for Phonological Coding contrasts with the nonsignificant
heritability for Orthographic Coding, and the .05 confidence
intervals for the two coding skills' heritabilities do not overlap.
This result suggests that the heritable variance in word recognition
might be associated with Phonological Coding and the nonheritable
variance with Orthographic Coding. To test this hypothesis, the
subjects' scores on the PIAT Word Recognition test were adjusted
separately for their relation to Phonological Coding and
Orthographic Coding, and the adjusted word recognition scores were
analyzed for their heritability. The results in Table 7 show that
in fact, Phonological Coding accounted for virtually all of the
heritable variance in PIAT Word Recognition, because the
heritability for PIAT Word Recognition was reduced to .01 after
adjusting for Phonological Coding. It appears that Orthographic
Coding accounted for at least part of the environmental variance,
because the heritability estimate increased from .4 to .7 for PIAT
Word Recognition adjusted by Orthographic Coding.

Table 7

DISABLED TWINS' DEVIATIONS FROM NORMAL MEANS, AND HERITABILITIES
FOR PIAT WORD RECOGNITION AFTER CONTROLLING FOR
PHONOLOGICAL OR ORTHOGRAPHIC CODING

| VARIABLE | MZ TWINS | | DZ TWINS | | HERITABILITY |
	PROBAND	COTWIN	PROBAND	COTWIN	(95% CONF.)
REC. ADJ. BY PHONOLOGICAL	−1.11	−0.60	−1.12	−0.61	.01 ± .39
REC. ADJ. BY ORTHOGRAPHIC	−1.54	−1.04	−1.67	−0.58	.70 ± .36

The lack of significant heritable variance for Orthographic
Coding suggests that the common environment shared by both MZ and DZ
pairs was most important in determining the subjects' knowledge of
the specific orthographic patterns for words. Common environmental
influences are likely to include the degree of print exposure in the
home and reading instruction in the schools. The results are
consistent with the speculation by Gough, Juel, and Griffith (1988)
that experience in reading specific words is the primary factor
influencing the development of word-level orthographic codes. Of
course one could imagine a brain injury that randomly induced a non
heritable "surface-dyslexic" syndrome in MZ and DZ twins through the
disruption of visually based orthograhic images. However, if
neurological damage was the cause of poor Orthographic Coding in our
subjects, we might expect correlated deficits in our measures of
visual-perceptual skills, but none were found. Our results are
consistent with Frank Vellutino's (1979) point that
visual-perceptual deficits are not a causal factor in reading
disablility, even for the component of word recognition that might
plausably be associated.

In contrast with Orthographic Coding, Phonological Coding
loaded on a factor that included two measures of analytic language
skills. The first measure, Rhyming Fluency, required subjects to
generate all the rhymes they could think of in one minute to the
word "eel". The second measure, Phoneme Segmentation, required
subjects to strip the initial phoneme from each of 45 words, place
the phoneme at the end of the word, and add "ay". In the
reading-level-match comparison, the disabled readers were about a
half standard deviation lower in Phoneme Segmentation than the
normal subjects, suggesting a possible causal role by Bryant and
Goswami's (1986) reasoning. Rhyming Fluency was not significantly
different for the two groups, which Bryant and Goswami suggest has
neutral implications for causality.

Heritability analyses for our two analytic language tasks are
presented in Table 8. Even though Phoneme Segmentation correlated
with Phonological Coding at r = .68 after adjusting for age, the

heritability estimate of h_g = .36 was not statistically
significant. However, the heritability estimate for Rhyming
Fluency, which was correlated with Phonological Coding at r = .37,
was statistically significant. These mixed heritability results for
the analytic language tasks do not present a clear picture. It
seems likely to us that the underlying causal factor for the
disabled readers' heritable Phonological Coding deficit is a
weakness in analytic language skills that is also heritable, but
more consistent evidence is needed to support the hypothesis.

Table 8

DISABLED TWINS' DEVIATIONS FROM THE NORMAL MEANS, AND
HERITABILITITES FOR RHYMING FLUENCY AND PHONEME SEGMENTATION

VARIABLE	MZ TWINS PROBAND COTWIN		DZ TWINS PROBAND COTWIN		HERITABILITY (95% CONF.)
RHYMING FLUENCY	−0.92	−1.22	−1.15	−0.56	1.40 ± .87
PHONEME SEGMENTATION	−1.19	−0.77	−1.32	−0.57	.36 ± .59

Our reading–level–match and behavior–genetic analyses strongly
suggest specific deficits in Phonological Coding and related
analytic language skills for the average disabled reader. But
remember that there was substantial variance in disabled readers'
Phonological Coding, with some subjects reading nonwords as well or
slightly better than the matched normal subjects. Perhaps as a
result of this variance, two recent studies with relatively small
samples have not found a significant phonological deficit (Bruck,
1988; Stanovich, Nathan, and Zolman, 1988). Stanovich et al.
suggested that their null results may have been due to many of their
subjects not meeting the usual specificity criteria such as normal
I.Q. Since our disabled subjects included in the previous analyses
varied widely in I.Q. above the minimum of 90 on either the verbal
or performance scales, we decided to compare subgroups of children
with the same mean word recognition deficit, but who were relatively
high or low in full scale I.Q.. The high I.Q. group had a mean
full scale score of 108, and was reading substantially below levels
that would be expected from their I.Q. These subjects could be
viewed as more specifically reading disabled than the lower I.Q.
group with a full scale score of 93. The disabled readers in the
two groups were then compared with their reading–level–matched
normal subjects. In both the high and low I.Q.–reading discrepancy
groups there were similar and significant Phonological Coding
deficits, as well as similar and significant Orthographic Coding
advantages for the disabled subjects. Regression analyses across
our entire sample of 250 disabled readers above 90 in verbal or
performance I.Q. confirmed that Phonological Coding was not
significantly related to the subjects' I.Q.–reading discrepancy (r =
.13, p > .01).

The above null results prompted us to examine 29 disabled readers who had been excluded from our previous analyses because they did not meet the 90 I.Q. minimum criterion. Fletcher and Morris (1986) have persuasively argued that we might obtain a better view of the nature of reading disabilities by including such subjects in our samples. Many of the disabled readers below 90 I.Q. actually read words on the PIAT as well or better than expected from their I.Q., although their reading and listening comprehension tended to be quite low. This group of subjects with an average full scale I.Q. of 85 was compared with with a group of disabled readers matched on PIAT Word Recognition whose full scale I.Q. was 100, and who were reading at a level that was lower than expected from their I.Q. The low I.Q. subjects were significantly better in Phonological Coding. We still need to generate a matched normal sample for the low I.Q. subjects, but it appears from our analyses so far that they are not likely to show a Phonological Coding deficit. Perhaps these subjects are similar to the "garden variety" poor readers discussed by Stanovich et al. (1988) who seem to fit the developmental lag model.

Environmental factors may also determine whether a Phonological Coding deficit is found in reading-level-match studies (Morrison and Coltheart, 1988). Although in our study, Phonological Coding variance shared with the probands' deficit in PIAT Word Recognition was highly heritable ($h2g = .93$), additional analyses assessing the heritability of Phonological Coding independent from PIAT Word Recognition yielded a heritability estimate that was lower ($h2g = .40$). This suggests that environmental influences such as remedial phonics instruction can make a significant difference in Phonological Coding. The intensive remedial phonics program given to Bruck's (1988) disabled readers may have eliminated their deficit in decoding nonwords.

Pessimism concerning prospects for remediation may arrise from the small amount of environmental influence found for the relation between PIAT Word Recognition and Phonological Coding in our twin sample ($h2g = .93$). Even if this unusually high heritability estimate is accurate, it does not imply that some phonologically based remedial efforts are not worthwhile. The high heritability estimate for the relation between PIAT Word Recognition and Phonological Coding is contingent on the environmental range in our sample. More powerful remedial techniques may have greater influence than this high heritability would seem to suggest. We are currently taking our best shot at strengthening disabled readers' Phonological Coding, along with word recognition and comprehension, through the use of computer-based reading and segmented speech feedback (Olson and Wise, 1987).

References

Backman, J.E., Mamen, M., & Ferguson, H.B. (1984). Reading level design: Conceptual and methodological issues in reading research. Psychol. Bull., 96, 560–568.

Bruck, M. (1988). The word recognition and spelling of dyslexic
    children. Read Res. Q., 23, 51–69.

Bryant, P.E., & Goswami, U.C. (1986). Strengths and weaknesses of
    the reading level design: A comment on Backman, Mamen, and
    Ferguson. Psychol. Bull., 100, 101–103.

DeFries, J.C., & Fulker, D.W. (1985). Multiple regression analysis
    of twin data. Behav. Genet., 15, 467–473.

DeFries, J.C., Fulker, D.W., & LaBuda, M.C. (1987). Evidence for a
    genetic aetiology in reading disability of twins. Nature, 329,
    pp. 537–539.

Fletcher, J.M., & Morris, R. (1986). Classification of disabled
    learners: Beyond exclusionary definitions. In S.J. Ceci
    (Ed.), Handbook of cognitive, social, and neuropsychological
    aspects of learning disabilities. Hillsdale, NJ: Earlbaum,
    pp. 55–80.

Gough, P.B., Juel, C., & Griffith, P. (in press). Reading,
    spelling, and the orthographic cipher. In P. Gough (Ed.),
    Reading acquisition. Hillsdale, NJ: Erlbaum.

Morrison, F.J. & Coltheart, M. (1988). Understanding reading
    disability: Conceptual and methodological strategies. Paper
    presented at the AERA meeting in New Orleans, April 6, 1988.

Olson, R.K. (1985). Disabled reading processes and cognitive
    profiles. In D. Gray and J. Kavanagh (Eds.). Biobehavioral
    Measures of Dyslexia. Parkton, MD: York Press. pp. 215–244.

Olson, R.K., Foltz, G., & Wise, B. (1986). Reading instruction and
    remediation with the aid of computer speech. Behavior Research
    Methods, Instruments, & Computers, 18, 93–99.

Olson, R.K. & Wise, B. (1987). Computer speech in reading
    instruction. In D. Reinking (Ed.), Computers and reading:
    Issues for theory and practice. New York: Teachers College
    Press. pp. 156–177.

Rack, J.P. (1985). Orthographic and phonetic coding in
    developmental dyslexia. Br. J. Psychol., 76, 325–340.

Rack, J.P. (1986). An investigation of memory coding in
    developmental dyslexia. Ph.D. Thesis, University of London.

Snowling, M.J. (1980). The development of grapheme–phoneme
    correspondence in normal and dyslexic readers. J. Exp. Child
    Psychol., 29, 294–305.

Stanovich, K.E., Nathan, R.G., & Zolman, J.E. (1988). The
    developmental lag hypothesis in reading: Longitudinal and
    matched–reading level comparisons. Child Dev., 59, 71–86.

Vellutino, F.R. (1979). Dyslexia: Theory and Research.
    Cambridge, MA: MIT Press.

IV
Memory Functions and Language

18

The Role of Phonological Memory in Normal and Disordered Language Development

Susan E. Gathercole and Alan D. Baddeley

INTRODUCTION

In recent years a major focus of research into developmental changes in short-term memory has been on the role that it plays in the acquisition of reading skills. The findings which have emerged from a wide range of studies suggest that short-term memory skills are indeed highly related to early reading achievement and that the nature of this relationship is at least partly causal and not merely correlational (e.g. Wagner and Torgeson, 1987, for review).

However, the influence of phonological memory skills in the acquisition of reading skills appears to be confined to the relatively brief period when basic sound-symbol relationships are being developed (e.g. Ellis and Large, in press). Moreover, although reading is a crucial skill for individuals to participate fully in literate cultures, print provides a secondary rather than primary linguistic representation (Shand and Klima, 1981). In the present project, we are concerned with assessing whether phonological memory skills are also important in a more central aspect of linguistic development which spans a much longer developmental period, and indeed also extends into adulthood - the acquisition of vocabulary.

The processes underlying vocabulary development are important for a number of reasons. Firstly, vocabulary knowledge is crucial to any mode of linguistic communication, spoken or written. The capacity to learn is perhaps the most important function for a developing child, and one of the things that children must learn is the vocabulary of their native language. Also, measurement of vocabulary skills are extensively used as indices of general verbal abilities, in intelligence tests. The assessment of the determinants of vocabulary development could, therefore, have far-reaching theoretical and practical consequences. Since a critical component of the vocabulary acquisition is the long-term learning of phonological information, it seemed at least plausible to us

245

that short-term phonological memory skills may play an important
role in the development of vocabulary. As yet, however, little is
known about the role of phonological memory in this aspect of
linguistic development. The present project seeks to provide some
basic data on this issue.

There is already some evidence pointing to the importance of
the articulatory loop component of working memory in the
acquisition of vocabulary. The first of these concerns a patient
PV, who acquired a very specific deficit in auditory STM following
a stroke, a deficit that subsequent investigation suggested could
be interpreted as an impairment in the phonological storage
component of the articulatory loop (Vallar and Baddeley, 1984). In
a recent study, Baddeley et al (in press) showed that PV was
completely unable to learn associations between words and nonwords
in a task analogous to that of acquiring the vocabulary of a new
language. This result suggests that the short-term phonological
storage component of the articulatory loop may be important for
long-term phonological learning. Since such learning is essential
for the acquisition of new vocabulary in children, it may be
expected that a deficit in short-term phonological storage would be
associated with retarded vocabulary development.

This hypothesis was investigated in two lines of enquiry in
the present project. In the first set of studies, the short-term
memory characteristics of a group of language-disordered children
was evaluated, using the working memory framework to guide the
exploration of memory. One of the characteristics of children with
specific language deficits is poor vocabulary, so the possibility
being investigated here was that an impairment of the phonological
short-term store plays a central role in their retarded vocabulary
development. The second line of enquiry was a longitudinal study
which assessed whether a measure of phonological memory was
effective at predicting the vocabulary development of a large group
of children entering school. In other words, this study evaluated
whether individual differences in phonological memory provided the
basis for the distribution of individual differences in vocabulary
development of a normal cohort of young children.

PHONOLOGICAL MEMORY IN LANGUAGE-DISORDERED CHILDREN

The term development language disorder is applied to children
who demonstrate impaired acquisition of language in the absence of
any global intellectual deficit, or any other known aetiology (e.g.
Bishop, 1979). The profile of deficits established for children
with this type of specific language impairment include disturbances
in phonological and articulatory aspects of speech production,
deficient oral comprehension and impaired immediate memory.

We were concerned with evaluating whether the poor vocabulary
development of language-disordered children reflects a central

deficit of the articulatory loop component of working memory. Although it is already known that language-disordered groups have impaired short-term memory abilities, the precise nature of this deficit is unclear. In terms of the most recent formulation of the working memory framework (Baddeley, 1986), the poor memory span of language-disordered children could reflect either poor central executive functioning or an impaired articulatory loop, which in turn could arise from either or both deficient phonological short-term storage or articulatory rehearsal. In our study, we attempted to examine the specific nature of the short-term memory deficit in a group of language-disordered children, by using the experimental techniques developed in the context of the working memory framework.

A group of six language-disordered children were selected for investigation in our study. The group, whose ages ranged between seven and nine years showed a pattern of poor vocabulary, reading and comprehension performance, but normal range nonverbal intelligence. The nonverbal controls were matched with the disordered children on nonverbal scores. As this control group had age-appropriate vocabulary and reading abilities, however, their scores on these tests were superior to those of the disordered group. The verbal controls were about two years younger than the language-disordered group, and had matched vocabulary and reading scores. Their nonverbal skills, though, were poorer than those of the disordered children with whom they were matched.

A range of different verbal tests were administered to the language-disordered group and the two sets of matched controls. Here our main concern is with the tests of immediate phonological memory. In two serial recall experiments, the influences of phonological similarity and syllabic length of the memory items on recall were compared across the three groups. In terms of the working memory framework, the presence of a phonological similarity effect is taken as evidence that information is being fed into the phonological store, while the presence of a word-length effect would suggest spontaneous subvocal rehearsal. So, if the language-disordered children were failing to make normal use of the phonological store, they should show a lesser similarity effect than the controls. A diminished word-length effect would indicate that they were failing to use the articulatory rehearsal process (Vallar and Baddeley, 1984).

In both of the experiments, the child's task was to reproduce the sequence of a list of spoken words by pointing to pictures in an array in the order in which they remembered them. This spatial recall method was favoured over the more conventional procedure of oral report as it circumvented the possible confounding effects of output problems of the language-disordered children. The memory lists in each condition consisted of four lists at each of five different lengths ranging from two to six items. The lists were presented in ascending length, and all lists were administered to all children. List presentation was always auditory.

In the first experiment, the memory lists were either
constructed by sampling from a set of phonologically distinct words
or from a set of phonologically similar ones. It was found that
the language-disordered children were generally poorer at recalling
memory lists than either of their matched control groups, but that
they were sensitive to phonological similarity to a comparable
degree at list lengths where performance was not restricted by
ceiling or floor effects. Table 1 illustrates this pattern of
results, showing the mean percent of distinct and similar items
recalled by each of the three groups in four-item lists. The
language-disordered children correctly recalled fewer items in both
types of list than either control group, but were nonetheless
sensitive to phonological similarity.

A similar configuration of results was obtained in the word-
length experiment. Illustrative data from this experiment are
shown in Table 1. The memory performance of the language-
disordered group was indeed lower than that of the two control
groups, but all three groups recalled fewer items in the lists of
long than short words. The magnitude of both the word length and
phonological similarity effects did not differ statistically across
the three groups.

The language-disordered group, then, have a clear short-term
memory deficit, as their memory performance was at a lower level
even than that of the younger children of matched verbal skills in
both experiments. The presence of a word length effect in the
recall of the language-disordered children, however, establishes
normal use of articulatory rehearsal in this group. Consistent
with this, other data not reported here had established that the
disordered group were no slower at articulating than the verbal
control children.

Table 1. Mean percent words correctly recalled by each
          group at list length 4 in serial recall
          experiments.

Group	Phonol. Distinct	Phonol. Similar	Short (1-syll)	Long (3-syll)
LDG *	62	35	66	40
Verbal controls	87	43	97	60
Nonverbal controls	86	54	93	68

* Language-disordered group.

Their sensitivity to phonological similarity also indicates that the phonological short-term store is functioning. The lower overall memory performance of the language-disordered group, however, indicates that this system operates less effectively for these children than for the children with normal language function. The precise form of the phonological memory deficit is as yet unclear, although some speculations about its nature are made in a later section of this paper.

One further type of phonological memory test also produced results which dramatically distinguished between the language-disordered children and the two control groups. Two experiments used a nonword repetition task, in which the child heard an unfamiliar phonological item on each trial, and was required to repeat it back immediately. Accuracy of repetition was scores. It was found that the language-disordered group were much poorer at repeating back spoken nonwords than both the verbal and nonverbal control groups. For example, in one study where 40 nonwords were presented to each child, the mean number of items correctly repeated was 21.0 for the disordered group, 31.8 for the verbal controls, and 33.6 for the nonverbal controls. This difference did not reflect perceptual deficits of the language-disordered children, as we had already established that they were no poorer at discriminating pairs of spoken items which differed by one phonetic feature than the other children. We view this pattern of results as providing further convergent evidence that our sample of language-disordered children have a deficit in phonological short-term memory.

It is interesting to note that the performance profile of the disordered group on these memory tests corresponds closely to that of the patient PV discussed earlier (Baddeley et al, in press). Once again, an association between phonological short-term memory skills and vocabulary learning has been demonstrated, such that poor phonological memory appears to be accompanied by difficulties in the long-term learning of phonological information. This association is certainly consistent with the notion that this component of memory plays an important role in vocabulary development.

The association between phonological memory skills and vocabulary learning established so far have, however, been correlational in nature. It is tempting to infer causality on this basis, but, of course, it must be acknowledged that the relationship may run either way. For example, it could be that the extent of childrens' vocabulary is a critical determinant of their phonological memory skills; as the number of works in the vocabulary increases, so may the sophistication of their phonological coding strategies. The second line of enquiry was therefore designed to evaluate the causal hypothesis that phonological memory skills play a critical role in the long-term learning of verbal information.

A further aim of this part of the research programme was to determine whether or not the relationship between memory and vocabulary acquisition also extends to populations of normal language function, or whether it only distinguishes between normal and linguistically-impaired groups.

PHONOLOGICAL MEMORY IN YOUNG CHILDREN

In this study, we were concerned with evaluating whether individual differences in phonological memory skills mediate vocabulary development in young children with no known language problems. Our choice of an appropriate methodology was guided by recent discussions about the most useful techniques of testing causal hypotheses in a developmental context (e.g. Jorm, 1983). The most powerful technique appears to be a longitudinal approach, which can provide a good estimate of which factor influences which by establishing whether one precedes the other chronologically. A longitudinal study of a large group of pre-reading four-year olds entering school was set up. Each year measures are taken of a range of their cognitive capacities, including vocabulary, reading, nonverbal skills and phonological memory. The phonological memory measure chosen here was the nonword repetition test which has provided such a good basis for distinguishing the language-disordered children from the controls in the earlier study.

One important point which should be emphasised here is that none of the children participating in the study obtained positive scores on a reading test when they entered school. This is critical, as any relationship between phonological memory performance and subsequent vocabulary scores could be mediated by reading abilities in a reading population. Specifically, as it is already known that phonological memory skills influence subsequent

Table 2. Relationships between vocabulary scores at Age 4
(corresponding Age 5 values shown in parentheses)
and other variables at the same time of testing.

Measures	Correlation Coefficient	Simple Regression (% Variance)	Stepwise Regression (% Variance)
Chronological Age	.218 (.007)	5* (0)	5* (0)
Nonverbal Intelligence	.388 (.164)	15* (3)	13* (0)
Nonword Repetition	.525 (.492)	27* (24*)	15* (21*)
Reading	- (.227)	- (5*)	- (0)

* p<.05

reading success (Mann, 1984), it could be that better readers will develop a more extensive vocabulary. Hence any relationship found between phonological memory and vocabulary could not be interpreted causally. This problem was, however, avoided here by the use of nonreaders, ruling out the possibility that reading mediates a relationship between memory and vocabulary.

So far we have collected data on the first two years of the longitudinal project, and the patterns of association which are emerging are encouraging for our hypothesis that the phonological short-term store plays a critical role in the long-term learning of verbal information. Consider firstly the correlational data; that is, the patterns of associations between scores on the different tests at the two times of testing. These are summarised in Table 2. At both ages four and five, the highest correlate of vocabulary scores was performance on the nonword repetition test, accounting for 27% of the variance at age 4, and 24% at age 5. Moreover, when the variance accounted for in the vocabulary scores by age and nonverbal intelligence is taken out in the stepwise regression, nonword repetition still accounts for a highly significant 15% of the variance at age 4, and 21% at age 5. At both ages, therefore, nonword repetition scores provide a better predictor of vocabulary scores at that time than even nonverbal intelligence.

In order to assess the causal hypothesis that phonological memory skills are the basis for subsequent vocabulary development, however, it is necessary to look at the associations between vocabulary scores at age 5 and performance on the other variables one year previously, at age 4. The results are summarised in Table 3.

Results from the simple regression show that nonword repetition scores at age 4 are indeed highly related to vocabulary scores one year later, accounting for 33% of the variance.

Table 3.   Relationships between vocabulary scores at Age 5 and scores at Age 4.

Measures	Correlation Coefficient	Simple Regression (% Variance)	Multiple Regression (% Variance)
Chronological Age	.007	0	0
Nonverbal Intelligence	.322	10*	10*
Vocabulary	.607	37*	30*
Nonword Repetition	.572	33*	8*

* p<.05

Not surprisingly, however, vocabulary scores at age 5 are most
highly related to vocabulary performance in the previous year.
This pattern of associations raises the possibility that the high
association between nonword repetition and subsequent vocabulary
scores in merely mediated by an association between repetition and
vocabulary at a particular time. This possibility, however, is
ruled out by the results of the stepwise regression shown in Table
3. Even when the variance accounted for by the previous year's
vocabulary scores is taken out, age 4 repetition scores still
account for a significant 8% of the variance in age 5 vocabulary.

The findings to emerge so far from this longitudinal study
establish a clear relationship between phonological memory and
vocabulary. Not only are nonword repetition performance and
vocabulary scores highly associated at the two times of testing,
but repetition at age 4 is a significant predictor of vocabulary
skills one year later, suggesting that phonological short-term
storage is continuing to be important in learning new words. Thus
there is good evidence that the relationship between phonological
memory and vocabulary is causal rather than merely correlational.
Furthermore, these results establish that the relationship accounts
for differences in vocabulary knowledge in individuals with normal
language function, as well as for differences between normal and
disordered language samples.

THE MAIN FINDINGS

Results from two projects designed to evaluate the
relationship between phonological memory skills and aspects of
language function in young children are reported in this paper.
The first set of studies compared the memory characteristics of a
group of children with disordered language development with groups
with normal language function. The second line of enquiry assessed
the relationship between memory and vocabulary knowledge in a large
cohort of children with no known language problems. In both cases,
a close association was found between phonological memory and
vocabulary knowledge. The evidence from the study of the language-
disordered children indicated that this group have an impairment of
the phonological short-term storage component of working memory.
Results from the longitudinal study establish that scores on a
measure of phonological memory - nonword repetition performance -
provide a good predictor of subsequent vocabulary development.
Thus taken together, our findings support the view that the
phonological memory skills tapped by nonword repetition play an
important role in this index of language development.

WHY SHOULD PHONOLOGICAL MEMORY SKILLS PLAY A ROLE IN VOCABULARY ACQUISITION?

The contention here is that phonological short-term memory may

mediate the long-term storage of phonological information that is
necessary for vocabulary development. Why should this be? Well,
the process of acquiring a new word for a child must involve, at
least in the initial stages, the phonological representation of an
unfamiliar spoken form. Indeed during the earliest stages of
language development when a child's experience of language is
restricted to speech inputs, these initial stages will involve the
immediate repetition by the child of an unfamiliar spoken
phonological form. From this perspective, it should not be too
surprising that simple nonword repetition skills provide such a
good indication of subsequent vocabulary success, as nonword
repetition is a critical aspect of the complex processes involved
in the permanent acquisition of a new vocabulary entry. And
phonological short-term storage is clearly a crucial aspect of the
task of nonword repetition; without any maintenance of the
phonological specification, how could articulation be even
attempted?

Of course, the process of vocabulary development must involve
more than just mediation by phonological short-term memory. Some
semantic encoding must accompany the successful long-term learning
of a word, and representations of information in other sensory
domains will, in many cases, also be involved. Our proposal is
simply that the phonological process will always be involved, and
so that individual differences in phonological memory skills will
necessarily have important consequences for the rate of vocabulary
development.

An implicit feature of our view is that differences between
children with varying levels of vocabulary knowledge are
quantitative rather than qualitative in nature. Two specific lines
of evidence support this notion. Firstly, the relationship between
phonological memory skills and vocabulary development embraces both
individual variation with a population of children with normal
language function, and the group differences observed between
language-disordered children and their controls. Secondly, a
detailed analysis of the nonword repetition data has revealed that
both controls and language-disordered children are similarly
affected by changes in the phonological complexity of the nonwords.
Correspondingly, if the cohort in the longitudinal study is divided
into those with high vocabulary scores and those with low ones,
each group shows the same sensitivity to phonological complexity.
On this basis, it seems likely that phonological memory skills,
like vocabulary skills, can indeed be usefully conceptualised as a
continuum.

The precise nature of the variation in phonological memory
skills has still to be established, and on this point we can at the
moment only speculate. There are a number of possibilities. The
process of phonologically encoding acoustic events may vary in the
degree of noise and hence the discriminability of phonological
specifications at retrieval. Alternatively, the storage capacity

of the phonological store may differ across individuals.
Consequences of this could be either that a variable number of
items can be maintained, or that the degree of richness and
redundancy of the phonological representations is open to
variation. Or else, these phonological traces may decay at
different rates. A priority for future research is to develop
techniques which are appropriate for distinguishing between these
different hypotheses.

So far, we have not considered the mechanism by which a short-
term phonological representation becomes an attribute of a stable
conceptual representation. In fact how this process might arise is
unconstrained by the working memory framework which we have used to
guide the current research programme, as this does not specify the
processes involved in long-term learning. To do this, we would
have to look to other current formulations of learning.
Speculatively, one fruitful approach could be provided by recent
connectionist models which suggest the value of assuming
associative strengths of different weights between units. In
particular, Hinton and Plaut (in press) have distinguished between
fast weights that are easily built up but which dissipate rapidly,
and slower, much less labile weights. In such a system, an
impaired capacity to set up and maintain fast weights would lead to
retarded slow weight development, providing that the fast weight
deficit stems from a limitation in the network that underlies the
operation of both types of weights. Implementations which yield
such a network limitation may be valuable in providing insights
into the potential nature of phonological memory deficits.

SUMMARY

The present work establishes that phonological memory skills
do play a role in an important but little-understood aspect of
language development - the acquisition of vocabulary. Our
interpretation is that the dependence of vocabulary development on
these memory skills reflects the mediation of short-term
phonological storage in the process of long-term learning of new
words. It remains to be seen whether this relationship will
continue to hold for older children and adults. However, even if
the contribution of phonological memory in vocabulary development
is increasingly overshadowed by other factors such as general
intelligence and richness of linguistic background, the present
findings establish that during pre-school and early school years,
at least, these memory skills are crucially important in this
central aspect of language function.

REFERENCES

Baddeley, A.D. (1986). Working Memory. Oxford University Press,
Oxford.

Baddeley, A.D., Papagno, C. and Vallar, G. (in press). When Long-Term Learning Depends on Short-Term Storage. J. Mem. & Lang..

Bishop, D. (1979). Comprehension in Developmental Language Disorders. Dev. Med. & Ch. Neur., 21, 225-238.

Ellis, N. and Large, B. (in press). The Early Stages of Reading: A Longitudinal Study. App. Cog. Psychol..

Hinton, G.E. and Plaut, D.C. (in press). Using Fast Weights to Deblur Old Memories. In Proceedings of the Ninth Annual Conference of the Cognitive Science Society, Seattle, Washington, 1987.

Jorm, A.F. (1983). Specific Reading Retardation and Working Memory: A Review. Br. J. Psychol., 74, 462-464.

Mann, V.A. (1984). Longitudinal Prediction and Prevention of Early Reading Difficulty. Ann. of Dyslexia, 34, 117-136.

Shand, M.A. and Klima, E.S. (1981). Nonauditory Suffix Effects in Cogenitally Deaf Signers of American Sign Language. J. Exp. Psychol.: H.L. and M., 7, 464-474.

Vallar, G. and Baddeley, A.D. (1984). Fractionation of Working Memory: Neuropsychological Evidence for a Short-Term Store. J.V.L.V.B., 23, 151-161.

Wagner, R.K. and Torgeson, J.K. (1987). The Nature of Phonological Processing and its Causal Role in the Acquisition of Reading Skills. Psy. Bull., 101, 192-212.

19
Orthographic Structure, the Graphemic Buffer and the Spelling Process

Alfonso Caramazza and Gabriele Miceli

The notion of representation plays a fundamental role in information processing theories of the functioning of the brain. Theories of this type attempt to characterize cognitive abilities in terms of the sorts of representations that are computed in the course of intelligent behavior (e.g., reading). The flow of information through the cognitive system may be represented as $I \longrightarrow R1 \longrightarrow R2 \longrightarrow R3 \ldots \longrightarrow Rn \longrightarrow O$, where I and O stand for input and output, respectively, R stands for representation, and '$\longrightarrow$' stands for some type of process that transforms Ri into Ri+1 (or, alternatively, computes Ri+1 from Ri). The core claim in this theoretical framework is that a cognitive process may be thought of as a set of operations carried out over different types of representations. Nontrivial theoretical claims in this framework require that we specify in some detail the structure of the hypothesized representations and the nature of the operations that are applied to these representations in the course of processing.

The task of developing reasonably well–articulated theories of cognitive processing has proven to be very difficult. Most information processing models of cognitive tasks go no further than the mere identification of the several levels of representation suggested by a "common sense" analysis of those tasks. This is no less (nor more) true for models of spelling than it is for models of other cognitive processes. Thus, models of spelling typically, though not always, assume a cognitive architecture roughly as that shown in Figure 1, but do not provide any more information about the nature of the hypothesized processes and representations than that which is suggested by the flow diagram itself. For example, there is no more detailed theory about the structure of the orthographic lexicon than the nominal fact that the information processed at that level of the system consists of orthographic representations.

The research reported here was supported by grants from NIH (NS 22202) and the Seaver Institute to the first author. This support is gratefully acknowledged. The ideas concerning orthographic representation presented here were stimulated by L.B.'s beautifully systematic performance and by discussions with members of the Cognitive Neuropsychology Laboratory, especially Bill Badecker, Caroline Carrithers, and Mike McCloskey. Andrew Olson and Jean–Roger Vergnaud explained to us some of the intricacies of computers and phonological theory, respectively. We are indebted to all of them.

Still, if a measure of a model's adequacy were the success it has when used as the basis for making sense of the various forms of cognitive disorders that result from brain–damage, then the model of spelling schematically depicted in Figure 1 should be considered a reasonable first approximation of the cognitive mechanisms involved in spelling. This model provides an adequate explanatory framework for the various types of acquired dysgraphias, so long as we restrict attention to relatively general features of patients' performance—e.g., presence or not of semantic errors (writing 'chair' in response to the stimulus /teybl̩/), whether or not spelling errors consist principally of phonologically plausible responses (writing 'taybel' in response to the stimulus /teybl̩/), and so forth. The various patterns of dissociation and association of symptoms in dysgraphic patients can adequately be explained as resulting from damage to one or more of the components of processing that comprise the proposed model of spelling. For example, patients have been described whose performance can be explained as reflecting selective damage to the orthographic output lexicon, the phoneme–to–grapheme conversion component, the semantic component, the allographic conversion component, the phonological buffer, or the graphemic buffer.

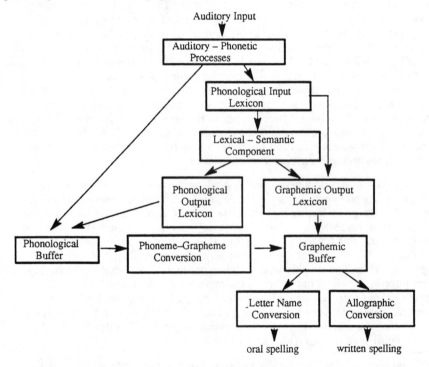

Figure 1: Schematic diagram of the spelling process

Although the model's success in accounting for relatively gross features of dysgraphic disorders constitutes strong support for the overall architecture of the model, it remains woefully underspecified, especially with regard to the processing structure of its component parts. Whatever the reason for this situation, it is not for lack of relevant empirical observations. Indeed, as we hope to show for at least one component of the spelling system, the detailed analysis of dysgraphic patients' performance allows us to articulate considerably stronger claims about the structure of orthographic representations than are made by current information processing models of the spelling process.

In this paper we will address two interrelated issues. First, we will briefly review recent research which shows that the graphemic buffer may be damaged selectively. Second, we will show that a detailed consideration of the spelling errors produced by a patient with apparently selective damage to the graphemic buffer reveals important properties of the lexical–orthographic representations that are temporarily held in the graphemic buffer.

THE GRAPHEMIC BUFFER AND ITS SELECTIVE IMPAIRMENT

The motivation for proposing the existence of a buffer in an information processing system is relatively straightforward: storage in a temporary memory is postulated at that point in the flow of information where a representation contains sub–units that must be processed sequentially (or, alternatively, where a set of independent representations must be processed simultaneously). In the spelling process a graphemic buffer is postulated because the graphemic representations activated in the orthographic lexicon as well those computed by the phoneme/grapheme conversion component consist of sets of graphemes (abstract letter representations) which must be processed sequentially for conversion into specific visuo–spatial patterns for written spelling, or into letter names for oral spelling. The graphemic buffer occupies a central position in the spelling process (see Figure 1): it mediates between the processes that compute graphemic representations (the orthographic lexicon and the phoneme/grapheme conversion component) and more peripheral output processes (letter name and allographic conversion component). Selective damage to the graphemic buffer should have widespread but clearly identifiable consequences for spelling.

The strategic location of the graphemic buffer in the spelling process and the fact that the buffer stores graphemic representations severely constrain the type of errors that may be expected to result from damage to this component of the spelling system. Damage to the graphemic buffer should result in the following pattern of performance: 1) there should be errors in all spelling tasks, independently of modality of input (e.g., spelling–to–dictation vs. written naming) or modality of output (written vs. oral spelling); 2) spelling performance should not be affected by lexical factors (e.g., grammatical class, word frequency, etc.) or lexicality (familiar vs. unfamiliar words/nonwords) since the damage is at a point beyond which these factors play a role in processing; 3) errors should only reflect properties of the representation that is affected by the damage: graphemic structure; 4) errors should be qualitatively (and quantitatively?) similar for familiar and unfamiliar words; and, finally, 5) there should be a marked effect of word length on performance—longer words being more difficult to spell than shorter words.

This richly articulated pattern of performance was first clearly documented by Caramazza et al. (1987; but, see also Hillis & Caramazza, in press; Miceli et al.,

1985; Posteraro et al., in press). Their patient L.B. made spelling errors in all
tasks, independently of modality of input or output; his errors were exclusively
transparent deformations of the graphemic structure of the stimulus and were
unaffected by lexical factors; he showed a healthy word length effect, being able to
spell correctly all two–letter stimuli but only 30% of 8/9–letter words; and, the
pattern of errors for word and nonword stimuli (operationally standing in for
unfamiliar words) was essentially identical. To better appreciate the strength of the
results, it may be useful to present some of them here.

    L.B.'s errors consisted almost entirely of letter substitutions (svolta ->
svonta), additions (taglio -> tatglio), deletions (nostro -> nosro), and transpositions
(stadio -> sdatio). This fact is in itself already quite important since dysgraphic
errors may take distinctly different forms: some patients make semantic or other
lexical errors, some make phonological errors, while others make various
combinations of these error types. In other words, the exclusively orthographic
nature of the error types in L.B.'s performance indicates that the locus of
impairment in the spelling system is at a level where graphemic structure is
represented. An equally striking feature of L.B.'s performance is the distribution of
error types for words and nonwords: the proportion of substitution, deletion,
addition, and transposition errors were identical for words and nonwords (see
Figure 2). The distribution of errors as a function of relative position of letters in
words and nonwords was also identical for the two types of stimuli (see Figure 3).

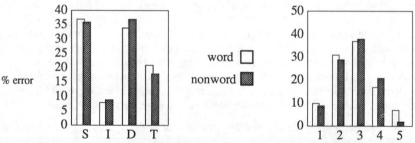

Figure 2: Distribution of substitution (S),
insertion (I), deletion (D), and transposition (T) errors for words and nonwords.

Figure 3: Distribution of errors for
words and nonwords as a function
of relative position in letter string.

    These results, showing that the representation type affected by the damage is
graphemic in nature and that familiar and unfamiliar words are affected identically
by the damage, together with the other results showing a marked length effect and
impaired performance independently of modality of input or output, strongly invite
the conclusion that L.B. has a selective "functional lesion" to the graphemic buffer.
Since L.B.'s spelling performance is explicable by hypothesizing a specific
transformation of (functional lesion to) the proposed model of spelling, we may
take the reported results as support for this model. We are reinforced in this
conclusion by the observation that the model of spelling proposed here can also
account for other well–documented patterns of dysgraphia by assuming damage to
other parts of the system. In other words, our confidence in the "correctness" (or
usefulness) of a model does not depend only on whether it can serve to explain a

specific form of impairment but, crucially, on whether it can account for the diverse patterns of deficits found in different patients.

Still, if we want the component processes that comprise the model of spelling proposed here to be more than the maligned "black boxes" of the critics of the information processing paradigm, we will have to articulate in greater detail the nature of the processes and representations that characterize the components of the system. We can be helped in this difficult task by attempting to explain not only relatively general features of patients' performance, but also increasingly finer details of their performance. In this latter task, we will have no choice but to articulate ever more detailed hypotheses about the nature of cognitive representations and the processes that support them. An example of such a development is provided by our effort to explain certain features of the spelling performance of patients with putative damage to the graphemic buffer.

THE STRUCTURE OF GRAPHEMIC REPRESENTATIONS

Let us suppose that the analysis presented for L.B. is correct; that is, let us suppose that he has suffered selective damage to the graphemic buffer. On this hypothesis, we may take the distribution of spelling errors produced by L.B. to reflect properties of (only?) the abstract letter sequences that are temporarily held in the graphemic buffer. Consequently, if we can explain the distribution of spelling errors produced by L.B. by appeal to damage–induced perturbations of hypothesized structural properties of graphemic representations, we will have provided empirical support for the hypothesized structural properties; that is, we will have provided empirical support for some hypothesis about the nature of the graphemic representations computed in the course of spelling.

Recall that L.B.'s spelling errors could be exhaustively described in terms of letter substitutions, deletions, additions, and transpositions—an error classification scheme that only appeals to orthographic features of words. Furthermore, since the distribution of these errors was only affected by the "orthographic" parameter of word length and by the relative position of letters in words, we may conclude that the representation affected by the deficit concerns an ordered set of abstract letter representations.

If graphemic representations were assumed to specify only the identity and the order of letters that comprise a word, then the only variation in the distribution of errors resulting from damage to graphemic representations should concern these two parameters—letter identity and order. That is, damage to the graphemic representation should result either in the loss of letter identity or order information, or both. On this view, and without additional constraints, we would predict that damage to the graphemic representation should result in errors such as those we have reported for L.B.—letter substitutions, deletions, additions, and transpositions. Furthermore, on this impoverished view of graphemic representations we would also expect, for example, that errors should just as likely result in the substitution of consonants for vowels or vowels for consonants as to result in the substitution of vowels for vowels or consonants for consonants. Thus, we should not only find errors such as 'tavolo' (table) —> 'tasolo' or 'tavelo' but also errors such as 'tavolo'—> 'tavslo' or 'taeolo'. This expectation is based on the fact that the conception of graphemic representation developed to this point fails to distinguish between consonants and vowels—the only information specified is individual letter identities and their order. However, as it turns out, L.B. (but also other patients with putative damage to the graphemic buffer) appears not to substitute consonants for vowels or vowels for consonants. In fact, upon close scrutiny his performance reveals a rich set of orthographic constraints on the distribution of spelling errors.

In the course of preparing an earlier report of L.B.'s spelling impairment (Caramazza, et al., 1987), we had noted several apparently inexplicable features in his performance. The most obvious was a remarkable consistency in substitution errors: consonants were substituted for consonants and vowels were substituted for vowels. Other features discordant with our simple view about the structure of graphemic representations were the fact that transposition errors appeared to involve exclusively either consonants or vowels (e.g., 'tavolo' —> 'talovo') and that there appeared to be disproportionately fewer errors on double–consonant (geminate) words (e.g., canna (cane)) than words of the same length but without double letters (e.g., canta (sing)). None of these features in L.B.'s performance was consistent with the view that the representations held in the graphemic buffer specified only letter identities and their order. We decided to explore this issue in greater detail.

To obtain a reliable corpus of errors we asked L.B. to spell several thousand words (>4000) over a period of several months. Here we will focus on just a few aspects of the results, enough to motivate the claim that graphemic representations share many structural properties with phonological representations (a detailed discussion of the results is available in Caramazza & Miceli, in preparation). Specifically, our data strongly suggest that graphemic representations, just like phonological representations (see for example, Clements & Keyser, 1983), should be considered as linked, tiered structures: one tier each for abstract letter identities or graphemes, consonant/vowel (CV) structure, and ortho–syllabic structure, respectively.

THE CV LEVEL OF REPRESENTATION.

There are several aspects of L.B.'s performance which would remain inexplicable unless we assume that graphemic representations specify an autonomous level for CV structure.

1. **Substitution errors**. One important source of evidence concerns the distribution of substitution errors. L.B. made 643 substitutions, 276 involving vowels and 367 involving consonants. Essentially all substitutions respected CV structure—in 640 of the 643 errors (99.5%), consonants were substituted for consonants and vowels for vowels. To explain this pattern of performance we must assume that L.B. had access to information about CV structure even when information about a specific abstract letter identity was unavailable. With this assumption, we would then be able to explain substitution errors as 'repairs' of representations in which the CV tier correctly specifies the CV structure, but the letter identity tier fails to specify one or more of the graphemes in the

representation. Thus, for example, if the damaged representation of 'tavolo' failed to specify the identity of the third letter but correctly specified that it is a consonant, subsequent components of processing (letter name or allographic conversion) could use the CV level information to produce a consonant: the 'repair' is constrained by CV level information.[Φ] A schematic representation of this process is shown in Figure 4. Were we not to assume an autonomous CV level of representation, the striking regularity in L.B.'s substitution errors would remain unexplained.

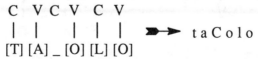

Figure 4. In this figure the substitution of a consonant, C, in the third letter position is driven by information at the CV tier.

2. Transposition errors.

Another aspect of L.B.'s performance which strongly argues for a multidimensional graphemic structure that includes a CV level of representation is the distribution of transposition errors. These errors also appear to be influenced by CV structure. Restricting attention, for the moment, to the subset of stimuli with regularly alternating CV structure (e.g., tavolo, cugino (cousin), etc., but not sedia (chair)), L.B. made 75 transposition errors in spelling these words. All the errors involved exchanging consonants for consonants (e.g., denaro—>derano) or vowels for vowels (e.g., decine—>dicene). As in the case of letter substitutions, this constraint on the distribution of errors can only be explained by assuming that CV structure is specified autonomously. With this assumption, if the letter identity level failed to specify correctly the order of some letters, the 'repair' resulting from subsequent processes would have available the CV structure information to order the letter identities. Thus, for example, if the graphemic representation for the word 'tavolo' were damaged so that the letter identities [T], [V], [L], [A], [O], and [O] were correctly specified, but the only order information available was that the first two positions were occupied by [T] and [A], then the possible 'repairs' that could result given information about CV structure are the correct response 'tavolo' and the transposition error 'talovo'.

3. Double–letter word errors.

There is approximately a 20% difference between L.B.'s spelling accuracy for double–letter words (78%; 114/146) and non double–letter words (57%; 579/1024). To explain this difference in spelling accuracy, as well as qualitative features of spelling errors for double–letter words, we may have to assume that CV structure is represented autonomously in the graphemic representation.

[Φ] Note that by 'repair' we simply mean the default computation that is possible given an under-specified representation. In the present case, if the letter identity information at one position in a graphemic string is, for whatever reason, not available, but the CV information is available, then the latter information will be used to compute a representation at the next level of processing. In this case, however, since the only information available concerns CV status, the letter that is produced may be any consonant for the consonant feature and any vowel for the vowel feature.

With respect to the quantitative difference in performance, a possible explanation is that letter identity information for double letters is specified only once. Letter doubling would then be represented by associating the single letter identity with two positions at the CV level. In this representational format there are fewer letter identities represented for double–letter words than comparable non double–letter words; for example, the respective representations for stella and stanco are:

As is apparent, the representation for stella specifies only 5 letter identities ([S], [T], [E], [L], and [A]), whereas stanco specifies 6 letter identities ([S], [T], [A], [N], [C], and [O]). And, since L.B.'s performance is strongly influenced by the parameter of word length, we may attribute the discrepancy in levels of spelling accuracy for the two types of words to the number of letter identities that are specified in their respective graphemic representations—5 vs. 6 graphemes. If, however, we are going to explain the discrepancy in performance for these two types of stimuli by appealing to differences in the size of their corresponding abstract letter representations in the buffer, we will then have to assume that the doubling of the letter is indicated by specifying two CV units or timing slots at the CV level—that is, we would be committed to the hypothesis that graphemic representations contain an autonomous CV level.

Qualitative aspects of error performance with double–letter words also generally support the proposed representational format. Although not exceptionless, transposition errors involving double letters behaved just like transposition errors with single letter exchanges; that is, consonants were exchanged with consonants. For example, we found errors such as crollo (crumble)—>clorro and scappa (run away)—>sacca. This type of error suggests that information about letter identities has been damaged independently of information about the CV structure of the word, which for this patient appears to be relatively spared. Consistent with this interpretation is the fact that in this corpus of errors we did not find errors such as crollo —> crrolo, where the letter identities remain in their relative word position and the doubling occurs at some other part of the word. The occurrence of this latter type of error would have required, contrary to what seems to be the case for L.B., that information about the CV structure of the word was damaged while information about letter identities and their order was spared.

THE ORTHO–SYLLABIC LEVEL OF REPRESENTATION.

The results I very briefly reviewed in this last section focused on features of L.B.'s performance which show that separate CV and letter identity tiers are needed in order to account for some aspects of the distribution of errors in his spelling performance. Other aspects of L.B.'s performance, as we will see below, show that a theory of graphemic representation that specifies only CV and letter identity tiers leaves unexplained a substantial part of his performance. A further level of representation—the ortho–syllabic tier, which specifies the syllabic organization of the graphemes that comprise a word—must be added to the graphemic representation in order to account for these other aspects of L.B.'s performance. Several aspects of L.B.'s performance are relevant to this issue. Here we discuss just one source of evidence for the hypothesis (see Caramazza & Miceli, in preparation, for detailed description).

The distribution of errors as a function of the orthographic structure of words. L.B. was asked to spell two sets of 6–letter words: one set consisted of regularly alternating CV sequences (e.g., tavolo), "regular CV" for short, and the other set consisted of various other orderings of CV sequences (e.g., intero, stanco, nostro, onesto, and so forth), "nonregular CV" for short. On the assumption that a graphemic buffer deficit results in the underspecification of graphemic representations, in our patient affecting primarily but not exclusively the letter identity tier, and on the further assumption that the only structure specified at the graphemic level is CV and letter identity information, we would expect spelling performance to be unaffected by the syllabic structure of a word. That is, we would not expect the syllabic structure of a word, whether it is "regular" or "nonregular", to affect either the overall level of spelling accuracy or the distribution of error types. For both types of CV strings, the 'repair' of underspecified letter identity information would proceed under the control of the CV tier information leading, where this information is available, to the replacement of consonants for consonants and vowels for vowels for both the "regular CV" and "nonregular CV" strings. Our results disconfirm this overly simple hypothesis.

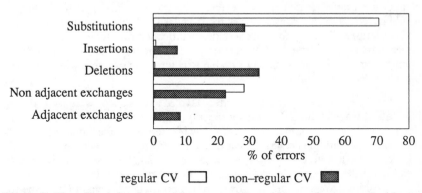

Figure 5: The effect of orthographic structure on writing performance: Incidence of various error types in incorrect responses to regular and non–regular CV stimuli.

The overall levels of accuracy for "regular CV" and "nonregular CV" words were significantly different—73% (1300/1777) and 57% (579/1024), respectively. This large difference in accuracy levels is accompanied by an even more striking difference in terms of the distribution of error types associated with the two orthographic structures. The only errors made for the "regular CV" words consisted of letter substitutions and (non–adjacent) exchanges (e.g., 'tavolo'—>

'talovo'); there were (almost) no deletion, insertion, or (adjacent) exchange errors (for "regular CV" words the latter type of error would have required exchanging a consonant for a vowel as in, for example, 'tavolo' —> 'taovlo', violating CV structure information specified at the CV tier level). In marked contrast, "nonregular CV" words in addition to substitution and (non–adjacent) exchange errors also led to insertion, deletion and (adjacent) exchange errors. These results are summarized in Figure 5, where it may be seen that the two distributions of errors are markedly different. What can account for these striking differences in error distributions?

As already noted, a two–tier hypothesis of the structure of graphemic representations cannot account for the reported results. To account for our results we must assume, at the very least, that graphemic representations specify syllabic boundaries in addition to CV and letter identity information. We can schematize the structure of graphemic representations as follows, where σ stands for syllable (for a similar proposal see Badecker, 1988): Φ

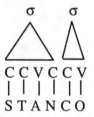

Damage to this type of representation, when it principally affects the letter identity level but also, though less severely, the CV and ortho–syllabic levels, would have less drastic consequences for "regular CV" structures than "nonregular CV" structures.§ That is, given local underspecification of a representation, it is easier to reconstruct "regular CV" sequences than "nonregular CV" sequences if graphemic representations specify syllabic structure. An example will help clarify this claim.

Suppose that the representations for 'tavolo' and 'stanco' were to be damaged in identical ways at the CV and letter identity levels, as schematically shown in Figure 6. In the case of the "regular CV" word, 'repair' of the damaged representation with the constraint that it respect information specified at the syllabic level can only lead to a "regular CV" structure. This is because the only default location for the obligatory vowel demanded by information at the syllabic tier is the fourth position. With the default vowel in this position, the default CV value for

---

ΦVarious hypotheses about the structure of the syllabic tier may be entertained. Depending on how richly structured we make the ortho–syllabic tier, we may find that the CV tier becomes totally redundant. In this latter case, the level of representation we have called the CV tier could instead correspond to a timing tier that specifies only a series of locations. Unfortunately, space limitations prevent us from considering alternative formulations in this chapter. (see Caramazza & Miceli, in preparation, for a more detailed discussion).

§This expectation need not go through for severely damaged representations where there may be insufficient structure for default decisions in the course of 'repairs'.

the third position is a consonant, leading to a "regular CV" sequence. By contrast, the damaged "nonregular CV" sequence allows different default solutions in 'repair'. A default vowel may be placed either in the third or fourth position, allowing 'repair' solutions that violate the original CV structure; another 'repair' solution available for this graphemic string is to leave the non–vowel position blank—that is, produce a consonant deletion error. In other words, there are major differences between "regular CV" and "nonregular CV" words in terms of the types of 'repair' solutions that are possible when defaults are driven by ortho–syllabic information—syllabic level information helps recover more of the "regular CV" structure than "nonregular CV" structure.

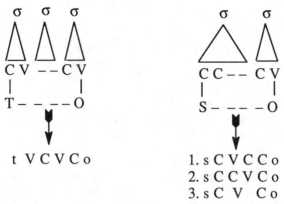

Figure 6. This Figure shows the default solutions obtained for equally impaired "regular CV" and "nonregular CV" words when defaults are driven by syllabic structure.

Consider along these lines the case of deletion errors in L.B.'s spelling performance. Why are there no deletion errors for "regular CV" words? And, when deletion errors occur for "nonregular CV" words, what gets deleted?

Vowel deletions may only occur when letter identity information about a vowel is unavailable and 'repair' fails to insert a vowel in the appropriate location. For "regular CV" sequences, a "repair" failure to insert a vowel can only occur when vowel information is damaged at the letter identity and CV tiers <u>and</u> syllable information is missing. This entails that vowel deletion errors for this type of word can only occur in the context of deletion of a whole syllable. Indeed, the only deletion error produced by L.B. involved the deletion of a whole syllable (cugino —> gino). If vowels are not deleted in "regular CV" words, a consonant will be introduced by default in non word–initial positions. Since there were essentially no errors in word initial position, there were no opportunities for L.B. to make consonant deletion errors either.

The situation is quite different for "nonregular CV" words. L.B. produced a large number of deletion errors (see Figure 4). However, by the hypothesis developed above, these deletions should not involve vowels <u>when they are the only vowel in a syllable</u>. The data strongly confirm the hypothesis. As predicted, of the 141 deletion errors the great majority were consonant deletions (91%; 128/141).

Of the 13 vowel deletion errors, only one (stagno —> stgno) violates the vowel insertion default solution predicted by the hypothesis. The remaining vowel deletion errors involved two–vowel contexts (e.g., compie —> compe; giugno —> gugno) where deletion of one of the two vowels is a permissible default in the 'repair' process. That is, our hypothesis allows us to provide a motivated account for 140 of the 141 deletion errors produced by L.B. in spelling 6–letter words! The hypothesis that there is an ortho–syllabic tier in the graphemic representation is strongly supported by the results we have briefly reviewed.

CONCLUSIONS

When results are very clear, conclusions may be brief.

It has been shown in a series of empirical reports on the structure of certain dysgraphic disorders that a plausible model of the spelling process will have to include a working memory component or buffer which temporarily stores graphemic representations. The further detailed analysis of the spelling performance of patients with selective damage to the graphemic buffer has allowed us to constrain, in highly specific and important ways, claims about the structure of graphemic representations—graphemic representations are highly structured, specifying not only an ordered set of abstract letter identities, but also CV and syllabic structure. This theory of the structure of the orthographic representations that are computed in the course of spelling is a natural extension of the proposed cognitive architecture of the spelling process. Therefore, we may interpret our success in providing a motivated explanation of the fine details of L.B.'s dysgraphic performance as providing the strongest support yet for the functional architecture of the spelling process schematically represented in Figure 1.

REFERENCES

Badecker, W., (1988). Representational properties common to phonological and orthographic output systems. Unpublished manuscript.

Caramazza, A., and Miceli, G. (in preparation). The structure of orthographic representation.

Caramazza, A., Miceli, G., Villa, G. and Romani, C. (1987). The role of the graphemic buffer in spelling: Evidence from a case of acquired dysgraphia. Cognition, 26, 59–85.

Clements, G. and Keyser, S. (1983). CV Phonology: A Generative Theory of the Syllable. MIT Press, Cambridge.

Hillis, A. and Caramazza, A. (in press). The graphemic buffer and mechanisms of unilateral spatial neglect. Brain and Language.

Miceli, G., Silveri, M.C. and Caramazza, A. (1985). Cognitive analysis of a case of pure dysgraphia. Brain and Language, 25, 187–212.

Posteraro, L., Zinelli, P. and Mazzucchi, A. (in press). Selective impairment of the graphemic buffer in acquired dysgraphia: A case study. Brain and Language.

20
Grammatical Capacity and Developmental Dyslexia: Issues for Research

Mary-Louise Kean

INTRODUCTION

The capacity to read and write competently involves the interaction of two distinct cognitive systems, one directed to the processing and representation of visual information and the other addressed to the processing and representation of language, typically language realized in the vocal-auditory mode. In the average child these capacities develop spontaneously as the child interacts with his or her environment. The child of five or six is an essentially mature analyzer of visual experience; at the same age, the child is a very competent, though still not fully mature, language user, capable of producing and comprehending novel utterances of considerable grammatical complexity and subtlety. It is at this same approximate age that the child is viewed as ready to embark on the course to fluent mastery of the written language. Given the child's level of linguistic and visual competence, it might be presumed that reading and writing skills would be relatively easy to acquire: after all, the written language is just another type of representation of something the child already knows, his or her native language. But mastery of the written language typically requires work and a level of explicit effort which is not required for normal language acquisition or visual maturation. Most children, of course, succeed admirably and unexceptionally at the task of developing a command of written language; however, for some otherwise average and motivated children the task requires Herculean efforts, and for yet others the written language is a Sisyphean boulder.

A written language is a cultural creation. We may view societies without a written language as "primitive", but we do not view the members of such societies as functionally deviant members of the species just because they have no written language. While the emergence of a written language is a function of socio-cultural phenomena, we do presume that the capacity to develop some orthography is well within the grasp of the members of any society.

269

That is, having a written language is not necessary for normal
human beings in the sense that having a native vocal-auditory or
sign language is, but an intrinsic ability to create and master a
written language is taken to be an ability characteristic of
typical human beings.

There are a host of cognitive abilities which are easily within
the grasp of average people - tapping in time to music and singing
tunes on key, learning mathematics, reading and following maps,
etc. -and for each of these abilities, as with the ability to
master a written language, there are individuals who depart from
the norm, some who are strikingly gifted in one area or another and
some who, by the same token, are surprisingly inept. Understanding
of such variations in abilities is of critical importance to the
development of explanations for both their typical realization in
people and, more generally, the range of individual differences
which are characteristic of the normal population. Within this
context, the study of individuals whose capacity to gain competence
over the written language is selectively circumscribed is just one
facet of a more general issue for research.

An average individual's ability to command the written language
may be compromised for a host of reasons. In adults, who were
previously literate, a brain lesion may lead to striking
impairments in reading and writing skills (Coltheart, Patterson,
and Marshall, 1980; Patterson, Marshall, and Coltheart, 1985). In
children, the acquisition of reading and writing skills may be
initially poor for maturational reasons, but in such cases the
child can be expected to "catch up" in due course. Against such
cases where orthographic competence has been or will be attained,
one can contrast the developmental dyslexic, an individual who is
otherwise as exceptional or unexceptional as any other average
individual but who nonetheless fails to achieve the expected level
of proficiency with the written language.

Two considerations give the study of the human ability to
master a written language particular prominence. First, linguistic
capacity is a cardinal feature of the species, and competence with
the written language of one's linguistic community seems intimately
tied to that capacity. The study of how command of an orthography
is gained, therefore, has the potential of shedding light on
linguistic capacity per se and how that capacity can integrate with
other cognitive capacities. By the same token, understanding
seemingly selective disruptions of the ability to command a written
language may also shed light on these issues. Second, we live in
societies where universal literacy is becoming increasingly
expected of individuals. In industrial societies competence with
the written language is becoming increasingly essential for
participation in the work force and as a means of access to the
culture. A selective curtailment in the ability to command the
written language can then extract a cost to the society and limit
an individual's opportunities to realize his or her potential. It

is with the first of these issues that I will be concerned here.

A host of data provide compelling evidence that normal human beings enter the world with a biological endowment which impels them to acquire the language of their speech community. The data range from the observation of language acquisition is remarkably consistent across languages to the observation that natural languages do not vary arbitrarily from each other and that many logically possible structur-al alternatives are not encountered in the languages of the world. Studies of adults with acquired disorders of language have provided extensive data that the left cerebral hemisphere, in particular cortical neural systems in the perisylvian region, plays a critical and selective role in supporting normal mature linguistic capacity. While it is evident from the aphasias that focal lesions in left hemisphere language areas can impair linguistic capacity in all modalities of language use, there is virtually nothing known of the relation between ontogenetic variation in these cortical regions and the realization of linguistic capacity. Neuroanatomical research over the last decade by Galaburda and his colleagues (Galaburda and Kemper, 1978; Galaburda, 1984; Geschwind and Galaburda, 1987) has consistently provided evidence that anomalies in neural maturation are to be found in the brains of developmental dyslexics, anomalies which involve language areas in the left hemisphere. Thus, consideration of linguistic capacity in developmental dyslexia is also of potential importance to the study of the biological foundations of language.

LINGUISTIC CAPACITY IN DYSLEXIA

Because of the intimate relation between linguistic capacity and mastery of a written language, the question is immediately posed as to whether dyslexia is a consequence of a more fundamental anomaly in linguistic capacity. A variety of researchers have suggested that dyslexia is a consequence of limitations in phonetic processing capacities (Liberman, 1983; Mann, 1986). The scope of such data are compelling, and it is accepted here as fact that developmental dyslexics are atypical in there ability to process the speech stream, at least in childhood. Beyond the level of phonetic processing, a variety of lines of research have provided data which are consistent with the notion that developmental dyslexics also have atypicalities in morphological and syntactic representation. Vellutino (1979) argues that developmental dyslexics have a basic problem with word encoding which arises out of more complex linguistic problems. In support of this hypothesis, he cites studies showing difficulties in areas of syntax and morphology as well as deficiencies in knowledge of phonological representations. Vogel (1975) provides evidence that developmental dyslexics do not exhibit as reliable a level of performance on tasks which require sensitivity to inflectional and derivational morphology as average readers. Whitehouse (1983) provides data indicating that developmental dyslexics do not perform at a typical level on the Token Test.

There is, however, a fundamental linguistic problem with these studies of morphology and syntax. In each case the data from these studies of English speaking dyslexics can potentially be explained in terms of phonetic processing. It is a central property of English that inflectional and derivational morphemes (e.g., past tense -ed and -ness, respectively) are relatively unstressed. Additionally, function words (e.g., the, is, and on) are also typically relatively unstressed in sentences. For all individuals, unstressed items are phonetically less salient than stressed ones. If developmental dyslexics are less efficient or somehow compromised in their capacity to carry out phonetic processing, then it would not be particularly remarkable if they showed apparent evidence of morphological and syntactic difficulties where task success specifically requires attention to such unstressed items.

As the phonetic analysis of verbal experience is seemingly necessary for establishing appropriate representation of the phonology and lexicon of a language and such representations provide the foundation for the development of a mature morphology and syntax, a limitation in phonetic processing might well be sufficient to lead to anomalies in linguistic representation at higher levels of analysis. However, research on the acquisition of sign language by deaf children of deaf parents, provides evidence that lexical, syntactic and semantic development are relatively insensitive to modality properties of the representation of linguistic stimuli (Klima and Bellugi, 1979). Thus, the existence of some modality specific constraint on the linguistic capacity of developmental dyslexics does not entail that there will be any central anomaly in the grammatical representation or processing. [It is, of course, also of relevance to the issue of understanding dyslexia, that the deaf also have difficulties in mastering written language (Locke, 1978)].

While the data available are consistent with the hypothesis that a compromise in phonetic processing is the essential underlying linguistic feature of developmental dyslexia, they do not provide compelling evidence that there is no morphological or syntactic involvement. First, one can only rule out such grammatical involvement on the basis of studies where a phonetic processing limitation is not a candidate explanation of anomalous findings. Second, studies of dyslexics are almost invariably carried out with children. Children are on a developmental trajectory, and the data of development can only be meaningfully interpreted with reference to the product of the developmental course. We should be no more prepared to make claims about linguistic capacity in developmental dyslexics on the basis child language data than we are to make claims about the grammatical structure of typical mature human linguistic capacity on the basis of acquisition data.

Several years ago, I reported two preliminary studies which had been carried out with a small group of self-selected adult developmental dyslexics (Kean, 1984). The goal of those studies was to see if there was sufficient evidence to warrant a detailed analysis of syntactic capacity in developmental dyslexia. In one study, subjects were asked to carry out a reaction time task which involved identical word monitoring; a target word was heard, followed by a sentence containing the word, and the subject had to press a reaction time key as soon as he or she heard the target word in the sentence. The data were analyzed in terms of response accuracy and latency to targets from various syntactic categories. The dyslexic subjects' error rates were not different from those of college students and non-dyslexic adults from the community for all categories except determiners (e.g., the and this), where their error rates jumped from the normal 5% to about 20%; reaction times for items in this category were also significantly longer. Such data are, of course, consistent with the hypothesis of a phonetic processing limitation, and, therefore, like the studies noted above shed no light on the issue of syntactic capacity in developmental dyslexia.

The second study involved grammaticality judgments. Subjects heard a sentence and said whether or not the sentences were grammatical or not; as two subjects may make the same judgment for different reasons, each response was systematically probed. While in the main the subjects performed on a par with various groups of adult controls, a number seemed to have rather striking anomalies in their responses to sentences such as those in (1) and (2).

(1)   John told Bill to mow the lawn, and he did it.
(2)   John promised Bill to mow the lawn, and he did it?

All subjects agreed that both sentences were "good", but a number of the dyslexic subjects seemed to find the sentences ambiguous, responding to the question, "Who mowed the lawn?" with "You can't tell," rather than "Bill" for (1) and "John" for (2), the normal responses. On the basis of this result, I conjectured that developmental dyslexics had anomalies in at least some areas of grammatical representation involving referential dependencies.

In recent work Neil Elliott and I have attempted to investigate this conjecture with a similar judgment task for which we have developed a set of 180 sentences involving various grammatical and ungrammatical uses of pronouns, reflexives, and the reciprocal (each other). To date we have tested 14 adult developmental dyslexics on these mate-rials, and each performs as well or better than our college student control group. While we did not test reading or writing abilities in this group ourselves, for each subject we had an independent diagnosis of dyslexia based on testing by qualified education therapists. Thus, while the original work suggested that we might find anomalies in this area

of grammar, recent more extensive (though still preliminary)
research provides no evidence of any grammatical anomaly in adult
developmental dyslexics. Such data do not, however, demonstrate
that there is no anomaly in morphological or syntactic
representation in dyslexia; it is possible that the method used is
not sensitive enough to pick up differences or that, while there
are no anomalies in this aspect of linguistic capacity, anomalies
do exist in other areas of grammar. It is clear, however, that at
this point there are no data which provide evidence of explicitly
morphological or syntactic deviations in the grammars of children
or adults with developmental dyslexia.

GRAMMATICAL CAPACITY - THE RELEVANCE OF DYSLEXIA DATA

     Linguistic theory makes a strong claim to being a functional
biological theory. If that claim has significant empirical
content, then we would anticipate that variation in the biological
substrate of that capacity would affect its realization. Galaburda
and his colleagues have consistently reported that there are
anomalies of cortical development in left hemisphere language areas
of male dyslexics; they have further consistently found hemispheric
symmetry in the typically asymmetrical areas of the temporal lobe
in both female and male. Both these findings suggest that the
patterns of local and interhemispheric connectivity in dyslexics
deviate from the norm. The failure to date to find any compelling
evidence of anomalies in grammatical capacity in developmental
dyslexics might be taken then as undermining the biological claims
of linguistic theory, at least in their strongest form. Such a
conclusion is not, however, warranted at this time.

     While it is certainly the case that there is no evidence of
grammatical anomaly in developmental dyslexia in the areas of
morphology and syntax, the scant research which has been done to
date and the fact that that research has for the most part been
carried out with children hardly conspire to make the currently
available findings compelling. It is clear that more detailed
research using carefully designed stimuli and more sensitive tasks
must be undertaken. Consideration of the implications of the
potential results of such studies indicate why the study of
dyslexia is of such interest for linguistics.

     First, let us assume that no anomalies in morphological or
syntactic capacity emerge in children or adults with developmental
dyslexia. From a theoretical point of view this would lend strong
credence to the theory of modularity and the autonomy of the
components of the grammar. As we know from the study of sign
language, how the signal is encoded and "phonologically"
represented does not influence the syntax of a language. What is
essential, it would seem, for the language learner is that there be
sequences which can be systematically categorized as discrete
morphemes. The syntax and the rules of word formation are

seemingly impervious to the internal content of that representation. Biologically, such a finding would suggest either that the levels of neuroanatomical analysis we have available are not the appropriate ones for characterizing the functional structure of the linguistic system or that there are brain areas which play a critical role in support of linguistic capacity of which we are unaware; certainly both possibilities might be true. Alternatively, it might suggest that there are degrees of structural freedom within the system which are consonant with the development of normal linguistic capacity. The robustness of linguistic capacity across "normal" individuals with rather glaring individual differences in perceptual and cognitive abilities makes this a viable possibility. Whatever the case, the data would provide important information for the development of a serious analysis of the biological foundations of linguistic capacity.

The second alternative which might be considered is a finding of seeming anomalies in the grammatical development of children while adult dyslexics' performance is unremarkable. It would be incoherent to suggest that the course of language acquisition in dyslexia is consistently anomalous in some area(s) but that normal mature linguistic capacity is nonetheless attained. The course of language acquisition in any subpopulation might, however, deviate from the normal trajectory at some point(s) in time and in some particular areas, with the output of the course of acquisition being essentially normal. Thus, the finding from any group of children who are poor readers that they deviate from the norm would be of importance to the theory of acquisition. Such deviations might arise because in some stages of acquisition the content of phonological representations is of significance, because of transitory short term memory limitations, or for a host of maturational reasons. It would be of considerable interest to understand the range of perturbations the system can tolerate in development without having the outcome compromised. The third possible alternative is, of course, that there are systematic deviations in the course of language acquisition and in the mature linguistic capacity of developmental dyslexics. From the perspective of linguistic theory, the formal characterization of those deviations and their relation to the formal structure of typical linguistic capacity would be of significance. The question would also arise as to what components of the neural substrate are responsible for those deviations. On the basis of data available to date, only male developmental dyslexics show anomalies in cortical ontogeny (A.M. Galaburda, personal communication). If, then, male dyslexics but not female dyslexics were shown to have anomalies in linguistic capacity then that would suggest that essential aspects of normal linguistic capacity are supported by detailed local neural circuitries. On the other hand, if both male and female developmental dyslexics showed patterns of anomaly in linguistic capacity, this would suggest that interhemispheric connectivity and its consequences for local circuitries would be the critical variable. In either case, given formal analyses of

the structure of linguistic capacity in the dyslexic and
non-dyslexic populations, our ability to address serious questions
about the biological basis of linguistic capacity would be greatly
enhanced.

At this point we are only at the start of exploring the
questions raised by the study of grammatical capacity in
developmental dyslexia. The results to date in this area have been
anything but exhilarating, but the potential interest of any result
has significant implications for our understanding of human
linguistic capacity and its biological foundations. Because of the
promise of this line of research, we are undertaking further
studies with the group of adult developmental dyslexics who work
with us. With my colleague Virginia Mann, we hope to study
phonetic and phonological processing in this population, research
which will allow us to assess the degree to which limitations in
those areas are persistent or maturational. We also plan to
investigate ourselves not only reading capacity in the population
but also spelling abilities through writing to dictation and free
writing tasks. As some of our subjects are well-educated
professionals, we do not anticipate that all will show severe
limitations in reading skills, but we do anticipate that spelling
problems will be more persistent and evident. We will, of course,
also be pursuing research on grammatical capacity in this group.
This work will involve moving from reliance on the off-line
judgment task to on-line tasks such as word monitoring. The
results of these studies have the promise of opening new avenues
for understanding linguistic capacity.

REFERENCES

Coltheart, M. Patterson, K. and Marshall, J.C. (1980) Deep
Dyslexia. Routledge & Kegan Paul, London.

Galaburda, A.M. (1984) Anatomical Asymmetries. In Cerebral
Dominance: The biological foundations. Harvard University Press,
Cambridge.

Galaburda, A.M. and Kemper, T. (1978) Cytoarchitectonic anomalies
in Developmental Dyslexia: A case study. Annals of Neurology, 6,
94-100.

Geschwind, N. and Galaburda, A.M. (1987) Cerebral Lateralization:
Biological mechanisms, associations, and pathology. MIT Press,
Cambridge. Klima, E. and Bellugi I. (1979) The Signs of Language.
Harvard University Press, Cambridge.

Kean, M-L. (1984) The Question of Linguistic Anomaly in
Developmental Dyslexia. Annals of Dyslexia, 34, 137-151.

Locke, J.L. (1978) Phonemic Effects in the Silent Reading of Deaf and Hearing Children. Cognition, 6, 175-187.

Liberman, I.Y. (1983) A Language Oriented View of Reading
Disabilities. In Progress in Learning Disabilities, Vol. 5. (ed.
H. Mykelbust). Grune & Stratton, New York.

Mann, V.A. (1986) Why Some Children Experience Reading Problems:
The contribution of difficulties with language processing and
phonological sophistication to early reading disability. In
Learning Disabilities: Some new perspectives. (eds. J.K.
Torgesen and B.Y. Wong). Academic Press, New York.

Patterson, K.E. Surface Dyslexia: Neuropsychological and Cognitive
Studies of Phonological Reading. Earlbaum, Hilldsale.

Vellutino, F.R. (1979) Dyslexia: Theory and research. MIT Press,
Cambridge.

Vogel, S.A. (1975) Syntactic Abilities in Normal and Dyslexic
Children. University Park Press, Baltimore.

Whitehouse, C.C. (1983). Token Test Performance by Dyslexic
Adolescents. Brain and Language, 18, 224-235.

21
Morphological Awareness in Dyslexia

Carsten Elbro

INTRODUCTION

According to a simple analysis, to read is to employ the principles of writing in order to reconstruct the meaning of a text. This means that dyslexic students may be lacking the prerequisites that are necessary in order to use the principles of writing. So before we start looking for these missing prerequisites it would be a good idea to consider the principles of writing.

Alphabetic writing systems, like the ones used in English or Danish, are usually described as morpho-phonemic, because the representations of the words are in accordance with a combination of a morphemic and a phonemic principle. These two principles may be said to control the way words are written. And in order to become a reader, the child will have to learn to make use of these two principles.

According to the phonemic principle each phoneme in spoken language is represented by a grapheme (letter). In cases where the phonemic principle dominates, words are said to be 'regular' or 'phonetic', they are 'written as they sound', e.g. ice, scandal, and life. The phonemic principle does not lead to any simple phonetic alphabet, because it works together with a number of orthographic conventions which governs the representation of vocal length, assignment of stress and so forth. The final -e in life is, for instance, not representing a final vowel [lɪfɪ], but the length of the preceding vowel [laɪf].

When words are not 'regular', the most common reason is that the morphemic principle is overriding the phonemic principle. One example is the inflectional suffix -s which is spelled in the same way regardless of variations in pronunciation as in books [buks], pens [penz], and horses [hɔsɪz]. In these and many other cases the morphemic principle is so pervasive that children are learning it fast and fluent readers hardly notice it. In other cases we may waver between the phonemic and the morphemic principle with words such as please -> pleasant/-*plesant, appear -> *appearent/apparent, and British -> Britishism/Brit-

279

icism.

Morphemes are the smallest units of meaning and expression, and according to the morphemic principle a morpheme is written in the same way regardless of phonemic variations. Due to the morphemic principle it is possible for a reader or listener to understand many compounds and derivatives that he or she may not have heard or read before. This applies especially to words with a transparent and conventional morphological structure, such as un/put/down/able (from the blurb of Fay Weldon's novel 'The hearts and lives of men'), con/-form/ity, and mis/re/collect/ion/s.

In order to come to master the principles of writing, the learning is facilitated if the student has some awareness of the units that are represented in writing. If the student cannot mobilize an awareness of the phonemes of spoken language, the significance of the letters will remain obscure to him or her. Therefore, phonological awareness is of critical importance to the responsiveness to initial reading instruction (Bradley & Bryant, 1985; Mattingly, 1972; Olofsson, 1985; Lundberg, this volume).

Correspondingly there are reasons to believe that morphological awareness is important to reading development. Morphological awareness or metamorphological abilities may be defined as abilities to shift perspective from language use to reflections upon the constituent morphemes themselves.

At least two conditions should be met if we are to take seriously this hypothesis concerning the importance of morphological awareness: firstly, morphemes should be psychologically real at least at some level, and secondly, it should seem plausible that readers use morphological decomposition strategies in reading.

Concerning the psychological reality of morphemes, Berko (1958) showed in a classical experiment that children at the age of 5:6 - 7 years were able to apply morphological conventions to words they had not heard before. For instance they could add plural inflections to new words like wug and get wugs, and produce the past tense form ricked from rick. The experiment have been replicated a number of times (Berry, 1977; Derwing, 1976; Vogel, 1977; Wiig et al., 1973), and the results have indicated that inflection of nouns and verbs precede inflections of adjectives and most derivations (Selby, 1972).

It may be discussed to what extent tests like these involves awareness of morphemes. Correct answers do not necessarily indicate a high degree of morphological awareness, but may reflect morphological skills which are working automatically. On the other hand, one way to be sure to find a correct answer is to search for analogies among real words and then transform the pattern of inflection, derivation or compounding to the pseudo-words. And this strategy requires morphological awareness.

In the second part of her study Berko (1958) investigated morphological awareness more directly by asking children to explain the
structure of compound words, e.g. blackboard. She did not ask what a
blackboard is, but "why do you think a blackboard is called a blackboard?" The results indicated that the children were aware of few
morphemes other than those that contained a salient feature or a major
function of the word. Hence some of the children explained that a
blackboard is called so because it is black, but they rarely explained
the last part of the word.

Together these results indicate that children at the age of 6
master the most common morphological rules for inflection, derivation,
and compounding, but that they are not spontaneously aware of the
morphemes of complex words.

An indirect argument for the psychological reality of inflections
can be found in the organization of dictionaries. Usually dictionaries do
not have separate entries for all inflected forms of the same word. It
is unnecessary to list inflected forms because the inflectional system
works automatically and because inflected forms are semantically
transparent.

On the other hand dictionaries usually have separate entries for
derived forms of the same root, because the derivation system does not
work with the same regularity. To read is called read/ing, not *read/ion
or *read/ment; we say un/just but in/justice, un/melodious but in/har-
monious and so forth. And derivations are not as semantically transparent as inflections, for example, un/grace/ful is not the same as dis/-
grace/ful and the difference is unpredictable. However, experiments
have indicated that students in 4th to 8th grade are able to define
derived words from knowledge of their roots through morphological
generalization (Freyd & Baron, 1982; Wysocky & Jenkins, 1987). And
with fluent readers, words with productive derivation suffixes such as
-ness, -er, and -ment seem to be stored in the mental lexicon both as
roots and whole words (MacKay, 1978; Bradley, 1980). But again this is
not the same as to be aware of the morphological components and
relationships between words, especially not if the words mirror genuine
morphological relations: vocal - vociferous, applaud - plausible, and
Peter - petrify are related, i.e. they share the same roots, but promise
- promiscuity, male - malicious are not.

Ohala & Ohala (1985) gave pairs of words like the above to linguistically naive adults and asked them to decide which of the pairs
could be thought to have the same ancestor, i.e. share the same root.
Since the words seemed both semantically and phonologically related,
subjects were unable to distinguish between real relatedness and
pseudo-relatedness. Maybe the results had been different if the
derivational suffixes of the experiment had all been productive (currently used to form new words) and not parts of latin loanwords.

A possible conclusion is that separate mental representations of
roots and derivational suffixes may be of greater importance to the

economy of the mental lexicon as regards the semantic description of
words than to the number of lexical entries (Henderson, 1985).

The second requirement for the importance of morphological
awareness to reading acquisition is that it should seem probable that
readers make use of a morphological decomposition strategy in reading,
i.e. that morphemes are important to the reading process. Luckily, there
are both theoretical and empirical reasons to believe this: Some words
are so long that they cannot be perceived in one fixation. They have to
be identified in smaller parts. In these cases an analysis in morphemes
has the advantage that the units bear directly on the meaning of the
word. Another argument is that it is economical to have orthographic
entries to the lexicon for morphemes rather than whole words. In
Danish, for example, there are approximately four times as many
different words as there are stems. Finally, a number of studies have
indicated that, apart from the post-lexical processing of constituent
morphemes, the identification of complex words involves a pre-lexical
decomposition by which potential morphemes are separated (Elbro, 1986;
Jarvella & Snodgrass, 1974; Jarvella et al., 1986; Smith & Sterling, 1982;
Taft, 1981).

We can now move on to the more direct evidence for the importance of morphological awareness to reading acquisition and to dyslexia.
A number of studies have discovered a positive correlation between
morphological abilities as measured by abilities to inflect and derive
new words (cf. Berko, 1958) and success in reading (Brittain, 1970; Wiig
et al., 1973). These studies have investigated morphological abilities,
however, and not necessarily morphological awareness. Other studies
have indicated that dyslexic readers have difficulties in particular with
closed class morphemes such as inflectional suffixes (Bryant & Impey,
1986; Henderson & Shores, 1982; Temple & Marshall, 1983).

To my knowledge, only a single prediction study has been carried
out. Tornéus (1987) asked 71 Swedish children in kindergarten to
explain the meaning of pairs of invented compounds such as grass bee
and bee grass (both are one word in Swedish). When the same children
were later tested on measures of reading in first, second, and third
grade she found a correlation between metamorphological skills found in
kindergarten and later reading skills.

On this basis it seems a reasonable hypothesis that one of the
causes of dyslexia may be poor metamorphological skills. However, this
hypothesis does not say anything about which aspects of the reading
process that are affected in particular by the poor metamorphological
skills. Considering dyslexic readers' difficulties with inflections, a
reasonable hypothesis may be that morphological awareness is related in
particular to accuracy in reading inflections. The experiment to be
reported was concerned with these two hypotheses.

THE EXPERIMENT

Subjects

The metamorphological abilities and reading abilities of severely dyslexic teenagers were assessed in an experiment using a reading level design. 26 developmental dyslexic teenagers aged 13:7 - 17:3 years (mean 15:3) were selected from a special school for dyslexics who have been unresponsive to remediation in normal schools and whose reading difficulties were found to be specific, i.e. to exist despite conventional instruction and normal intelligence, and despite the absence of grave neurological, sensory, and emotional disturbances (cf. Critchley, 1970). The reading age of each of the dyslexic subjects was at least 3 years below chronological age. The dyslexics received remedial teaching in small groups of 4 to 5 by different teachers each using different approaches to remedial teaching.

The dyslexic teenagers were matched by 26 normal readers of the same reading age as measured by a standard silent reading test with sentences (number of correctly read sentences within 5 minutes, Nielsen et al., 1986) and of same IQ as measured by the Raven progressive matrices (Raven, 1958). The 26 normal readers were selected from 2nd and 3rd grade classes in a public and a private school. They were aged 8:4 - 10:11 years with a mean age of 9:4 years. As a second control group 13 normal readers of approximately the same chronological age and IQ as the dyslexic teenagers were selected (Table 1).

Materials

There were five tests of morphological awareness:
1. Sentence analysis (s-ana). The task was to count the number of words in sentences which were orally presented and accompanied by illustrations to support comprehension and memory. The sentences were constructed to test awareness of "function" words and compound words,

Table 1. Characteristics of the three groups of the reading level design.

	N	Age	Sentence reading	Raven score	Raven percentile
Dyslexic teenagers	26	15:3	33.5	44.3	50-75
2nd-3rd grade normal readers	26	9:4	33.2	31.2	50-75
8th grade normal readers	13	14:7	–	46.8	50-75

separately. This was accomplished by selecting some sentences with
long compound words and others with many non-prominent "function"
words, i.e. pronouns, prepositions, articles, and other words belonging
to closed classes. If a subject was not aware of "function" words he or
she would be likely to miss some of them, and, correspondingly, if a
subject was unaware of the conventions of compound formation, he or
she would be inclined to count one compound word as two words or
more. There were 18 sentences with between 2 and 9 words each.
Subjects were asked to repeat each sentence after the experimenter in
order to make sure that the sentence was perceived and could be
reproduced. Then the subjects were asked to name one word at a time
and count on the fingers or by means of filing cards.

2. Inflection, derivation, and compound formation with pseudo-
words (affix) (Figure 1). This test was inspired by the original test by
Berko (1958) and later developments (Berry, 1977). The tasks covered
the most productive types of inflections, derivations and compounds in
Danish. 18 items out of a total of 24 concerned inflections.

3. Morphological analysis and reversal (m-rev). This test consisted
of 20 compound words. The task was to reverse the order of the
elements of the compound words, e.g. mailbox -> *boxmail . The
difficulty of the task varied due to the degree of semantic transparency
of the compound words and to the fact that some of the root-mor-
phemes were only allomorphs to free morphemes, e.g. three in three-
pence).

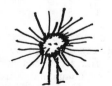

Yesterday I saw a sput.

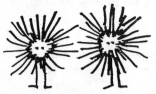

Later I saw another sput.
I saw two of them.
I saw two _____.

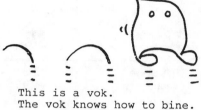

This is a vok.
The vok knows how to bine.
What would you call a vok
that knows how to bine?
It is a _____.

Figure 1. Inflection and compound formation or derivation of new
words.

4. Morphological synthesis (m-syn). 44 words consisting of two morphs each were presented to the subjects, one morpheme at the time with main stress on each morpheme and half a second's pause between the morphemes of each word. The task was to decide whether or not the two spoken morphemes formed a real word or not. Five types of words were employed: compounds consisting of two open class morphemes (e.g. dining table, one word in Danish), compounds of one closed class morpheme and one open class morpheme (up...side), derivatives of meaning (un...belief), derivatives of word class (good...ness), and inflections (high...est).

5. Morphological completion (m-compl). The subjects heard either the first or the last morpheme of a complex word and were asked to say a whole word containing the morpheme. The morphemes chosen for this task were mostly 'monogamous', i.e. they occur in combination with only one other morpheme (e.g. -whelm in overwhelm), and the 'polygamous' morphemes were not particularly 'promiscuous'. The morphemes to be added by the subjects were high frequent like over- in overwhelm. There were 16 items.

Originally, a test requiring explanations of compound words was also planned for the experiment (cf. Berko, 1958). A test asking for definitions of neologisms was also tried, e.g. "what do you think a paper-coat would be if such a thing existed?" After a pilot study these tests were given up, however, partly because the answers were difficult to score and partly because there seemed to be great differences among subjects as to the degree of explication they considered necessary. It was found that a subjects failure to provide a correct etymological response was not necessarily indicative of a lack of cognizance of morphological relationships (cf. Derwing, 1976).

Procedure and scoring

All subjects were tested individually in sessions lasting approximately 20 minutes. The tasks were administered in the same order to all subjects. Answers to all items were scored as either correct or incorrect. In cases of possible doubt whether a particular answer should be considered correct or not, a group of normal, linguistically naive adults acted as models. This was necessary with the test of inflection, derivation and compound formation with pseudo-words. The answers of the normal adults were decided to be the possible choice of correct answers.

Results

Results showed that in three of the five tests of metamorphological abilities the dyslexic teenagers were outperformed by the reading-age-matched normal readers (differences in s-ana and m-rev were significant with $p < 0.01$, and m-compl with $p < 0.05$, Mann-Whitney two tailed test) (Figure 2). No reliable differences were found with the other two tests ($p > 0.5$). The dyslexic teenagers were also outperform-

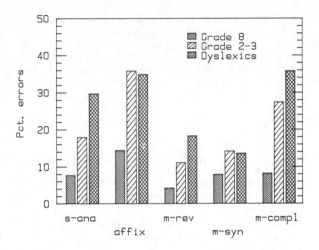

Figure 2. Metamorphological abilities as measured by tests of sentence analysis, affixation, morphological reversal, synthesis, and completion.

ed on a mean score giving equal weights to all five tests ($\underline{p}$ < 0.01). The chronological age matched controls consistently outperformed the other two groups (all differences between dyslexics and controls were significant with $\underline{p}$ < 0.001, except m-syn with $\underline{p}$ < 0.01). No significant effects of sex were found in any of the three groups (cf. Berko, 1958).

The difference in sentence analysis scores between the dyslexic subjects and the reading-age-matched controls was mostly a result of differences in the number of words missed. This indicates that the dyslexic readers had a greater tendency to miss 'function' words when counting words than normal readers ($\underline{p}$ < 0.01). And this result supports the notion that dyslexic readers have pronounced difficulties handling closed class morphemes. The lack of differences between the dyslexic group and the normal 2nd and 3rd graders on the test of affixation of new words may reflect the fact that the dyslexic teenagers had had several years of formal instruction in grammar whereas only one of the normal classes had begun with grammar.

The no-difference result in morphological synthesis may reflect two things: firstly, the test may have been too easy to detect relevant differences, and secondly, the scores may to a large extent be dependent on vocabulary, and in this area the dyslexic teenagers may take advantage of their higher age and more linguistic experiences.

Morphemes in reading

In order to gain insights into the actual use of morphological awareness in reading the dyslexic group and the reading-age-matched normal readers were asked to read 20 nonsense words and 148 real words of varying length and morphological structure (for a closer description of the words, see Elbro, 1986 and 1988). Each word was printed in lower case 24 point Times on a separate filing card. Subjects were tested individually, there were no time limits, and all responses were tape recorded.

The results showed that the normal readers read 73.3% of the words correctly whereas the dyslexic readers read only 52.6% correctly (p < 0.001). This result stresses the primacy of the decoding difficulties among the dyslexic readers since the two groups performed equally well on the standard sentence reading test.

The accuracy of the reading of inflections was measured as the percentage of all reading errors in which only the inflection was misread no matter whether it was misread, omitted, or inserted in words without inflections. As expected, the dyslexic subjects made significantly more errors on inflections than the normal controls (12.1% against 7.4%, p = 0.01).

Of particular interest was the connexion between metamorphological skills and reading skills. Since the metamorphological tests tended to correlate with Raven score, subjects were analyzed in groups according to the Raven scores.

As appears in Figure 3, scores in the tests of metamorphological abilities correlated with accuracy in reading in both groups of subjects. However, the differences between the groups with high and low metamorphological scores were only significant for the groups with a Raven score above the median. So morphological awareness did not appear to

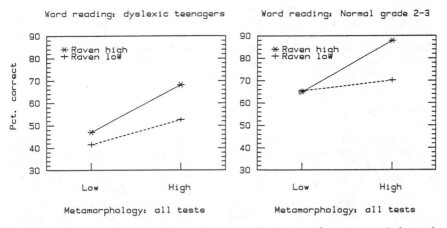

Figure 3. Accuracy in word reading as a function of metamorphological skills (above or below median) and Raven (above or below median).

Reading inflections

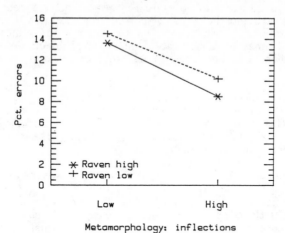

Figure 4. Accuracy in reading inflections as a function of awareness of inflections (above or below median) and Raven (above or below median).

be used automatically, since only the readers who were probably the most reflexive seemed fully to use their abilities.

Figure 4 shows the corresponding relations between awareness of inflections and the percentage of reading errors hitting only the inflections. The measure of morphological awareness is the number of correct responses to the 18 items with inflections in the affix test with new words. The relations between the reading of inflections and the other measures of metamorphological abilities were less pronounced. And there was no corresponding relationship in the normal group. It should be noted that the correlation between metamorphological abilities and reading accuracy with inflections seemed to be independent of the Raven scores. These results are interesting because they indicate a specific link between awareness of a certain type of morphemes and the reading accuracy with the same type.

DISCUSSION

The results of the experiment indicate that severely dyslexic students are not as morphologically aware as normal readers of the same age and intelligence and in some respects neither as morphologically aware as reading-age-matched normal readers who are several years younger. Since a reading level design is rather powerful (Backman et al., 1984), these results indicate that poor morphological awareness is at least connected with the causes of dyslexia. Poor reading abilities do not alone explain the low morphological awareness of the dyslexic readers, since the normal and dyslexic readers were reading at the same level according to a standard reading test.

Although further insights into the causes and effects of metamorphological abilities will require prediction and intervention studies, a closer look at the performance of the dyslexic readers may reveal some of the origins of the difficulties. The dyslexic students displayed greatest difficulties with the tests of sentence analysis, reversals of morphemes and morphological completion of words, whereas they performed on the same level as the reading-age-matched normal readers on tasks requiring morphological synthesis, and inflection, derivation, and compound formation of new words.

The three tests which proved most difficult for the dyslexic students seem to differ from the other two tests in respect to the demands they pose on working memory. All three tasks require subjects to keep closed class morphemes in memory while some other linguistic activity is being carried out. In sentence analysis subjects had to remember both open class and closed class words while they counted the number of words, and in this case the dyslexic students displayed difficulties with closed class words in particular. The morphological reversal task and the completion task also both required the subjects to remember the bound morphemes while they manipulated them or searched for other morphemes to produce a real word.

Conversely, the affixation test required subjects to remember new words, while searching for a proper affix, but all words were meaningful because they corresponded to things, actions, and properties which were illustrated, and all new words belonged to open classes. And the test of morphological synthesis only posed minimal demands on memory, since the items were presented in the correct order with a pause of only half a second. The results would probably have been different, if, for instance, three or four morphemes had been presented together and subjects had been asked to use them to produce as many real words as possible. Closed class morphemes and not yet identified bound morphemes share the common feature of abstraction. The characteristic of closed class morphemes is not that they lack semantic content, but that their meanings are very general and thus abstract. In a class consisting of a limited number of members, each member has to cover a greater field than in classes with a potentially infinite number of members.

Dyslexic readers have been reported to fail to use syntactic clues for decoding and comprehension (Steiner et al., 1971; Weinstein & Rabinovitch, 1971). Since syntax is to a large degree signalled by closed class morphemes (i.e. function words and affixes), this failure may be a result of problems with closed class morphemes. The sentence reading of the subjects was not analyzed, however, so this idea remains an open possibility.

The comparisons of morphological awareness with reading ability indicated that one thing is to be aware of the morphemes of words, another thing is to use this awareness in reading. Only the most reflexive readers seemed to benefit substantially from their metamorphological abilities in reading accuracy and reading of inflections (see also Freyd & Baron, 1982). This result may reflect the fact that the teaching of morphemes has been limited to a restricted set of inflections in order to support accuracy in spelling and has failed to point to regularities which may be useful in reading. While some students are more apt at using what they actually know, others must have the potential uses of their knowledge demonstrated.

Provided that the above reasoning is correct, the implications for the teaching of reading to dyslexic and beginning readers are promising. Teaching may be most effective when it just has to point out to the student what he or she already knows.

REFERENCES

Backman, J.E., Mamen, M. & Ferguson, H.B. (1984). Reading level design: Conceptual and methodological issues in reading research. **Psychological Bulletin, 96**, 560-568.

Berko, J. (1958). The child's learning of English morphology. **Word, 14**, 150-177.

Berry, M.F. (1977). **The Berry-Talbott developmental guide to comprehension of grammar.** Rockford, IL.

Bradley, D. (1980). Lexical representation of derivational relation. In M. Aronoff & M.-L. Kean (eds.), **Juncture. A collection of original papers.** Saratoga: Anma Libri, 37-55.

Bradley, D. & Bryant, P. (1985). **Rhyme and reason in reading and spelling.** IARLD, Ann Arbor: University of Michigan Press.

Brittain, M.M. (1970). Inflectional performance and early reading achievement. **Reading Reasearch Quarterly, 6**, 34-48.

Bryant, P. & Impey, L. (1986). The similarities between normal readers and developmental and acquired dyslexics. **Cognition, 24**, 121-137.

Critchley, M. (1970). **The dyslexic child.** London: Heineman.

Derwing, B.L. (1975). Morpheme recognition and the learning of rules for derivational morphology. **The Canadian Journal of Linguistics, 20**, 38-66.

Elbro, C. (1986). Morphemes in the reading process. In K. Trondhjem (Ed.), **Aspects in reading processes - with special reguards to hearing-impaired students.** Twelvth Danavox Symposium. Copenhagen, Denmark: Danavox, pp. 167-185.

Elbro, C. (1988). **Current subtypes of dyslexia questioned: Information processing at various levels in dyslexia.** Paper presented at The 4th International Conference on Systems Research, Informatics, and Cybernetics. Baden-Baden, August 15-21, 1988.

Freyd, P. & Baron, J. (1982). Individual differences in acquisition of derivational morphology. **Journal of Verbal Learning and Verval Behavior, 21**, 282-295.

Henderson, A.J. & Shores, R.E. (1982). How learning disabled student's failure to attend to suffixes affects their oral reading performance. **Journal of Learning Disabilities, 15**, 178-182.

Henderson, L. (1985). Toward a psychology of morphemes. In A.W. Ellis (ed.), **Progress in the psychology of language, Vol 1.** London: Lawrence Earlbaum Associates, pp. 1-91.

Jarvella, R.J. & Snodgrass, J.G. (1974). Seeing ring in rang and retain in retention: On recognizing stem morphemes in printed words. **Journal of Verbal Learning and Verbal Behavior, 13,** 590-598.

Jarvella, R.J., Job, R., Sandström, G. & Schreuder, R. (1986). **Morphological contraints on word recognition.** Department of Psychology, Umeå University, Umeå, Sweden.

MacKay, D.G. (1978). Derivational rules and the internal lexicon. **Journal of Verbal Learning and Verbal Behavior, 17,** 61-71.

Mattingly, I.G. (1972). Reading, the linguistic process, and linguistic awareness. In J.F. Kavanagh & I.G. Mattingly (Eds.), **Language by ear and by eye. The relationships between speech and reading.** Cambridge, Mass.: MIT, pp. 133-148.

Nielsen, J.C., Kreiner, S., Poulsen, A & Søegård, A. (1986). **Sætningslæseprøven SL6o.** Copenhagen: Dansk Psykologisk Forlag.

Ohala, M. & Ohala, J. (1985). **Psycholinguistic studies in phonology.** Lecture at the University of Copenhagen, April, 1985.

Olofsson, Å. (1985). **Phonemic awareness and learning to read: a longitudinal and quasi-experimental study.** Department of Psychology, University of Umeå, Umeå, Sweden.

Raven, J.C. (1958). **Standard progressive matrices. Sets A, B, C, D, and E.** London: H.K. Lewis.

Selby, S. (1972). The development of morphological rules in children. **The British Journal of Educational Psychology, 42,** 293-299.

Smith, P.T. & Sterling, C.M. (1982). Factors affecting the perceived morphemic structure of written words. **Journal of Verbal Learning and Verbal Behavior, 21,** 704-721.

Steiner, R., Wiener, M. & Cromer, W. (1971). Comprehension and syntactic responses in good and poor readers. **Journal of Educational Psychology, 62,** 506-513.

Taft, M. (1981). Prefix stripping revisited. **Journal of Verbal Learning and Verbal Behavior, 20,** 289-297.

Temple, C. & Marshall, J. (1983). A case study of developmental phonological dyslexia. **British Journal of Psychology, 74,** 517-533.

Tornéus, M. (1987). **The importance of metaphonological and metamorphological abilities for different phases of reading development.** Paper presented at The Third World Congress of Dyslexia. Crete.

Vogel, S.A. (1977). Morphological ability in normal and dyslexic children. **Journal of Learning Disabilities, 10,** 41-49.

Weinstein, R. & Rabinovitch, M.S. (1971). Sentence structure and retention in good and poor readers. **Journal of Educational Psychology, 62,** 25-30.

Wiig, E.H., Semel, E.M. & Crouse, M.A.B. (1973). The use of English morphology by high-risk and learning disabled children. **Journal of Learning Disabilities, 6,** 59-67.

Wysocky, K. & Jenkins, J.R. (1987). Deriving word meanings through morphological generalization. **Reading Research Quarterly, 22,** 66-81.

22
Information-Processing Obstacles in Reading Acquisition

Torleiv Höien, Ole F. Leegaard and Jan P. Larsen

INTRODUCTION

Reading depends on decoding and comprehension. The reading problems of the dyslexic child seem primarily to be associated with the decoding process. Convincing evidence has been accumulated to suggest that the major obstacle confronting the dyslexic child is in decoding single words (see reviews by Gough & Tunmer, 1986; Stanovich, 1982).

Decoding Strategies

Various strategies may be used to decode single words, and two of them seem to be of special importance: the orthographical strategy and the phonological one. The orthographical strategy involves direct access to the printed word's meaning and phonology on the basis of the word's visual–orthographical representation. The orthographical strategy is considered to be capable of recognising familiar words but not letter arrays, which, although conventially spelled, are not known words. The phonological strategy has to be used when reading either unfamilar words or nonwords. The reader uses knowledge of spelling–sound correspondences to translate the written word into an internal phonological representation, which is then used to understand the word. The phonological strategy is considered to be capable of translating words which contain standard spelling-to-sound correspondences, but not those which contain atypical or irregular spellings.

In order to become a proficient reader, both strategies have to be acquired. Some readers seem primarily to rely on one single strategy when decoding words, and it is important to understand why other strategies are not used. Non-use does not always indicate non-competence in using the specific strategy. A reader may have

293

acquired a given strategy, but for various reasons does not use this strategy when reading. Subjects differ in their strategic emphasis on the use of particular processing routes. In general, however, the failure to use a strategy often indicates that relevant competence has not yet been sufficiently acquired. Among dyslexic children, for example, some are not able to recognize words on a direct visual basis. Others meet obstacles when trying to use phonological information for word recognition. A specific strategy dysfunction may be caused by obstacles connected with different component processes necessarily involved during the decoding process.

We assume that the behaviours from which reading and spelling competence are inferred are the products of a set of underlying psychological processes, and that, in cases of dyslexia, certain of these processes operate in an atypical or defective manner.

Process Analysis

A testing procedure called process analysis may be useful in diagnosing the impaired or abolished decoding strategy. Process analysis gives information about what decoding process or processes are not functioning adequately. A model of the normal reading process is the basis for the analysis. The applied method is standard in experimental cognitive psychology. It involves assessment of the effects on speed and accuracy of response of systematic variations in factors considered relevant to the operation of the decoding strategies.

The process-analytical principle was originally formulated by the Russian neuropsychologist Luria (1976) but in more recent years language researchers in the West have also argued for a process-analytical classification of language disorders, especially as regards reading disorders (Marshall, 1984; Caramazza, 1984; Coltheart, 1984; Ellis, 1987; Seymour, 1987; Høien, 1986). There are, however, two conditions that have to be fulfilled before one can make a process-analytical interpretation of an abnormal reading pattern. First one has to have a model of the normal reading process. Secondly, one has to have a method of examination that makes it possible to measure each component of the reading prosess.

Several word-processing models have been published which are all alike in principle, even though they are formulated differently, (e.g. Coltheart, 1981; Warrington & Shallice, 1980; Marshall, 1984).

In the following we will describe a model of word-processing, which is basically a variant of the traditional dual-route model. After outlining the model we will demonstrate how this model may be utilized in a process-analytical description of two cases of dyslexia.

A Model for Word Decoding

To describe those component processes which appear essential for a functional analysis of the basic decoding strategies, it seems necessary to postulate co-operating systems concerned with the representation of meaning and phonology, and the representation of print and writing. We can refer to the first two systems as "a semantic system" and "a phonological system". The semantic system is postulated as the basis for understanding the word's meaning. The phonological system is the speech production system which contains a vocabulary store and provides the phonemic level of speech representation. The third system will be referred to as a visual-orthographical system, which is specialized for the handling of print, and is, beyond some peripheral level, functionally distinct from visual processing required for the analysis and identification of objects. The three systems also have to be connected with each other with pathways or channels of communication. Finally, we assume that each system can be divided into a definite number of independent processes.

In Figure 1 our hypothetical word decoding model is outlined showing the orthographical and phonological strategies. The circles indicate decoding processes and the arrows represent the flow of information from one processor to another.

The orthographical strategy is supposed to depend on the activity of the following processes: Visual analysis, grapheme identification, visual-orthographical word-recognition, semantic activation and phonological word-recall.

Visual analysis (VA) is a visuo-spatial process, an experiencing of the word, not as a string of letters, but as a graphic form of a certain size and shape. Grapheme identification (GI) is a fast, automatic process, where the word's letters are indentified simultaneously without the subject attending to them one at a time.

This information is then used to search through the orthographical memory, the reader's acquired knowledge about how words are spelled. If the reader is familiar with the spelling of the presented word, then the relevant visuo-orthographical knowledge is activated and he/she will recognize the word. This visuo-orthographical word-recognition (OR_1) often happens before the word-perception is finished. If the word is well-known and expected in the context, then information about the word's length and shape and first few letters and perhaps final letter are enough for the word to be recognized (Taylor & Taylor, 1983). The activated orthographical information is now semantically processed (SA), whereby the word's semantic representation in the lexicon is activated. This semantic information, together with the orthographical information, is used to search the phonological memory, where the reader's knowledge about how the word sounds is activated (phonological word-recall PR_2).

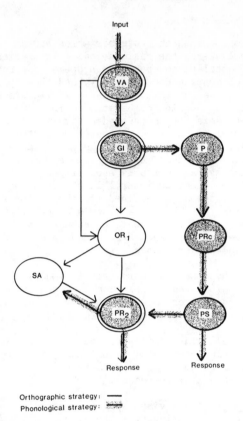

Fig. 1. Orthographical and phonological strategy

     If the reader does not know the visuo-orthographical structure
of the presented word, the word cannot be recognized directly. When
this happens, the word-recognition must be accomplished by the
phonological strategy, that is, by means of prior phonological
recoding of the letter string. This <u>prelexical phonological
encoding</u> is composed of at least three processes (Coltheart, 1984):
1) <u>orthographical parsing (P)</u>, wherein the string of letters is
divided into smaller orthographical segments, 2) <u>phonological
recoding PRc)</u>, wherein each of these orthographical segments is
recoded to a corresponding phonological segment, and 3) <u>phonolo-
gical synthesis PS</u>, where the phonological segments are blended to
make a sound-gestalt, a sound-image. This sound-image is used when
accessing the word's phonological identity in the lexicon.

These comments about specific processes behind the orthographical and phonological strategies inevitably contain an element
of speculation. However, they provide a framework within which the
cognitive processes of reading can be discussed. Such models have
proved useful in the analysis of acquired disorders of reading
because they lend themselves quite readily to explanation which are
stated in terms of the likely effect of a selective impairment of a
particular system or route (Shallice, 1981; Patterson, 1982). We
assume that such a process—analytical approach also is relevant
concerning investigation of developmental dyslexia. Therefore, we
will provide information about the prosess—analytical test battery
used when assessing our dyslexic subjects and the results of the
assessment.

METHOD

Two cases were diagnosed by means of a process—analytical test
battery devised by Høien (1988). The battery consists of five
tests and is carried out by means of a microcomputer (IBM AT).
This makes it possible to register precisely the reader's reaction
time; that is, the time it takes from the word is presented until
the answer is given. The reaction time tells us something about
the degree in which an ability is automated. The computer also
calculates the score and the reaction time in percent and z—value
in relation to population norms.

The test battery was designed to assess the decoding strategies the reader employs when reading word lists (test 1), how <u>well
the orthographical and phonological strategies function</u> (tests 2
and 3) and how well the separate processes that make up the
orthographical and phonological strategy, function (tests 4 and 5.)

Assessing the Decoding Strategies

The test consists of two lists of words (lists A and B). List
A contains 126 words which vary systematically along the dimensions
of length (three, five or seven letters), concrete versus abstract
meaning, frequencies of occurrence, and according to grammatical
class (content and function words). Each word is presented on the
computer screen with an exposure time of five seconds. The
reaction time is measured and the test—giver notes whether the word
is decoded correctly or incorrectly. The errors also form the
basis for a qualitative analysis. List B contains 42 words which
vary systematically along the dimensions of length (three, five and
seven letters) and regularity of their pronunciation (an index of
the degree to which the letters contained in a word receive a
conventional pronunciation).

Assessing the Orthographical Strategy

The test consists of 40 words which vary in regard to visual and linguistical dimensions. Each word is presented for a short stimulus time (100 milliseconds). The short exposure time makes it nearly impossible for the reader to employ the phonological strategy, and the result of the decoding therefore reflects primarily the ability to read orthographically. A qualitative analysis of the errors is made on the basis of the following categories: 1) visual paralexia, 2) phonological paralexia, 3) semantic paralexia, 4) the addition or deletion of suffixes, 5) neologisms and 6) other types of errors.

Assessing the Phonological Strategy

This test contains 42 non-words which are presented on the computer screen without any time limit. The non-words vary according to length (three, five or seven letters) and graphemic complexity (consonant clusters or not). When non-words are used as stimuli, the reader cannot employ the orthographical strategy. Non-words have no orthographical identity which can be activated directly through visual stimulation. There is of course the possibility of employing an analogy-strategy if the non-words have an orthography similar to real words. The non-words were, however, designed to foil this. The reaction time and accuracy are registered, and the pupil's method of decoding the non-words is noted.

Assessing the Processes Underlying the Decoding Strategies

The following tests were used to assess the processes underlying the orthographical strategy:

(1) Visual analysis. The test consists of two tasks. The first of these presents a string of letters on the screen, and the reader is asked to determine whether all the letters are the same or if there is one or more of them that are different. The arrays have either seven or eleven letters. The pupil strikes the yes-button if all the letters are alike and the no-button if they are not all alike. This part of the test tells us about the pupil's ability to process letters simultaneously. The statistical program calculates whether the position of the odd letter influences the score or the reaction time. If it takes the pupil longer to answer when the odd letter comes at the end of the array than, say, at the beginning, it indicates that he or she employs a sequential strategy when perceiving letters.

The second task presents two rows of letters simultaneously on the screen, one row above the other. The pupil is asked to decide whether the rows are the same or not. In items wherein the arrays

are different, the position of the different letter varies as in
the first section. It was assumed that if comparison is a serial
self-terminating procedure which progresses from left to right
across the array, then No reaction time will increase as a function
of the position of the odd letter.

(2) Grapheme identification. This test tells whether or not
the reader has acquired grapheme knowledge. Letters are presented
tachistoscopically on the screen, two at a time. The reader is
asked to decide if the letters belong to the same category or not
(for example, r-R or e-r). It is not possible for the reader to
answer correctly solely on the basis of a visual comparison of the
form of the letters.

(3) Visual-orthographical word-recognition (lexical decisions). Words and non-words are presented tachistoscopically on the
screen. The reader is asked to determine whether the stimulus is a
word or a non-word. The non-words are constructed in such a way
that they are either orthographically acceptable or unacceptable.
The acceptable non-words are combinations of letters that are
plausible, they might have been real words (example: SLART). The
orthographically unacceptable non-words are composed of letters
chosen at random (example: RTBSL). One would expect that the
reader would find it more difficult to discriminate real words from
the orthographically acceptable non-words than from the
unacceptable non-words. If the reader makes as many errors on both
types of non-words, it indicates faulty orthographical knowledge.

(4) Phonological word-retrieval. The ability to retrieve
words phonologically is examined with the aid of a two-part test.
Part one tests phonological retrieval after semantic input, while
part two tests phonological retrieval after orthographical input.
In part one, 20 pictures of objects are shown one at a time on the
screen. The reader is asked to name them as quickly as possible.
The answers are scored and the reaction time is registered. In
part two, the test-giver reads a word aloud. Then another word is
presented tachistoscopically on the screen, and the subject is
asked to determine whether or not the two words rhyme.

(5) Semantic activation. 40 words are presented on the screen
in a random order. 20 of the words belong to the category "things
that grow", while the other 20 are "things that do not grow". The
reader is asked to perform a semantic categorization and assign
each word to one of the categories. The computer registers the
score and the reaction time.

Assessing the Processes Behind the Phonological Strategy

The tests assess the processes that are important for the
employment of the phonological strategy. The phonological strategy
is built upon these processes: (1) Visual analysis, (2) grapheme

identification, (6) orthographical parsing, (7) phonological recoding (prelexical) and (8) phonological synthesis. The first two processes were discussed in connection with the orthographical strategy.

(6) Orthographical parsing. This test consists of two tasks: a) finding the syllables and morphemes in words, and b) finding the syllables in non-words. The reader is presented with words and non-words and is asked to divide them into syllables and/or morphemes. The accuracy score and reaction time is registered.

(7) Phonological recoding. In this test, all the letters of the alphabet are presented on the screen, both as capital letters and as small letters. The pupil is asked to say what sound they make. The accuracy score and the reaction time is registered.

(8) Phonological synthesis. This test consists of ten words and ten non-words. The phonemes in each item are pronounced separately by the test-giver, and the subject has to synthesize them. The words and non-words vary in degree of graphemic-phonological complexity.

This test battery was used assessing two dyslexic children in grade 3. The test results of those two dyslexic subjects are compared with the data obtained among all the children (80) in 3 randomly selected classes, grade level 3, in Stavanger, Norway.

CASES OLE AND PER

Ole and Per were diagnosed by their school psychologists as suffering from **auditory dyslexia**. An assessment of their ability to employ reading strategies (tests 1, 2 and 3) makes it clear that both boys master the orthographical strategy but have difficulty employing the phonological strategy .

Ole's problem with the phonological strategy can be traced primarily to a basic weakening of the ability to perform phonological synthesis, while Per's problem seems to be the result of poorly automated letter knowledge. Both pupils have in addition a minor weakening of the ability to parse letter string efficiently.

Ole scored significantly poorer on the verbal section of the WISC-R than on the performance section (the difference was 28). He also had a retarded language development and still has some difficulty articulating correctly phonologically complicated words. It is therefore reasonable to assume that Ole's reading disorder primarily is the result of a general linguistic and/or meta-linguistic deficency. We found that Ole's reading disorder was precedented in the family history.

Per has difficulty with phonological recoding. This is seen clearest in the testing of his ability to read letters. He confuses b–d–p and has a slow reaction time for all categories of letters. This shows clearly that his knowledge of letters is not sufficiently automated. This poor automation leads to difficulty with phonological synthesis, even though he does not have any weakening of the synthesizing process itself. There are some indications that Per has specific problems associating orthographical segments with their phonological equivalents. When reading aloud words presented tachistoscopically, he read significantly better content words than function words, and concrete nouns were easier for him to decode than abstract nouns. As noted, this indicates a weakening of the connection between the orthographical and phonological identities of words. When decoding content words, Per can support the phonological encoding with semantic information. When reading letters and function words he does not have the semantic clues to rely on, and his errors and slow reaction time reveal his disorder.

It was reported that Per had difficulty learning the names of the colors, and that he is not progressing normally as regards the learning of the multiplication table by rote. Moreover, we found that he scored significantly poorer on the coding test than on the other sections of the WISC–R. We know that a low score on the coding test often occurs with persons suffering from dyslexia, and that difficulties with the names of colors and with the multiplication table are not unusual for people with dyslexic problems. We therefore pose the question here if there might be some connection between a weakening of the association of the orthographical and phonological identities and the problems with other types of associative learning mentioned above.

Ole and Per were classified as auditory dyslexics. The process analysis revealed that the reading disorders these two pupils are experiencing, which at first seem quite similar, can be traced to two different causes: a weakening of the phonological recoding and a weakening in the phonological synthesis. The result seems to support our presumption that dyslexic subjects may possess individual processing characteristics, and that a classification in sub-types of dyslexia does not provide sufficient information. On these grounds, we would argue that a more sensible procedure to adopt in the analysis of dyslexia is one in which descriptions are given for each individual, indicating which elements of the processing system are present or limited. Such descriptions should provide a good knowledge basis to build upon when planning remedial programs.

REFERENCES

Caramazza, A. (1984). The logic of neuropsychological research and the problems of patient classification in aphasia. Brain and Language, 21, 9-20.

Coltheart, M. (1981). Disorders of reading and their implications for models of normal reading. Visible Language, 15, 245-86.

Coltheart, M. (1984). Acquired dyslexias and normal reading. In Dyslexia: A global issue. (eds. R.N. Malatesha and H.A. Whitaker). Martinus Nijhoff, Haag.

Ellis, A.W. (1987). Intimations of modularity, or, the modularity of Mind: Doing cognitive neuropsychology without syndromes. In The cognitive neuropsychology of language. (eds. M. Coltheart, G. Sartori and R. Job). Lawrence Erlbaum, London.

Gough, P.B. and Tunmer, W.E. (1986). Decoding, reading, and reading disability. Remedial and Special Education, 7 , 6-10.

Høien, T. (1986). Diagnosing Word Decoding Problems: A Process-analytic viewpoint. In Aspects in Reading. (ed. K. Trondheim). Danavox Symposium, Copenhagen.

Høien, T. (1988). Processanalytic decoding test (only in Norwegian version). Stavanger Teacher College, Stavanger.

Luria, A.R. (1976). Basic problems of neurolinguistics. Mouton, Haag.

Marshall, J.C. (1984). Toward a rational taxonomy of the acquired dyslexias. In Dyslexia: A global issue. (eds. R.N. Malatesha and H.A. Whitaker). Martin Nijhoff, Haag.

Patterson, K.E. (1982). The relation between reading and phono-logical coding: Further neuropsychological observations. In Normality and pathology in cognitive functions. (ed. A.W. Ellis). Academic Press, London.

Patterson, K.E., Marshall, J.C. and Coltheart, M (1985). Surface dyslexia. Neuropsychological and cognitive studies of phonological reading. Lawrence Erlbaum, London.

Seymour, P.H.K. (1987). Developmental dyslexia: A cognitive experimental analysis. In The cognitive neuropsychology of language. (eds. M. Coltheart, G. Sartori and R. Job). Lawrence Erlbaum, London.

Shallice, T. (1981). Neuropsychological impairment of cognitive processes. Br. Med. Bull., 37, 187-92.

Stanovich, K.E. (1982). Individual differences in the cognitive process of reading. Journal of Learning Disabilities, 15, 485–493.

Taylor, I. and Taylor, M.M. (1983). The psychology of reading. Academic Press, New York.

Warrington, E.K. & Shallice, T. (1980). Wordform dyslexia. Brain, 103, 191–211.

V
Visual Analysis and Saccadic Strategies in Reading

23
Comments on Eye Movements

Ragnar Granit

At the 1980 Dyslexia Conference here in Stockholm, John Stein and Susan Fowler presented evidence to the effect that disturbance of oculomotor control is a characteristic feature of dyslexia in children. The elegant new method of recording eye movements, developed in a Polish-Swedish cooperation between Jan Ober and Per Uddén, has confirmed their findings. Thus, at least in a considerable number of cases, the binocular symmetrical eye movements in reading are replaced by a measure of independence of the saccadic patterns in the two eyes.

Recalling now that the eyes have several types of movements at their disposal and that oculomotor control is a precision instrument of a high order, the first question to raise is whether merely the saccadic movements are disturbed in dyslectics and thus are leaving the other types of movement intact. This seems to me an urgent question to answer by experimentation whether disturbed oculomotor control is a causative factor in dyslexia or merely one of its symptoms.

An easy introduction to ocular motility as a controlled event is to consider the reflex instalment of foveal vision after a turn of the head, the so-called VOR, the vestibulo-ocular reflex. This is what happens: the velocity-sensitive semicircular canals respond with a burst of impulses fed forward to the vestibular nuclei and thence to oculomotor nuclei which respond purposively by eliciting a corrective muscular contraction restoring foveal vision. Since the velocity-responsive burst precedes the excursion of the eyeball, how is the correcting controller in the brain informed about the final position of the eyeball in the head movement? The forward process is lacking a feedback to the vestibular nuclei. Masai Ito in his monumental monograph on the cerebellum says he does not know, but refers to the important centre for ocular motility in the reticular formation as a possibility. The idea at the back is that side-path activity may lengthen the discharge time beyond the vestibular burst-time.

Ito himself has direct evidence for a side-path through the cerebellar flocculus acting through the climbing fibres which are carrying information on the retinal slip to the cerebellar oculomotor output. However, while this side-path does exist and is acting in the postulated way, floccular ablations do not lead to a breakdown of the VOR, only to some reduction of its gain. Another idea is that the VOR-forward process converting head position to corrected eye position is provided with an internal integrator prolonging the effect of the brief burst from the velocity signalling vestibulum.

The extensive literature on the VOR refers to experiments on guinea pigs, cats, and monkeys, all of them with a poor outfit of muscular receptors compared with man and ungulates. Our eye muscles as well as neck muscles cooperating in the VOR belong to the spindle-richest in the body. And we have long had evidence from an Oxford team consisting of Sybil Cooper, Daniel, and Whitteridge that the spindle afferents project to all the sites that could be relevant for localization of oculomotility. The message from the spindles is maintained throughout the muscular act, their sensitivity is adjustable by the gamma motor control system and, above all, they are much faster in action than any retinal signal from the slip that has to spend some 20 msec in traversing the neuronal layers of the retinal centre.

The inventiveness of the model-makers is spurred into top performance by their efforts to neglect the well-documented existence of a gamma-spindle system that evolution has developed into such perfection in man. It is now 35 years since Kaada and I showed it to be at the disposal of most of the central stations engaged in motricity. Under gamma control the muscle spindles have proved to be extremely sensitive and to operate in conjunction with motor acts, a principle known as alfa-gamma linkage for limb muscles.

Those willing to accord the afferent spindle message a role in slow motor acts are likely to make saccades an exception. But in this regard there is a basic likeness between VOR and saccades. The saccadic movement does not either possess that component of maintenance of motor activity to the end point of a saccade, that we found characterizing VOR. Again there arises the same question: how does the brief saccadic burst of spikes inform motor control centres of the range of the resulting movement of the eyeball? Again the model-makers are willing to provide us with answers based on side-paths and integrators. Again I will remind them of the possibility that fast and highly sensitive information arriving from the ocular spindle afferents, which avoid the delay passage through the retinal nervous centre, should be perfectly capable of solving the problem.

If the slow message across the retinal slip actually is the prime message, why is it so unimportant where it is proved to exist, by Ito, as entering the flocculus? And what about colliculus superior shown by Miss Apter already in 1945 to possess a point-to-point projection of the retina. To this structure arrive impulses from the oculomotor afferents, from the neck afferents, from the frontal eye fields. Ablation of colliculus superior seriously impaired the generation of unrewarded saccades while only a minimal deficit was induced in reward-conditioned saccades.

Here now I have presented three cases in which the postulated information from the range of the retinal slip has (i) been proved to exist but not to be relevant for saccadic control, (ii) been postulated to exist but shown irrelevant for reward-conditioned saccades while (iii) required for unrewarded saccades. There is more that meets the eye in these complexities. To me they suggest that the information from the retinal slip is too slow to be decisive in a process of fast control.

The fast muscular information from the spindles is widely available in centres controlling ocular motility. It seems to me quite likely to have established any number of connexions with motor acts simply by being practiced daily in the life of the individual. In ocular motricity subconscious purposive learning is required to explain records such as those of Yarbus in which saccadic movements are shown to explore the human face by concentrating on contours and other salient markers. We are not aware of the whole systematic process of saccadic exploration at top gamma-spindle sensitivity.

References

Apter, J.T. (1945). Projection of the retina on Superior colliculus cats. J.Neurophysiol., 8, 123-134.

Cooper, S. and Daniel, P.M. (1949). Muscle spindles in human extrinsic eye muscles. Brain, 72, 1-24.

Cooper, S., Daniel, P. and Whitteridge, D. (1953). Nerve impulses in the brain stem of the goat. Short-latency response obtained by stretching the extrinsic eye muscles and jaw muscles. J.Physiol., 120, 471-490.

Granit, R. and Kaada, B.R. (1952). Influence of stimulation of central nervous structures on muscle spindles in cat. Acta Physiol. Scand., 27, 130-160.

Ito, M. (1984). The Cerebellum and Neural Control. Raven Press, New York, 580 pp.

Stein, J.F. and Fowler, S. (1982). In Dyslexia, Wenner-Gren Center Symposium 1980, Stockholm. (ed. Y. Zotterman). Pergamon Press, Oxford, p. 49-63.

Whitteridge, D. (1959). The effect of stimulation of intrafusal muscle fibres on sensitivity to stretch of extraocular muscle spindles. Quart.J.Exp.Physiol., 44, 385-393.

Yarbus, A.I. (1967). Eye Movement and Vision. Plenum Press, New York.

24
Hemispheric Interactions in Saccadic Responses to Bihemifield Stimuli

Yehoshua Y. Zeevi

INTRODUCTION

The nonuniform sampling and processing (Fig. 1), with the highest density in central fovea vision and gradual decrease with eccentricity, necessitate sequential foveation of areas of interest or newly-appearing targets. Consequently, measurements of eye movement responses to simple nonlexigraphic stimuli provide effective means for studying visual-oculomotor mechanisms involved in the acquisition of visual information. Indeed, major contributions to the understanding of saccadic programming involved in the programming of such mechanisms have resulted from studies employing single point stimuli (Westheimer, 1954; Young and Stark, 1963; Robinson, 1973).

Considering the unilateral retinotopic mapping of the visual field, in a contralateral mode of organization, it is of special interest in the context of the Rodin Symposium to determine how the segregation of visual information from the left and right hemifields affects the interactions which ultimately result in saccadic responses. In order to place the image of a visual target on the fovea, the saccadic system responds to a spatial error signal comprised of retinal error and information concerning extraretinal eye position (Young, 1962; Robinson, 1973, 1975; Hallett and Lightstone, 1976 a,b; Mays and Sparks, 1980). What happens then when there is more than one point target and hence more than one spatial (position) error signal? Are there built-in preferences that will select one of the point stimuli and give it a higher priority so that the response will be toward it? This question becomes most interesting when a bihemifield stimulus is presented symmetrically about the visual axis.

To better understand the interhemispheric interactions that take place prior to the execution of a saccade, we focus on lateral (direction) and eccentricity-dependent preferences revealed by experiments employing unihemifield and bihemifield dual-target stimuli. We first review some relevant results of experiments with double-step (single target) stimuli, and then present the results of experiments with dual-target stimuli. The latter were originally conducted at the Massachusetts Institute of Technology (Wetzel and Zeevi, 1982; Zeevi et al. 1983, 1988) and then further elaborated at the Technion (Hason and Zeevi, 1986; Venis et al. 1988; Venis and Zeevi, 1988) to investigate the interactions between laterality- and eccentricity-dependent preferences. Finally we comment on the relevance of these studies to the understanding of a certain type of developmental dyslexia (Hermann et al. 1986a,b).

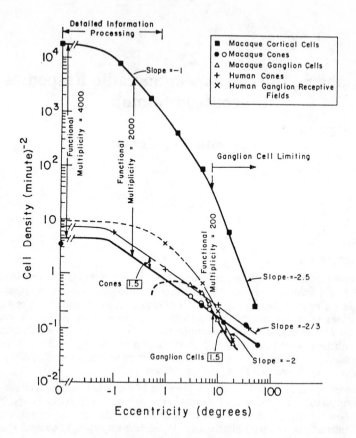

Fig. 1.   Distribution of cells over the visual field in primates indicating nonuniform
           sampling (by cones) and processing (at the level of cortical cells), with the
           highest density in the central fovea and the corresponding cortical area
           (Kronauer and Zeevi, 1985).

Double-Step Stimuli

Many previous studies have used double-step stimuli in which a point target is displaced to a given position and remains there for a period of time before being displaced to
another position (Fig. 2a). When the second step involves a displacement of the target
from one visual hemifield to the other, the trajectory is termed "crossed". Wheeless et al.
(1966), Komoda et al. (1973), Levy-Schoen and Blanc-Garin (1974), Becker and Jurgens
(1974, 1979), and Findlay and Harris (1984) used crossed double-step stimuli to study
bihemispheric interactions. They found that if the response is to the second step, its latency
is slightly greater than the latency to single targets. Becker and Jurgens (1974, 1979)
extracted from their experiments an amplitude transfer function (ATF) which describes the
amplitude of the saccadic response. To construct the ATF, they measured the time interval
from the appearance of the second step until the start of the saccadic response,   and found

that this time interval (denoted by D in Fig. 2a) is correlated with the saccadic response direction and amplitude. Findlay and Harris (1984), and Deubel et al. (1984) have since confirmed the validity of the ATF, and defined its characteristics and temporal position.

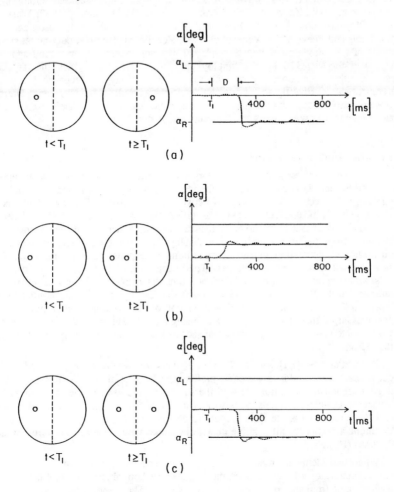

Fig. 2   Schematic representation of the spatial (left) and temporal (right) structure of visual stimuli.

    a)   A "crossed" double-step stimulus in which at $t=0$ the point is translated from the primary gaze position to the left, and at time $t < 200$ ms it is crossed to the right hemifield.

    b)   A unihemifield dual target stimulus with a delayed inner (closer to the fovea) target.

    c)   A bihemifield dual target stimulus, illustrating a response to the delayed target. This type of response indicates preference to the right.

SACCADIC RESPONSES TO DUAL TARGETS

Experiments with stimuli composed of as few as two point-light sources are sufficient to explore interesting organizational principles of the visual-oculomotor system
(Levy-Schoen, 1969; Zeevi and Peli, 1979; Zeevi et al., 1979; Findlay, 1982; Wetzel and
Zeevi, 1982; Zeevi, et al. 1983; Ottes, et al. 1984; Deubel et al. 1984; Hason and Zeevi,
1986; Venis and Zeevi, 1988; Venis et al. 1988; Zeevi et al. 1988). A dual-target stimulus
consists of two single-point targets displayed, but not necessarily appearing simultaneously, over the visual field. We employ dual-target stimuli in which the targets are
presented either simultaneously or with one of them delayed. Eccentricity-dependent
preferences were investigated using unihemifield stimuli (Fig. 2b), and laterality-
dependent preferences as well as possible asymmetries in the dynamics of interhemispheric interactions were assessed using bihemifield stimuli (Fig. 2c).

Dual Target Unihemifield Stimuli

Two classes of responses to dual-target unihemifield stimuli have been reported.
Findlay (1982) and Deubel et al. (1984) found that their subjects saccaded unimodally to a
point slightly less eccentric than midway between the two targets. Findlay called this type
of response the "global effect". Zeevi et al. (1983), Hason and Zeevi (1986) and Zeevi et
al. (1988) observed that their subjects saccaded towards either one of the two targets but
exhibited a strong preference for the target displayed closer to the initial fixation point (i.e.
the inner target), generating an asymmetrical bimodal response pattern. Ottes et al. (1984)
were able to elicit both response modes. Their subjects exhibited unimodal responses for
targets with a small separation (10 deg) and bimodal responses for targets with a large
separation (30 deg). Venis et al. (1988) found that the type of response is idiosyncratic.
Findlay (1982) noticed that the standard deviation of the amplitudes of responses to two
targets was larger than that of responses to a single target. He found that one contribution
to this was a tendency for the amplitude of saccades to two targets to vary with the latency
of the saccade.

Zeevi et al. (1983), Hason and Zeevi (1986) and Zeevi et al. (1988) delayed the inner
target appearance in order to offset its preference. Zeevi et al. (1983, 1988) found that,
with simultaneous presentation, 95% of the saccades were towards the inner target. With
the inner target delayed 100ms, 50% were towards the inner target, and, at 160ms delay,
only 10% were towards the inner target. Since for zero delay the preference is already
95%, the data points for all positive delays (i.e. inner target leading) are virtually at the
100% level (Fig. 3).

When two identical unihemifield targets appear simultaneously or with short (less
than 40ms) intertarget delay, the saccadic response has normal latency, i.e. it is not significantly different from that of a single target response. The response latency is not influenced by the separation of the targets (Findlay, 1982; Hason and Zeevi, 1985), nor by their
brightness (Deubel et al. 1984; Ottes et al. 1984), but it is influenced by the relative
appearance time of the targets. Zeevi et al. (1983) found a significant increase in response
latency (both inner and outer target responses combined and latency always measured from
the leading target's appearance) of about 20ms when the inner target was delayed from 60
to 120ms. Hason and Zeevi (1985) found that the saccadic latency to the lagging target,
measured from its appearance time, linearly decreased with increasing intertarget delay, up
to approximately 40ms, at an intertarget delay of 100ms.

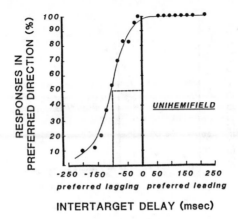

preferred lagging   preferred leading

INTERTARGET DELAY (msec)

Fig. 3   Percentage of saccadic responses to preferred (inner) target as a function of
the intertarget delay (T_1 illustrated in Fig. 2b). Positive delays indicate that
the preferred target appeared first.

Dual Target Bihemifield Stimuli

A bihemifield stimulus consists of a single target that bifurcates into two targets, one
appearing in each hemifield (Fig. 1c). Four factors are known to influence the target to
which the subject responds: the subject's directional preference; relative target eccentricity; relative target brightness; and relative appearance time of the targets. Findlay (1980,
1982), Zeevi et al. (1983, 1988), Hason and Zeevi (1985) and Venis et al. (1988) have studied the influence of these factors on saccadic response. If a target bifurcates into two
simultaneously appearing targets of equal eccentricity and brightness, subjects exhibit a
directional preference which is manifested in a higher probability of response to the preferred hemifield, ranging from 60 to 100% (depending on the subject). The mean percentage of response in the preferred direction for all (nondyslexic) subjects was about 80%.
No relationship has been found between this preference and handedness or other aspects of
hemispheric dominance. For this reason data were analyzed with respect to response
preference rather than absolute direction.

Several investigators have studied how various stimulus-related factors influence
directional preference. Findlay (1980, 1983) showed that it is possible to offset directional
preference by increasing the size (effectively the brightness) of the target projected onto
the non-preferred hemifield, or by decreasing its eccentricity. Hason and Zeevi (1985) confirmed that directional preference can be offset by decreasing the eccentricity of the target
projected onto the non-preferred hemifield. Zeevi et al. (1983, 1988) demonstrated that the
percent of preference varied as a function of the delay between the appearance of the two
targets. Shown in Fig. 4 is the percentage of responses in the preferred direction plotted as
a function of the delay between the leading and lagging targets (with respect to the preferred direction). The continuous curve was drawn by eye through the data and intersects
the ordinate (representing zero delay) at about 80%. This is representative of the mean
response preference obtained in one set of experiments with six subjects. The amount this
curve must be shifted along the delay axis in order for it to intersect the ordinate at the
chance level of 50% is approximately 50ms (see dashed lines).

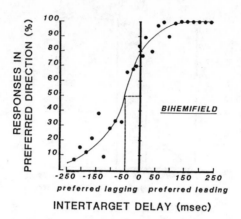

Fig. 4   Percentage of saccadic responses in the preferred direction plotted as a func-
          tion of intertarget delay (T_1 illustrated in Fig. 2c). Positive delays indicate
          that the target presented in the preferred visual hemifield appeared first. The
          dashed lines indicate the delay required to offset the directional preference
          (Zeevi et al. 1988).

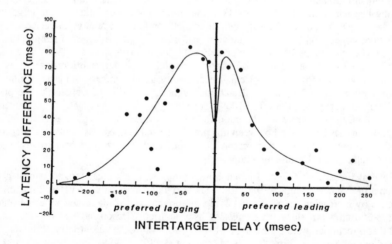

Fig. 5   Latency difference, indicating the increase in response time to bihemifield
          stimuli as compared to latency of response to single targets, plotted as a
          function of intertarget delay. Positive delays indicate that the target present-
          ed in the preferred hemifield appeared first. The data are pooled over both
          the preferred and nonpreferred direction of responses (Zeevi et al. 1988).

Compared with responses to single targets, there was an increase in latency when two targets were presented — one in each visual hemifield. It should be noted that for some subjects there was a small but statistically significant difference in response latency to single targets presented to the left and right hemifields. Therefore, the latency of the rightward and leftward responses to the bihemifield targets were corrected by subtracting from them the latency to the single targets presented in the corresponding direction. In all cases latency was measured from the onset of the leading target.

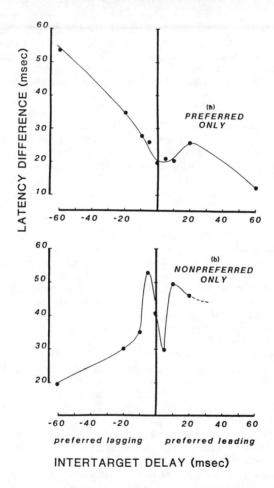

Fig. 6   Latency difference, indicating the increase in response time to bihemifield stimuli as compared to single targets, is plotted as a function of the intertarget delay (T_1 illustrated in Fig. 2c). Positive delays indicate that the target presented in the preferred hemifield appeared first. Shown in (a) and (b) are response latency data in the preferred and nonpreferred directions, respectively (Zeevi et al. 1988).

Shown in Fig. 5 is the latency increase, relative to the single target condition, as a function of the delay between the targets presented in the right and left visual hemifields. The responses in both the preferred and nonpreferred directions are combined. Note that all data points above the abscissa indicate increases in latency relative to the responses to single targets. The data point at zero delay indicates a latency increase of about 40ms in response to simultaneously presented bihemifield stimuli. This increase in latency, compared with response to unihemifield single or simultaneously presented dual target, was found to be highly significant. When the referred target leads (right side of Fig. 5), intertarget delays of up to 40ms give rise to an additional significant increase in response latency beyond that at zero delay. When the nonpreferred target leads (left side of Fig. 5), the additional increase for short delays is also significant. Further, the increase for short delays in this condition appears to extend over a somewhat wider range of intertarget delays than is the case when the preferred target leads. For longer delays in either direction the difference in response latency decreases and gradually approaches the single target response time represented by the abscissa.

The response preference data of Fig. 4 is suggestive of asymmetries in lateral interaction between the visual hemispheres. Such asymmetries are indeed supported by a different influence of the preferred target on the response latency to the nonpreferred target than vice versa (Fig. 6). Statistical analysis of the data shown in Fig. 6 indicates that responses in the nonpreferred direction have a significantly increased latency (of about 20ms for this group of subjects) compared to those in the preferred direction.

DISCUSSION

The data of Fig. 4 show that when the stimuli bifurcate such that the left and right field targets appear simultaneously, subjects exhibit a preference in one direction. The population average for this preference was found to be 84% for a group of eight subjects (Zeevi et al. 1983), 83% for a group of six subjects (Zeevi et al. 1988) and 72% for a group of five subjects (Venis et al. 1988). This laterality-dependent preference was in neither group found to be related to handedness. A delay of approximately 50ms in the presentation of the preferred target was required, for the group of subjects whose response data are shown in Fig. 4, to eliminate the preference shown by these subjects. This result indicates that in the sequence of events occurring prior to the execution of a saccade, about 50ms are allocated for decisions concerning direction of response. That is to say, to reach the chance level, representing an equal probability of response in either direction, requires that the stimulus in the preferred direction be delayed by this duration. It might be noted that conclusions of this kind may be drawn also from double-step experiments in which only a single target is on at any one time (Wheeless, Boynton and Cohen, 1966; Levy-Schoen and Blanc-Garin, 1974; Becker and Jurgens, 1979). The present data establish that analogous mechanisms are active when the stimuli are projected to both hemispheres simultaneously. In the unihemifield condition there is a strong preference to the inner target. As is the case for the preference in the bihemifield condition, the unihemifield preference can be eliminated by delaying the onset of the preferred target. The delay is about 100ms and is longer than the analogous delay required in the bihemifield condition presumably because an additional decision concerning response amplitude has to be made in this case (cf. Young, 1981).

The finding, that when two targets are distributed over both hemifields and presented simultaneously, there is a significant increase in response latency to the dual target as compared to the single target, is consistent with those of Levy-Schoen (1969) and Findlay (1982). A comparison of these results with those obtained in response to unihemifield dual-target stimuli suggests that the latency increase in the case of bihemifield stimuli is not due to the number of targets but rather to the fact that they are distributed over both hemifields. However, Ottes et al. (1984) showed that when stimuli are presented eccentrically over one hemifield and 15 deg from the horizontal meridian, there is an increase in latency even in the case of unihemifield stimulation. It is reasonable to assume that the interhemispheric interaction resulting from bihemifield stimulation requires extra processing time as compared to that required for unihemifield stimuli, but in view of Ottes et al. (1984) finding, it is unclear as to what spatial factors, other than distribution over both hemispheres, demand extra processing and why.

When the bihemifield stimulus is presented with a short intertarget delay there is a further increase in latency beyond that just described for simultaneously presented bihemifield stimuli. The increase in response latency to either the preferred or nonpreferred target occurs only if the second target precedes or follows the first by less than 60ms. The response latency data of Fig. 5 thus display two peaks which may result from the combined effect of two mechanisms.

The difference in shape of the lobes to the left and right of the ordinate in Fig. 5 is taken as evidence of an asymmetry in the effect of the disturbing target on responses in the preferred and nonpreferred directions. Separation of responses according to their direction show that the effect of bihemifield bifurcation on response latency in the nonpreferred direction is about twice as large as it is on responses in the preferred direction. The data in the lefthand portion of Figs. 6a and 6b show that the interaction occurring beyond the critical period is primarily due to the disturbing effect of the target, in the nonpreferred hemifield, on responses in the preferred direction (reflected by the latency of response in the preferred direction when the target to which the subject responds lags by 60ms (left-most data point in Fig. 6a). To complete this comparison would require data points for responses in the nonpreferred direction when the target in the preferred direction leads by 60ms. However, such responses are extremely rare and, in fact, none were obtained in the present study. It might be argued that the asymmetries in Fig. 6 discussed above could be due to asymmetries in saccadic response to even single stimuli presented in either the left or right visual fields (Rayner, 1978). We reiterate, therefore, that these data have been corrected for the intrasubject difference between left and right response latencies to single targets. Thus it is concluded that the existence of a response preference is due to interhemispheric interaction.

Considering the task of responding in one direction when targets are presented in both hemifields (thus stimulating both hemispheres), it is obvious that one hemisphere must predominate and suppress the counterhemisphere. We assert that the mutual interaction of the two hemispheres in this mode of operation requires inhibitory signals for suppression of one or the other hemisphere (Fig. 7). This concept was previously proposed in the context of interhemispheric interaction in higher cognitive functions and the orienting control mechanism (Kinsbourne, 1972, 1973), and a variant of it is incorporated into the model proposed by Becker and Jurgens (1979). According to Kinsbourne (1973), "Each hemisphere is in a reciprocal inhibitory relationship with the other, and the paired midbrain output facilities have a similar reciprocal relationship". Such a reciprocal inhibitory interaction could explain the non-monotonic dependence of latency difference on intertarget delay (see Figs. 5 and 6) if it is assumed to be one of two underlying mechanisms contributing to the form of the curve — the second being related to the probabilistic nature of the response preference depicted in Fig. 4. Referring again to the data of Figs. 5 and 6, the response latency for short intertarget delays is greater than that for simultaneously presented targets. This increase in latency difference can be explained by postulating an increase in the disturbing effect (i.e. interference) of the counterhemisphere on the hemisphere and midbrain controlling the response. The time course of the postulated interhemispheric interaction may be determined by dynamics analogous to those arising from mutual inhibition in simple neural networks (cf. Ratliff, 1965). It should be noted that the interference is greatest when the competing target appears within the critical period during which response direction is decided. The asymptotic decline in response difference towards the single target latency may be attributed to the fact that the critical period is not a fixed quantity but is instead probabilistic in nature. If mutual inhibitory interactions of the type described above are, in fact, involved in the processing of bihemifield visual stimuli, then one must conclude that there exists asymmetry in the inhibitory signals transmitted between the two hemispheres and paired midbrain facilities.

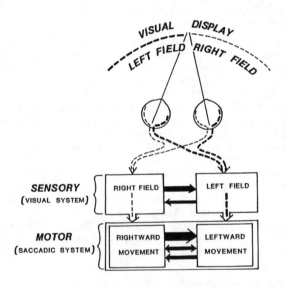

Fig. 7   A schematic diagram illustrating asymmetries in inhibitory lateral interactions between the hemispheres and paired midbrain facilities controlling saccadic responses. Asymmetries are depicted by arrows of various sizes.

A preliminary study with a small group of developmental dyslexics shows that response to simultaneous symmetric bihemifield stimulation lacks normal strong laterality in dyslexics. Also, the latency of responses to such bihemifield stimuli is significantly prolonged in dyslexics, while their responses to single targets are normal (Hermann et al. 1986a,b). This finding suggests that in addition to diminished lateralized specialization, interhemispheric coordination may also be altered in a developmental form of dyslexia. If this preliminary finding is further established, our paradigm may enrich the repertoire of objective techniques available to the clinician in his diagnosis of a certain type of dyslexia.

REFERENCES

Becker, W. and Jurgens, R. (1979). An Analysis of the Saccadic System by Means of Double Step Stimuli. Vision Res., 19, 967-983.

Deubel, H., Wolf, W. and Hausk, G. (1984). In: *Theoretical and Applied Aspects of Eye Movement Research.* (eds. A.G. Gale and F. Johnson). Elsevier Science, North Holland.

Findlay, J.M. (1982). Global Visual Processing for Saccadic Eye Movement. Vision Res., 22, 1033-1045.

Findlay, J.M. (1983). Visual Information Processing for Saccadic Eye Movements. In: *Spatially Oriented Behavior.* (eds. A. Hein and M. Jeannerod). Springer Verlag, New York.

Hallett, P.E. and Lightstone, A.D. (1976a). Saccadic Eye Movements Due to Stimuli Triggered During Prior Saccades. Vision Res., 16, 99-106.

Hallett, P.E. and Lightstone, A.D. (1976b). Saccadic Eye Movements to Flashed Targets. Vision Res., 16, 107-114.

Hason, B. and Zeevi, Y.Y. (1986). Interactions Between Laterality and Eccentricity-Dependent Priorities in Programming of a Saccade. EE Report, Technion, Haifa.

Hermann, H.T., Sonnabend, N.L. and Zeevi, Y.Y. (1986). Interhemispheric Coordination is Compromised in Subjects with Developmental Dyslexia. Cortex, 22, 337-358.

Hermann, H.T., Sonnabend, N.L. and Zeevi, Y.Y. (1986). Bihemifield Visual Stimulation Reveals Reduced Lateral Bias in Dyslexia. Ann. of Dyslexia, 86, 154-175.

Kinsbourne, M. (1972). Eye and Head Turning Indicates Cerebral Lateralization, Science, 176, 539-541.

Kinsbourne, M. (1973). The Control of Attention by Interactions Between the Cerebral Hemispheres. In: *Attention and Performance IV.* (ed. S. Kornblum). Academic Press, New York.

Komoda, M.K., Festinger, L., Phillips, L.J., Duckman, R.H. and Young, R.A. (1973). Some Observations Concerning Saccadic Eye Movements. Vision Res., 13, 1009-1020.

Kronauer, R.E. and Zeevi, Y.Y. (1985). Reorganization and Diversification of Signals in Vision IEEE Trans. SMC-15, 91-101.

Levy-Schoen, A. (1969). Determination et Latence de la Response Oculomotrice a Deux Stimulus. L'Annee Psychol., 69, 373-392,

Levy-Schoen, A. and Blanc-Garin, J. (1974). On Oculomotor Programming and Perception. Brain Res., 71, 443-450.

Mays, L.E. and Sparks, D.L. (1980). Saccades are Spatially, Not Retinocentrically, Coded. Science, 208, 1163-1165.

Ottes, F.P., Van Gisbergen, J.A.M. and Eggermont, J.J. (1984). Metrics of Saccade Responses to Visual Double Stimuli: Two Different Modes. Vision Res., 24, 1169-1179.

Ratliff, F. (1965). *Mach Bands: Quantitative Studies on Neural Networks in the Retina.* Holden-Day, San Francisco.

Rayner, K. (1978). Eye Movement Latency for Parafoveally Presented Words. Bull. Psychonomic Soc., 11, 13-16.

Robinson, D.A. (1973). Models of the Saccadic Eye Movement Control System. Kybernetik 14, 71-83.

Robinson, D.A. (1975). Oculomotor Control Signals. In: *Basic Mechanisms of Ocular Motility and Their Clinical Implications.* (eds. P. Bach-y-Rita and G. Lennerstrand). Pergamon, Oxford.

Stark, L. (1968). *Neurological Control Systems.* Plenum Press, New York.

Venis, M.A. and Zeevi, Y.Y. (1988). Timing of Events in Saccadic Responses: A Model. EE Report, Technion, Haifa.

Venis, M.A. and Zeevi, Y.Y. and Hason, B. (1988). Saccadic Responses to Two-Point Stimuli. EE Report, Technion, Haifa.

Westheimer, G. (1954). Eye Movement Responses to a Horizontally Moving Visual Stimulus. Archs. Ophthal., 52, 932-941.

Wetzel, P.A. and Zeevi, Y.Y. (1982). Eye-Movement Responses to Unidirectional and Bidirectional Bifurcating Targets. J. Opt. Soc. Am., 72, 1798.

Wheeless, L.L. Jr., Boynton, R.M. and Cohen, G.H. (1966). Eye-Movement Responses to Step and Pulse-Step Stimuli. J. Opt. Soc. Am., 56, 956-960.

Young, L.R. (1962). A Sampled Data Model for Eye Tracking Movements. Sc.D. Thesis, Massachusetts Institute of Technology.

Young, L.R. and Stark, L. (1963). A Discrete Model for Eye Tracking Movements. IEEE Trans. MIL., 7, 113-115.

Young, L.R. (1981). The Sampled Data Model and Foveal Dead Zone for Saccades, In: *Models of Oculomotor Behavior and Control.* (ed. B.L. Zuber). CRC Press, Boca Raton, Florida.

Zeevi, Y.Y. and Peli, E. (1979). Latency of Peripheral Saccades. J. Opt. Soc. Am., 69, 1274-1279.

Zeevi, Y.Y., Peli, E. and Stark, L. (1979). Study of Eccentric Fixation with Secondary Visual Feedback. J. Opt. Soc. Am., 69, 669-675.

Zeevi, Y.Y., Wetzel, P.A. and Young, L.R. (1983). Temporal Aspects of Eye Movement When Viewing Multiple Targets. AFHRL-TP-83-6, Air Force Human Resources Laboratory, Brooks AFB, Texas.

Zeevi, Y.Y., Wetzel, P.A. and Geri, G.A. (1988). Preferences and Asymmetries in Saccadic Responses to Delayed Bihemifield Stimuli. Vision Res., in press.

25
Sequential Vision and Reading

Göte Nyman

INTRODUCTION

The neural architecture of the visual system seems to be designed for parallel information processing, but its normal operation
relies on effective serial processes. Because the neural sampling
density and spatial sensitivity decrease towards the visual field
periphery, sequential eye movements are needed for optimizing the
collection of accurate spatial information from the whole visual
field. An ideal system using the saccade/fixation sequences might
be such that extracts the critical visual features from the fixated pattern in a minimum time and then executes a fast new saccade
spending only a neglible time in a state of saccadic attenuation.
The visual system parameters whose effects must then be optimized
to obtain the best possible performance, are the speed of saccades,
duration of the fixations, and the size of the foveal window from
which parallel information input is possible.

A saccade is one of the fastest neurally controlled events in
the visual system having the maximum velocity of about 600 deg/sec
for large saccades (Bronstein and Kennard, 1987; Van Opstal and Van
Gisbergen, 1987) which indicates that the saccadic speed is not a
significant capacity limiting factor for sequential vision. The duration of a fixation on the other hand, is relatively long, being in
normal reading about 200 msec on average (McConkie et al., 1985) although the variability can be very large, e.g. from 100 msec to
1000 msec for the same person (Rayner and McConkie, 1977). Single
letters or spatial patterns can be recognized when their duration
is only 50 msec or even less which leaves a considerable time period for the visual processing and the eye movement control. Hence,
the duration of fixations affects critically the fluency of sequential vision and reading. The span of the foveal window within
which the spatial details of a fixated pattern can be recognized
and words identified without eye movements is only about 10 letter
positions for normal text (cf. Rayner and McConkie, 1977), but it
is not well known how different image features are processed in

different parts of the fovea. There is clear evidence that contrast
sensitivity and visual acuity drop towards the visual periphery
(Weymouth, 1958; Koenderink et al., 1978; Virsu and Rovamo, 1979)
but the identification of suprathreshold image features within the
fovea and parafovea is a more complex phenomenon and it is not likely that only one type of a functional window would be used in foveal vision.

The dynamics of the visual sequence are apparently determined
by the optimization of the fixation duration so that the necessary
information can be extracted before the next saccade. These significant features might be, for example, spatial frequency, phase, orientation, or color, or some of their conjunctions. The programming
of the saccade depends on the integration of such feature information. But which image features need to be identified in order for
the visual system to be ready for the input of the next image in
the sequence?

A well-documented and useful way to characterize spatial patterns is to use their spatial frequency content and more specifically the amplitude and phase spectra. The visual system's ability
to process spatial and temporal information has been succesfully
described by this methodology (cf. Campbell and Robson, 1968; Breitmeyer and Ganz, 1977) although one must be careful in generalizing
the psychophysically obtained sensitivity measures to such complex
tasks as reading. However, we have made an observation that the
spatial phase spectrum of the compound sinusoidal gratings that
consist of a sum of two harmonic components, has significant effects on the recognizability of such targets when they are only
briefly presented. The waveform recognition improved monotonically
as a function of the fixation duration but only after a critical
duration the use of free eye movements gave a better performance
than a steady fixation did (Nyman et al., 1986).

To see if the relationship between the duration of fixation and
the timing of the eye movements is a more general property of the
serial processing we used letters instead of the gratings as stimuli. In the experiments reported here we chose to use only the letters "p" and "q" that can be discriminated on the basis of their
mirror symmetry, that is, they have identical power spectra but
different phase spectra.

METHOD AND RESULTS

In the first experiment the subjects fixated at the middle of
two letters or letter strings (see the insets of the figures) which
were separated by a gap of 1 deg or 2.5 deg. Two different experimental conditions were used: fixation and free eye movements, and
the task was to judge whether the two letter strings presented side
by side were identical or not. The order of p:s and q:s in each
string was randomized for each presentation so that the probability
of similar strings occurring was 0.50 and the probability of diff-

erent strings appearing was the same. Thus, guessing would give 50%
correct responses. The string lengths used were 1, 2, and 3 letters
the size of each letter being 0.2 deg x 0.4 deg with a spacing of
0.2 deg. This gave the width of 1 deg for the three-letter string.
The letters were black and on white (P4 phosphor) background that
had the luminance of 20 cd/m². The letter contrast was approximately 70%.

Figure 1 shows the effect of the stimulus duration on the discriminability of the two letter strings when the separating gap was
2.5 deg. Only a mariginal effect of stimulus duration was observed
for the two-letter string and no effect for the one-letter string.
When the three-letter stimuli were presented for 60 msec which was
the shortest duration for them, the subject performed at chance
level. It is well known that the so called lateral masking affects
the discriminability of individual letters in a string (Bouma, 1970).

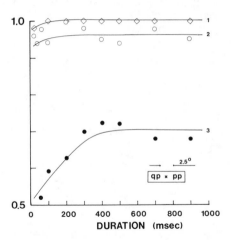

Figure 1. The effect of stimulus duration on the discriminability
of letter strings. The probability of a correct response in this
2AFC experiment is given on the ordinate where 0.50 denotes pure
guessing. The gap width as shown in the inset was 2.5 deg. During
the presentation of the stimuli the subject was not allowed free
eye movements but fixated at the cross between the strings. Notice
the saturation in the performance for the three-letter strings at
about 400 msec.

That this was indeed the case here was confirmed by a control experiment in which the subject fixated at the middle of two single
letters separated by a 5 deg gap. Even at the stimulus duration of
60 msec he could still perfectly discriminate the two letters. Thus
the deterioration in the discriminability of the three-letter string
was not caused by a drop in visual acuity or contrast sensitivity
outside the foveola.

There appears to be a relatively long integration time during
which new information is extracted from the fixated target, however.
This is shown in Figure 1 where the saturation in the discrimination
performance for the three-letter strings occurs as late as about
400 msec from the stimulus onset. As the control experiment showed
the critical individual features of each letter could be extracted
in less than 100 msec. Hence, this 400 msec must be used for processing the feature information from the whole string to form a
stable and ordered representation of the visual pattern. It is not
known which features are typically confused in the letter strings
but the use of mirrored stimuli reveals that the confusions might
be caused by the misjudgement of the feature locations and not by
a lack of sufficient feature information as such.

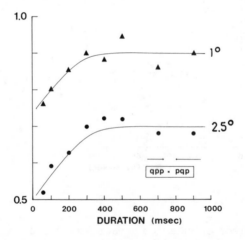

Figure 2. Discriminability of the three-letter strings as a function
of the stimulus duration and the string separation. Notice that decreasing the gap size improves the performance, i.e., weakens the
effect of lateral masking. However, the saturation point remains at
about 400 msec for both gap sizes. The effect is not caused by a
better visibility of individual letters which can still be perfectly
discriminated when presented alone while separated by a gap of 5 deg.

To see if the effect of lateral masking depends on the eccentricity we repeated the previous experiment with a narrower gap
of 1 deg. The results of this experiment are shown in Figure 2
together with the data for the 2.5 deg gap. Only the three-letter
strings were now used.

As can be seen from Figure 2 the two data sets follow a similar
course and the saturation point occurs at about 400 msec for both.
The guessing factor which gives the probability of a correct response when the subject bases his decisions on pure guessing was 0.50
in all the experiments reported here. However, for the 1 deg gap
the data at short durations would suggest a guessing factor of about.
0.75 which indicates that the subject had been able to use additional
information besides guessing, perhaps about the letters located
nearest to the fixation point.

In order to find out how the use of free eye movements affects
the discrimination of the letter strings we repeated the experiment
using the 1 deg gap but now allowing the subject to move his eyes
freely as best he could. Figure 3 shows the results from the two
conditions for the three-letter strings: fixation and free eye movements. Interestingly, the use of free eye movements gave a better
performance only when the duration was about 500-600 msec or more
for this subject, indicating that fixation was a better strategy
for optimal information input when the stimulus duration was shorter than this value. The data for the fixation situation has been

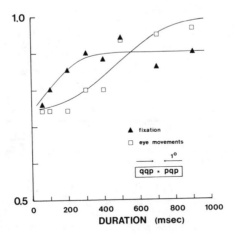

Figure 3. Discriminability of the three-letter strings when fixation and free eye movements were used. The continuous curve fitted
to the eye movement data has the form of a probability summation
function with a guessing parameter of 0.75

fitted by eye but the fit to the eye movement condition is based on the psychometric function that has been used to describe probability summation (Watson, 1979). It has the following form:

$$p = 1-(1- \gamma)\exp(-t/\alpha)^{\beta} \qquad\qquad (1)$$

where the parameters are α=580 msec, β=2.5, and γ=0.75 .

When the 2.5 deg gap was used in otherwise similar conditions and free eye movements, the time after which the eye movement condition gave a better performance corresponded well to that shown in Figure 3. However, the gain from the fixation during the initial rise of the function was not equally clear.

CONCLUSIONS

The visual processes underlying object recognition and eye movement control require a finite amount of time for execution and when the decision about the pattern must be made, all the critical features must have been extracted from the retinal image. The detectability of a spatial pattern improves with its duration and consequently, also as a function of the fixation duration. However, the detection of specific image features such as line or curve orientation or the fundamental spatial frequency, although significant for the visibility, may not be sufficient for the recognition of complex patterns such as character strings. Apparently, much of the fixation time is used for creating an ordered and stable spatial representation of the fixated target.

A correct discrimination of the letter strings that we used required specific information about the letter features and stable image topography. Clearly, lateral masking is able to disturb either or both of these visual factors. If the masking were a static and systematic phenomenon that disturbs the visual appearance of the letters then it should not have such drastic effects on the tasks where the subject performs a simple same/different discrimination in a spatially symmetric viewing condition. Hence it seems possible that the errors in discriminating between the simultaneously presented letter strings were caused by a difficulty in judging the relative location or orientation of the image features.

Our preliminary experimental data suggest a functional principle that partly determines the timing of eye fixations during normal viewing and reading. Clearly, the information about relative location or orientation of specific image features cannot be integrated visually as fast as simple spatial frequency and textural (cf. Bergen and Julesz, 1983) information can. In order to be able to localize the appropriate details of a fixated target the visual system needs a relatively long time, of the order of several hundred milliseconds. The process of spatial localization can also be conceived as the integration of spatial phase information. Theoretically, the importance of phase spectrum in signal processing and image representation is well known (Oppenheim and Lim, 1981; Piotrowski and Campbell, 1982). Although an appealing hypothesis, the idea that the relatively long fixations are used for collecting accurate phase information must be left open for further detailed studies.

REFERENCES

Bergen, J. R. and Julesz, B. (1983). Parallel versus serial processing in rapid pattern discrimination. Nature, 303, 696-698.

Bouma, H. (1970). Interaction effects in parafoveal letter recognition. Nature, 226, 177-178.

Breitmeyer, B. and Ganz, L. (1977). Temporal studies with flashed gratings: Inferences about human transient and sustained channels. Vision Res., 17, 861-865.

Bronstein, A. M. and Kennard, C. (1987). Predictive eye saccades are different from visually triggered saccades. Vision Res., 27, 517-520.

Campbell, F. W. and Robson, J. G. (1968). Application of Fourier analysis to the visibility of gratings. J. Physiol. (Lond.), 197, 551-566.

Koenderink, J. J., Bouman, M. A., Bueno de Mesquita, A. M., and Slappendel, S. (1978). Perimetry of contrast detection thresholds of moving sine wave patterns. J. Opt. Soc. Am., 68, 845-865.

McConkie, G. W., Underwood, N. R., Zola, D., and Wolverton, G. S. (1985). Some temporal characteristics of processing during reading. J. Exp. Psychol., Human Perception and Performance, 11, 168-186.

Nyman, G., Laurinen, P., and Campbell, F. W. (1986). Image processing in human vision: The analysis of spatial phase in peripheral vision. Acta Univ. Oul. A 179, 39-42.

Oppenheim, A. V. and Lim, J. S. (1981). The importance of phase in signals. Proc. IEEE, 69, 529-541.

Van Opstal, A. J. and Van Gisbergen, J. A. M. (1987). Skewness of saccadic velocity profiles: A unifying parameter for normal and slow saccades. Vision Res., 27, 731-745.

Piotrowski, L. N. and Campbell, F. W. (1982). A demonstration of the visual importance and flexibility of spatial-frequency amplitude and phase. Perception, 11, 337-346.

Rayner, K. and McConkie, G. W. (1977). Perceptual processes in reading: The perceptual spans. In: Toward a Psychology of Reading. (eds. A. S. Reber and D. L. Scarborough). Lawrence Erlbaum Associates, Hillsdale, New Jersey.

Virsu, V. and Rovamo, J. (1979). Visual resolution, contrast sensitivity, and the cortical magnification factor. Exp. Brain Res., 37, 475-494.

Watson, A. B. (1979). Probability summation over time. Vision Res., 20, 515-522.

26
Dyslexia and Reading as Examples of Alternative Visual Strategies

Gad Geiger and Jerome Y. Lettvin

INTRODUCTION.

We offer evidence that ordinary readers and dyslexics differ systematically in the distribution of certain perceptual properties over the visual field. These differences are laid to alternative strategies of perception. Our supposition is that any ordinary person possesses a file of visual tactics and can switch between them, depending on the type of task to be performed and the strategy used in performance. Tactics as well as strategies evolve as a result of practice that carries task performance from the novice level to the expert level.

The notion of a task entails that certain regions in the perceptual sphere be more salient than others, weighted by usefulness to the task that is being set appetitively. So, in reading, vision is most salient; in piano-playing, audition and kinesthesia are most salient; and so on. This weighting of perception does not alter the content of the representations offered to perception. Such weighting can be called "attention"; and it is clearly a tactic in the appetitive or goal-setting process.

Appetition, accordingly, affects perception in two ways. One way is by the external loop through the motor system acting against the world. The other way is by a direct action on perception itself, differentially weighting different regions of perceptual sphere with respect to the representations offered. That is, progress to expert performance involves learning what to attend in perception as much as what to do in action.

Ordinarily, what is meant by "visual attention" is the setting of a narrow zone in the visual field wherein perception is clear and distinct. Experimentally this can be made to occur anywhere within about a 10 degree radius around the foveal region. Practically, however, it usually means centering the axis of gaze on a part of the image in which detail of form and change in the detail is important. But this view ignores the bulk of our use of vision when we are not reading.

For example, take a sports broadcaster reporting a football scirmmage. Twenty-two men are engaged in a play that usually takes but a few seconds. Yet the broadcaster not only tells who carried the ball, but who was blocked and by whom, who committed a penalizable move, and in general, provides a

remarkable amount of information about the play. We must attribute to the
reporter an attention in which the exact detail along the axis of gaze is not
only mostly useless, but would distract from the more important patterns of
action distributed over a fairly wide angle in the field of view. The reporter
has learned the basic plays, and how they are embodied in configurations of
the players prior to the action. And so he reads, more easily than most of us,
the actual events as error with respect to what is predicted from the plan. In
this way he uses prior knowledge to reduce how much information he needs to
recount events in the scrimmage.

Without fussing about further refinement of this approach, we will identify
two simple broad strategies of vision and call them the "scribe" mode and the
"hunter" mode. In the scribe mode, attention is profoundly foveal, and objects
rapidly become less clear and distinct as their angular distance from the fovea
increases. In the hunter mode, attention is on the scene, and the gaze axis
mainly sets a point in the scene as a kind of a center around which events of
known character are expected. In short, if the visual task calls for high local
detail at a narrow region of a relatively stationary or slowly changing arrangement of objects in the field of vision, a scribe strategy is chosen. If the task calls
for ruleful relations between more widely spaced things, the hunter strategy is
chosen. This is an example of two task-determined strategies between which
the observer can switch.

The notion that what is attended is clear and distinct, while what is not
loses saliency, raises the issue, wherein lies the loss of saliency? The demonstration below provides the basis for an argument.

N   x   V H N E K

If you fix and hold your gaze on the x, the N on the left seems relatively
clear. The N on the right, imbedded among other letters, is not clear at all.
(That this is not a function of left versus right in the visual field can be shown
by turning the page upside down). The clarity of the solitary N on the left
testifies that visual acuity is adequate at that angular distance from the fovea.
Thus, the obscuring of the imbedded N has to be explained. The terminal
letters of the group can be identified – the further one, surprisingly, is more
definite than the nearer one. But it is as if the letters flanking the N prevent it
from being assigned a form. This property has been termed "lateral masking"
in the literature (e.g. Bouma,1970; Mackworth,1965; Townsend et al,1971).

Lateral masking increases in strength as the letters become more closely
spaced or if the group is moved yet further out in the peripheral field. Another
way of describing the impression of the letter string is that it has lost form and
has become a texture, more or less in the sense of B. Julesz. One has the feeling
that the perceived spatial order of the parts has been degraded while certain
statistics of the image remain, so that there are distinct edges and corners,
but where they lie with respect to each other and how they are connected is
somehow obscured. That this is not a loss of information in representational
processing can be shown by "demasking" the interior N. If the letter string is
flashed tachistoscopically with any figure except N flashed at the same time
at the fixation point, the masking of the N is quite strong. But, if an N of
the same font, size, contrast, and spatial orientation is flashed at the fixation
point simultaneously with the string, the interior N stands out.(Geiger and

Lettvin,1986). The same is true in varying degrees for all other upper-case letters, save the plain vertical bar, "I". In the steadily shown image, steadily attended at the fixation point, a quick small vertical movement of an imbedded laterally masked letter also demasks it.

What we suspected is that, among readers, the sharp increase of lateral masking with eccentricity of the letter string from the fixation point is a learned tactic. Since even a single letter, if more complex than a simple vertical bar, shows lateral masking between its parts, it is obviously subject to the same tactic. But is it a tactic or a built-in process in vision? Suppose someone is frozen to the hunter mode of seeing, would he show the same measures? Could these measures be changed by practise?

With tachistoscopically presented letters the shape of the decline in letter recognition with increing lateral displacement – the Aubert-Foerster law (1857) – has been taken as a sturdy and primitive observation for over a century. No one seems to have noticed that the subjects were predominantly readers. As is shown by the experiments reported here, dyslexics have a different shape to the recognition/displacement curve in the peripheral visual field. And as is also shown, the shape can be changed by designed practise.

In lateral masking, the reduction of form to texture has an odd quality. There are "features",by which we mean those primitives used to characterize forms. Let us suppose, for the moment, that they are the "textons" which Julesz and Bergen (1983) use for their description of texture elements. In perceiving a form, we see these component elements connected in a particular arrangement or spatial sequence. The form has handedness, orientation, and is clear and distinct. In perceiving the same arrangement texturized, we see the same component elements, but cannot assign them that connecting order which determines a form. If this transition between an aggregate, described statistically, and an arrangement, described geometrically, can be simply governed, that accounts for one of the tactics by which appetition directly affects perception. There is a control on conversions between form and texture vision. This does not introduce content into the representations offered to perception, but only weights how they are processed in perception.

The notion of task-determined control of perception can be realized by such a scheme. Returning to the scribe/hunter paradigm, the scribe, whose interest is confined to a narrow angle in the field of vision, practicing to become expert, introduces as a result of practice a degenerative lateral masking outside that angle. He limits his attention to the fovea, which is engineered for highest acuity. The hunter, who is concerned with the distribution of possible events over a wide angle in the field of vision, introduces, under practice, lateral masking in the fovea to suppress the excess of form resolution there. Instead he uses the fovea to set a center around which he attends patterns of related change.

Common experience of driving in traffic testifies to the alternation between scribe and hunter states – instants when one glances at a road sign versus stretches when one is concerned with the ambient flow of cars. But this is anecdotal. A more careful experiment was done by George Sperling (personal communication) two decades ago. It had earlier been shown that foveal vision is somehow compromised during a saccade. Sperling's experiment was this: A strobe light is coupled to the eye movements of a subject sitting in a dark room. It is the sole illuminant and flashes only in the middle of a large saccade. The subject finds it impossible to read even a newspaper headline when its image falls on the fovea during a saccade. (He quickly learns how to center the text on the fovea at the instant of the flash). The headline is there, but has the same textural quality that is observed in the eccentric letter strings of the previous demonstration. What is interesting is the result that after the subject tries to read for about a quarter-hour under this abnormal lighting, quite suddenly his reading ability returns as if the foveal "suppression" had been switched off. Many sources provide evidence for the proposition that practiced performance involves not only a change in the course of action, but also a change in the perceptions guiding that course. These changes can be attributed to practised task-determined strategies, and such strategies are usually mutually exclusive. Ivo Kohler (1962) as well as Richard Held and Alan Hein (1958) give good illustrative examples. Our concern, however, has been with tactics, such as regional form-texture conversion within the visual field. These seem to us to be quite as important as general strategies, and equally susceptible of appetitive control.

EXPERIMENTS.

In order to show the differences in visual strategy between ordinary readers and dyslexics, we designed two tests. In one, we measured how recognition of single letters falls off in the visual field with increase of angular distance from the axis of gaze. In the other we used strings of letters rather than singlets to note differences in lateral masking as eccentricity increases away from the axis of gaze.

The First Test: Form-Resolving Field (FRF)

The form-resolving field (FRF) is that portion of the visual field in which forms, presented tachistoscopically, are recognized to one degree or another. We operationally defined the FRF in the following way: In a test flash (as described below under "methods") the displayed letters are presented at some fixed angular size and contrast against a background of fixed luminance. Once the flash duration is chosen for a subject it is held constant for the run of measurements. The displayed letters are changed with every flash, and their angular distance from the gaze axis can be varied. Two letters are exposed in each flash, one at the fixation point (the center of gaze), the other at some angular distance in the peripheral field. The two letters are never the same. Both are to be identified by the subject immediately after the presentation. When about twenty such exposures of different letter pairs have been delivered at one eccentricity, the eccentricity is changed and a new series of twenty is presented. After the tests in all eccentricities are finished we plot the percentage of correct identification of the peripheral letters as a function of eccentricity. This plot is the FRF. It is not a measure of acuity, as will be evident later. What is at issue is the recognition of form rather than the resolving power.

Aparatus and Stimuli: Three slide projectors were focussed from behind on a framed translucent diffusing screen 35 cm. long and 23 cm. high. Each projector was set to give a uniform illumination across the screen at 180 cd/sq.m. as measured at the front of the screen. The projectors were operated in a time sequence. At first a fixation point is presented (by projector I). Except during a test this slide is constantly on. In a test the shutter in front of projector I shuts as that in front of projector II opens for short interval, T_1, to present the stimulus image. T_1 is followed by a second interval, T_2, when no projection plays on the screen. The stimulus duration is counted as the sum of T_1 and T_2. This sum is adjustable but never was longer than 10 ms. in the first test,(single letters to show the FRF), and it was 61 ms in the second test,(letter strings to show the effects of lateral masking). Following the interval T_2 the eraser goes on (projector III) for 2.5 seconds. In these tests the eraser consists of a blank lit screen. Following the eraser a new cycle starts after the subject reports.

No two letters on any slide were the same, and no two slides were the same. All eccentricities are given in terms of visual angle away from the fixation point.

Procedure: In the stimulus sequence the effective stimulus duration (from onset of the stimulus until the onset of the eraser) was adjustable in such a way that the best score of identification (at whatever eccentricity of the peripheral letter that gave the best score for the subject) lay just below 100%. This normalization procedure is best suited for form resolution since this normalizes sensitivity in form identification and not the sensitivity to contrast or lightness[1].

The stimulus exposure duration was set prior to the test itself. Once the best duration was determined for a subject it was fixed for that subject throughout the test at all eccentricities. After each stimulus presentation, the subjects reported what letters they had seen and which was at the fixation point, which in the periphery. The report was recorded and the next stimulus was given. Once all slides for all eccentricities had been presented, the percentage of correctlly identified letters at each eccentricity was determined.

The centering of the subject's gaze on the fixation point was visually monitored by the experimenter. This crude monitoring was sufficient, as some later instrumental verification has shown.

Subjects: All subjects were above 18 years old. All but two of them were completely unaware of the purpose of the tests until the testing was finished. Two groups were tested: ORDINARY READERS: This is a group of 10 ordinary readers (3 females and 7 males), all between 18 and 25 years of age with one exception. The subjects came from the general university-level student population. DYSLEXICS: This is a group of 10 dyslexics (2 females and 8 males) who did not have special tutoring within the last 3 years. They were between 20 and 58 years of age. All the dyslexics were diagnosed as such by their respective neurologists, psychologists and teachers. They all showed a normal level of comprehension of heard texts, but all had serious difficulties in reading.

Results of the Test: At the end of testing all the subjects, the scores of correct identification were gathered and averaged at each eccentricity for each separate group . These avereges are plotted in figure 1 to show the FRF's of the groups.

In general the FRF falls off with eccentricity from the center of gaze. However, there are obvious differences in the shape and the grading of the fall-off.

In the right hand side of figure 1 two curves are plotted; one for ordinary

---

[1] In another study we measured correct identification when stimuli exposure durations were equal for all subjects. The results were similar to the ones obtained with this normalization, but were less distinct.

readers and one for the dyslexics . From these curves we see that ordinary readers and dyslexics are significantly different at all eccentricities except at 5 deg. (we have performed the ANOVA and t-tests). Therefore it is safe to say that these are two distinct groups under this test.

The differences between the dyslexics and the ordinary readers are two-fold. Dyslexics identify letters further in the periphery than ordinary readers do. Also, dyslexics identify letters better at 5 deg. eccentricity than they do nearer to the center under the conditions of this test (i.e. a letter at the center and the second one in the periphery). This is in contrast with ordinary readers who identify letters best at the center and have an FRF that falls off mono-tonically to the periphery.

As this test is a measure of the form-resolving field we are able to say that ordinary readers have a narrower FRF than dyslexics do. The shape of the FRF in dyslexics shows a peripherally displaced peak. That is, lateral masking occurs near the center of gaze, a peak of "best vision" shows up in the near periphery, and the FRF falls off shallowly with further eccentricity. In contrast, among ordinary readers the FRF falls off steeply, smoothly and monotonically with eccentricity from the center of gaze. The implications are that ordinary readers are able to discern forms (single or aggregates) best at the center of gaze (fovea), whereas dyslexics discern aggregates of forms best in near periphery but have lateral masking at the fovea.

The left side of figure 1 shows no significant difference between ordinary readers and dyslexics. The shape of the fall-off of identification on the left is

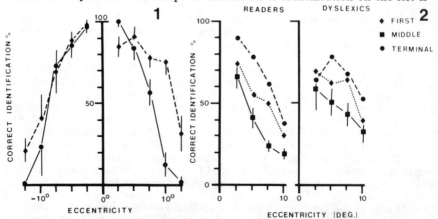

Figure 1. This figure displays the Form-Resolving Field (FRF) of ordinary readers ● and dyslexics ◆ . The measures are of % correct identifications of the letters at different eccentricities in the periphery. Vertical bars show the standard deviations. The scores for the letters presented at the same time at the fixation point are constant for all eccentricities (95%+or-4%) and are not given here.

Figure 2. The graphs show the strength of lateral masking as it varies with eccentricity. Ordinary readers are compared with dyslexics for correct identification of each letter in 3-letter strings that are presented at various ec-centricities. The score at each locus along the string is given separately.

monotonic and steep for both groups. But the fall-off is steeper on the right for ordinary readers than on the left, and for dyslexics is clearly much shallower on the right than on the left. We attribute the differences between left and right in ordinary readers to the conventions of reading. (The basis for this guess is that two readers, for whom Hebrew is the native language, have shown the opposite asymmetry.)

These measures of the form-resolving field are well correlated with ability to read. The reader has a narrow FRF and a most clear vision around the center of gaze, as is needed for usual reading (we do not talk here about speed reading). On the other hand, not having that kind of FRF seems connected with difficulties in reading, as manifest in the dyslexics.

As also can be seen, what the FRF measures is certainly not what is ordinarily meant by "acuity". We do not hold that there is a difference in peripheral acuity between ordinary readers and dyslexics. Instead the difference lies in the perception of forms and not in the resolving power, as is suggested by the figure used in the introduction.We suspect that the differences are accountable by different tactics in the distribution of lateral masking. With single letters (not "I") the parts of a letter exert masking effects on each other. We can call this self-masking. If ordinary readers and dyslexics differ in FRF we propose to explain the difference in terms of distributions of lateral masking and self-masking.

Experiments on demasking (Geiger and Lettvin, 1986) have shown that only "complex" letters are demasked (letters comprised of more than a single bar). Single bars can not be demasked, while annuli are not easily masked. Thus it is reasonable to think of parts of a letter masking one another in much the same way as one letter laterally masks another.

We have been mentioning that the lateral masking at the center of gaze, such as occurs in dyslexics, looks similar to the lateral masking in the peripheral field had by ordinary readers. It remains for us to show how ordinary readers and dyslexics differ in lateral masking.

The Second Test: Lateral Masking Between Letters in a String.

The apparatus and methods are the same as for the FRF test. The differences lie in the nature of the stimuli and the duration of the stimulus-exposures. In this test four letters are presented in each stimulus (instead of two as in the previous test). One letter is at the fixation point and a string of three letters is in the periphery. All letters in each stimulus display are unlike each other. As in the previous experiment no two slides are alike. The strings in the periphery are displayed at various eccentricities in the various slides. Duration of the stimulus exposure was 61 ms. for all subjects.

Figure 2 presents the data by which to compare nine dyslexics with five ordinary readers. At each eccentricity of the string we give identification scores for each locus along the string (first, middle and terminal letters).

Some general properties of lateral masking are seen in the plots for ordinary readers: Masking increases with eccentricity; it is least effective for the terminal letter of the 3-letter strings and strongest for the middle letter. These properties are generally preserved for the dyslexics. However, there are some differences. a. Near the center the masking of the first, middle and last letters are about the same for dyslexics and for readers; but at 10 deg. eccentricity the middle letter is significantly less masked for dyslexics than for readers. b. The variance of the masking of the middle letter at string eccentricity of 10 deg. is larger for the dyslexics.

Learning Visual Strategies.

The results of the two kinds of test, as described above, suggest differences between readers and dyslexics in the distribution of certain perceptual processes over the visual field. The differences become magnified when severe dyslexics are examined, like the case of a severe dyslexic, whose initial FRF is shown in figures 3 and the initial test for lateral masking gave the plots graphed in figure 4a.

In figure 4a we show, for this severe dyslexic, the initial results of measuring lateral masking as a function of eccentricity. At 2.5 deg. eccentricity his score for all the letters in the string was almost zero. At the same time his score for the fixation letter also went to zero, as if the mutual lateral masking was extremely intense in the region around the center of gaze. With respect to this test he acts as if he had little or no form vision of aggregates in the fovea and parafovea. However at 7.5 deg. and 10 deg. he performed as if there were little lateral masking and little loss of letter recognition (as evident also from the initial FRF in figure 3). In this respect he was superior to readers in his peripheral vision. Such a case might raise the suspicion of some organic deficit in retinal function at the fovea were it not for the fact that so long as the background was blanked up to 5 deg. away from the center of gaze, he had

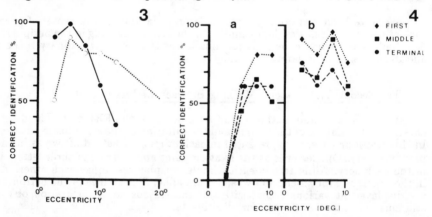

Figure 3: The initial plot of the FRF on a severe dyslexic is compared to the plot of the FRF taken four months later (solid line), after the practise described in the text.

Figure 4: a.) This graph of lateral masking against string eccentricity (done as in figure 2) plots the initial performance of the same severe dyslexic as in figure 3. b.) This graph shows the performance of the same subject four months later after the practise described in the text.

normal vision for single letters presented in the foveal field.

At this point, using the line of thought sketched in the introduction, we asked if it would be possible for this severe dyslexic to learn a new visual strategy that would permit him to read. Whatever set of visual strategies he possessed, if there were indeed such a set, excluded reading at and around the center of gaze. Thus no use of his existing set of strategies could be made in teaching him to read, because no reinforcement could occur in the foveal region. Since his FRF as well as his performance with the tests on lateral masking showed that his near peripheral vision had acuity adequate to reading, we decided to probe whether he could acquire a strategy for reading in the peripheral field of vision. If he could, and our tests measured something that correlated with visual strategy, then a retest after acquisition of the new strategy would show the change. Our hopes were based on the well-known phenomenon of speed-reading which implied that peripheral vision might be adequate to the task.

He was the first subject on which we tried the learning of a new strategy. The program we tried on him is described below in the protocols for training four dyslexics. It must be emphasized here that we were not and are not proposing a therapy. We are only testing the hypothesis that a new visual strategy can be learned if it does not compete in the domain of other firmly set strategies, i.e. it would not be advisable to train for foveal reading if the consequences of his existing strategies are that he masks in the fovea. He would than have no success by which to reinforce a new strategy by practise.

If, as we felt, the two tests, given above, measure some properties related to visual strategy, retesting after successful training, should it occur, would reflect the introduction of the new strategy.

He responded to the procedure, and, within four months went from a third grade reading level to about a tenth grade level. In practical terms he was able to take a job in which he had to read memos, bills of lading, and the like. When tested at the end of four months he showed the change in FRF given by the solid line in figure 3, and the change in lateral masking shown by figure 4b.. He can now make out letters in strings presented at 2.5 degrees eccentricity. His performance at that eccentricity is not as good as that of an ordinary reader or residual dyslexic, but is far better than in the initial test. Curiously, in now reporting the letters at that eccentricity, he stuttered (Geiger and Lettvin·,1987).

There is no point in describing further what the pictures make clear, and so we will go on to lay out the general method for testing the hypothesis.

We asked four of the dyslexics (part of the group of 10 and including the severe dyslexic just described) to participate in a program aimed at their learning a new strategy. After we characterized each of the 4 subjects with the two tests, we advised them to devote two hours every day to the performance of novel, direct, small-scale, hand-eye coordination tasks such as drawing, painting, clay-molding, model-building, etc.. The rationale for this practise comes from experiments performed by Held and Gotlieb (1957), Held and Hein (1957) and remarks by Helmholtz (1867) on how a person shifts spatial localization after viewing his hand through a prism. The general idea was to provide visual perception with a new space of operation as defined by the new tasks.

Along with this practise the subjects were to try reading through a window in the peripheral field. A sheet lay over the text to be read. It could be transparent and colored, or translucent, or opaque. On it lay a fixation point or mark. At the right of that mark a window was neatly cut to a size somewhat larger than the length and height of a long word in the text. The distance from the fixation point to the center of the window was set individually for each subject by using the eccentricity of the peak of the FRF and the eccentricity at which there was a drop in lateral masking of the middle letter in a string.

When the subjects intended to read they were to lay the window over the desired word or words in the text while gazing at the fixation point and try to read what lay in the window. Keeping gaze on the fixation point they then shifted the sheet so that the window lay over the next word, and so on. In this way the words in the window might be seen as form rather than texture, without interference from the ambience.

After a few months (2.5–4) with this combined practice we again measured the FRF curves for each of the four subjects. We measured the lateral masking curves afterwards on only the severe dyslexic described above. We also inquired about, but did not measure, their reading skills. Figure 5 shows the averaged FRF for the four subjects before and after the practice term. For comparison, the curve for ordinary readers (from figure 1) is also displayed.

We should remark that the four subjects were not chosen by us. They were the only candidates among the 10 original subjects who could afford the time to practise daily. We did not instruct or guide the subjects more then by occasional telephone conversation.

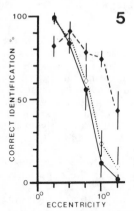
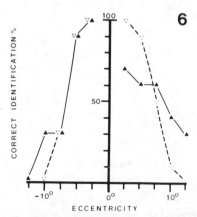

Figure 5. Graphed here is the effect of learning and practicing a new strategy. Plots of the FRF are averaged for a.) ordinary readers ● (taken from figure 2) ; b.) four dyslexics ◆ prior to the practise described in the text; c.) the same four dyslexics after that practise ◇ . The bars measure standard deviation.

Figure 6. Two strategies in one subject are measured within a few hours interval. One FRF was taken when he was in an alert phase (mostly in the morning) ▽ . The other FRF was taken 6 hours later when he was in a tired phase ▲ .

As seen in figure 5 there is a significant shift of the FRF from before practice to after practice. The shift is toward the FRF of ordinary readers. Ordinary readers do not vary significantly in FRF over time although we measured some over periods of 2 years and longer.

In general the reading performance of all the four improved much. The reading score of one went from 3rd grade before practice to 10th grade after practice. Another subject went from hardly reading at all (about 2nd grade) to reading fluently for half an hour at a time (difficult to estimate grade level). Another went from spells of slow reading for five minutes at a time to spells of reading fluently for hours at a time (So he reported). The fourth initially could only skim fast (like speed reading) with many errors. He had no ability to read slowly and with care. After the course of practise he was able to read "word by word" as well as by skimming.

Three of the four stopped practising after they had achieved some skill, and fairly quickly regressed in their ability ro read. This change was also reflected in their FRF's.

An Unusual Case. As a final note we want to describe an unusual case in some detail. This subject is a male 30 years of age. He has the peculiar complaint that while he can read facilely when he is "alert", he is unable to read or reads with great difficulty when he is "tired". When he is extremely tired he is able to "speed read" or skim a newspaper with good comprehension of the text, but he is unable to read in a "usual" way.

We interviewed him and tested him in two of his "phases", the alert one (mostly occurring in the mornings) and the tired one (in the same afternoons). We did not test him in the extremely tired phase.

When he was in the tired phase he appeared to be markedly dyslexic. He had high level of comprehension and intelligence. He seemed generally alert in his tired phase and without optical defects, but could hardly read. In the alert phase his reading was good for long spells of time (over an hour), with the usual speed of reading and with only an occasional stumble over an unfamiliar long word every now and then.

The measures of his FRF in these two phases are shown in figure 6. On the right side of the figure, one of the plots matches nicely the FRF of ordinary readers. These data were taken when he was in the alert phase. The other plot was taken when he was in his tired phase. It falls off shallowly with eccentricity and so extends further into the peripheral field. It resembles that of the dyslexics. On the left side of figure 6 the differences in the plots are small although a slight extension of the FRF into the periphery is evident for the tired phase.

Figure 6 shows a clear relation between measures of the FRF and the task-competence reported by the subject. In the light of his subjectively distinct states we can suppose him to be a conditional dyslexic whose states can be told by objective testing. He switches between these states for some not very obvious reason. In the tired state he is not fatigued—he uses the term to describe only his inability to read; otherwise he is alert and competent. That this is not a problem of acuity is driven home by the fact that these states are in the same individual. If his acuity is improved for peripheral vision, can the same change in optics worsen his foveal acuity, if one supposes that his physical optics have somehow altered? Alternatively, can one suppose that his retina has changed its connectivity somehow? Has he changed his linguistic ability? If so, what tests could be used to distinguish his clearly reported states? Has he altered the anatomical connections in his brain?

After we had made our measurements on this subject and explained to him our notion of task determined strategies, he succeeded in teaching himself to use the wide field (dyslexics') strategy when he was alert (in the morning). He did this because he knew that creative art work was easier for him when he was tired. When he needed to do creative work while he was alert he now could swicth voluntarily to the tired mode. The reverse shift, from being in the tired mode (wide FRF) to alert mode (narrow FRF), he is still unable to do. .

CONCLUSIONS.

We have presented evidence for the existence of alternative states or strategies in visual perception. These strategies can be tested by measuring recognition of figures or letters as a function of eccentricity from the gaze axis. They are also tested by measuring the strength of lateral masking as a function of the same eccentricity. By both these sorts of tests there are marked differences between ordinary readers and dyslexics in the peripheral field of vision. These differences cannot be laid to changes in visual acuity between subjects for two reasons: first, they can be altered by certain kinds of practise; second, they can be demonstrated in the same subject (one case) at different times of the same day.

In the strategy of the ordinary reader, best vision is around the axis of gaze. Lateral masking increases steeply with eccentricity from the gaze axis as does loss of letter recognition. In the visual strategy of the dyslexic there is masking around the center of gaze and best vision occurs a few degrees to the right of the gaze axis (if the language is English). Loss of letter recognition beyond that peak increases less steeply than for ordinary readers.

A dyslexic can be trained to read in the peripheral field of vision. This training does not challenge a prior strategy which masks letter strings in the foveal region. (Such masking does not allow that reinforcement needed to practise the foveal seeing of letter strings). When he is practised in reading by peripheral vision, the test signs of his visual strategy, when plotted, approach the plots found for ordinary readers.

The training of reading in the peripheral field is not to be construed as a therapy. It was done to probe the hypothesis that task-determined visual strategies can be learned, and that the presence of a new strategy can be detected by testing. While a therapy may possibly be based on this demonstration and the reasoning that led to it, we emphasize again that the demonstration was meant only to test a notion, not to cure a disorder.

REFERENCES.

Aubert, H. and Foerster, (1857) Beitraege zur Kenntniss des indirecten

Sehens. Graefes Archiv fuer Ophthalmologie 3(2), 1-47.

Bouma, H. (1970). Interaction Effects in Parafoveal Letter Recognition. Nature 226, 177-8.

Geiger, G. and Lettvin, J.Y. (1986). Enhancing the Perception of Form in Peripheral Vision. Perception 15, 119-130.

Geiger, G. and Lettvin, J.Y. (1987). Peripheral Vision in Persons with Dyslexia. N. Engl. J. Med. 316, 1238-43.

Held, R. and Gottlieb, N. (1958). Technique for Studying Adaptation to Disarranged Hand-Eye Coordination. Perceptual and Motor Skills 8, 83-86.

Held, R. and Hein, A.V. (1958). Adaptation of Disarranged Hand-Eye Coordination Contingent Upon Re-Afferent Stimulation. Perceptual and Motor Skills 8, 87-90.

Helmholtz,H.v. (1867). Handbuch der Physiologischen Optik. Vol.lll Leipzig; Leopold Voss.

Julesz,B. and Bergen,J.R. (1983). Textones, the Fundamental Elements in Preattentive Vision and Perception of Texture. Bell System Tech. J. 62, 1619-45.

Kohler, I. (1962). Experiments with Goggles. Sci. Am. 206, 62-72.

Mackworth, N.H. (1965). Visual Noise causes Tunnel Vision. Psychonomic Sci. 3, 67-8.

Townsend,J.T., Taylor,S.G. and Brown,D.R. (1971). Lateral Masking for Letters with Unlimited Viewing Time. Percep and Psychophysics 10, 375-8.

27
Reading with and without Eye Movements

Lawrence W. Stark and Christof C. Krischer

This chapter reviews the control of eye movements, including Hering's law with its rare and pathological static violations and its common and incidental dynamical violations. Two unusual protocols for reading eye movements, reading Chinese and zero eye movement reading, help to define basic concepts. We have included material about abnormal eye movements found in dyslexics, both those secondary to the basic linguistic abnormality and those that may be primary and provide clues about dyslexia, and finally a brief speculation on phonological-motor coding. The senior author wishes to dedicate this paper to the memory of his former student, Dr. Deborah Adler, whose research and thesis on eye movement patterns in dyslexic children has remained a substantial contribution to the field.

MULTILEVEL CONTROL OF EYE MOVEMENTS

Two different disciplines, neurology and bioengineering, have contributed to the concept of multilevel control of eye movements. The neurological origins stem from Hughlings Jackson. Recent bioengineering studies have added the concept of feedback sharing with input the control of the active feedforward path and thus forming a closed-loop feedback control system (Figure 1). The block of pulse-shaping algorithms for generating time-optimal saccadic trajectories would be 'jacksonian lower level' control. The block for the sampled-data control mechanism that initiates eye movement precedes this lower level block, but also lies in the forward loop path; it would be 'higher level' control (Young and Stark, 1963). Other blocks, out of the main control loop, that calibrate gains and calculate space constancy and perhaps lie in the cerebellum and parietal lobe respectively, would be 'highest level' controllers.

Saccadic trajectory. The rapid dynamics of saccadic eye movements (Figure 2) are driven by high frequency bursts of action potentials causing high muscle forces. Reciprocally innervated antagonist muscles are turned off in sequence during this

multipulse control and silent periods result. The high
accelerations and velocities permit, for example, 10-degree
saccades to reach final position in 30-40 ms (Cook and Stark, 1968;
Clark and Stark, 1975; Lehman and Stark, 1979).

Kinematics and Hering's Law for Versions and Vergences.
According to Hering's Law corresponding muscles of each eye receive
equal innervation (Figure 2). This simple control mechanism works
because there are four vertical muscles for each eye and because
extraocular muscles have wide insertions. Hering in 1868 (Bridgeman
and Stark, 1977), was able to demonstrate that the neurological
constraint defined in Hering's Law produces binocularly conjugate
or equal movements within the bifixation area.

Hering's Law was postulated for static aspects of binocular
coordination; the recently discovered multipulse control of
saccades are often in violation of Hering's Law in normal persons
(Figure 2), and mismatched pulse-steps lead to glissades (Bahill et
al, 1976).

Dual mode control.   Position errors, eccentric target images,
are controlled by saccades and velocity errors, retinal slips, by
smooth pursuit. Sampled-data saccadic movements play an vital part
in looking and reading and the sampled-data control features will
be discussed below. Smooth pursuit has been considered as a
sampled-data system, then as continuous control, and now perhaps as

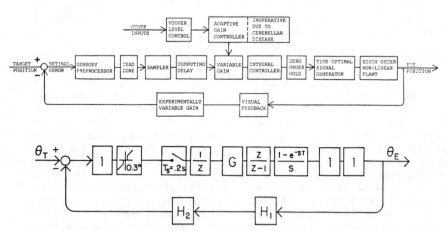

FIG 1   Block diagram   for Saccadic Eye Movement Control.
Upper diagram has verbal descriptions of each block, while lower
diagram has mathematical form with "s" as the LaPlace operator and
"z" as the z-transform operator; several blocks are simplified to a
value of 1. Note higher level blocks for adaptive gain in verbal
model are not represented in mathematical form (from Hsu, Krishnan
and Stark, 1976).

a sampled-data system with shorter periods than saccades.
Optokinetic nystagmus is a form of interrupted smooth pursuit, but
driven by flow field visual stimuli. These large fields can
generate velocities of up to 100 degrees/s (Stark, 1971).
Fixational eye movements are basically expressions of low amplitude
dual mode control and will be discussed further below.   Gaze
movements represent coordination of eye movements with head
movement; the latter has dynamical lags due to large inertia, but
is more amenable to predictive and schematic control. A variety of
gaze types occur; frequencies of these types vary with protocol
conditions and neurological disease.

   Highest Level Looking Eye Movements: Scanpaths. When we regard
ordinary complex scenes or pictures, we generate repetitive
sequences of saccades or "scanpaths" that check the subfeatures of

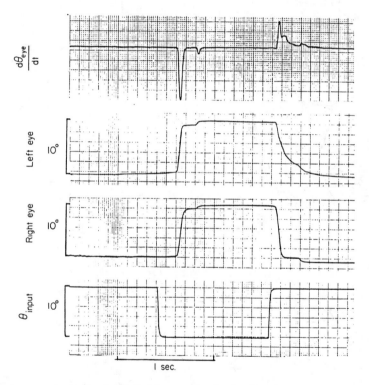

FIG 2   Dynamical Violations of Hering's Law.
Synchronous conjugate saccade is followed by a synchronous
conjugate corrective saccade; note high velocities (upper trace)
for both initial and corrective saccades. Then a similar saccade is
seen in right eye, but left eye shows an abbreviated saccade
followed by a glissade that persists through the corrective
saccade. Normal skilled reader (lws!) (from Stark, 1971).

SCANPATH THEORY

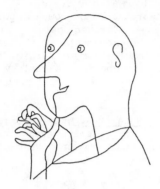
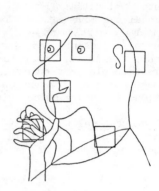

PICTURE WITH SUBFEATURES REQUIRING CHECKING FOVEATIONS

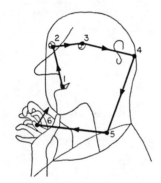
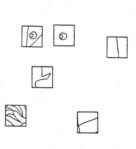

MOTOR AND SENSORY REPRESENTATION

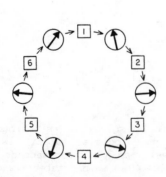
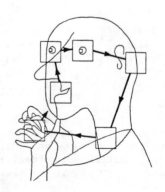

FIG 3   COGNITIVE MODEL CONTROLLING ACTIVE LOOKING

a particular picture (figure 3). This use of eye movements in active looking has been studied by Noton and Stark (1971) and Stark and Ellis (1981); their scanpath theory supposes that cognitive models in the brain drive the sequences of saccadic eye movements in a checking or pattern recognition phase of visual perception. Each person has a distinctive pattern for each picture he looks at. Yarbus (1967) demonstrated that when a particular picture is looked at by the same subject but with different intentions--such as to determine the social class of the individuals in the picture or to plan to redraw the picture--different scanpaths eventuate. Looking is an important function, tested throughout man's evolutionary history and kept at a peak of performance. Reading has rather been adapted by culture to fit man's looking and seeing abilities.

READING EYE MOVEMENTS.

Normal reading movements form a much more stereotyped pattern. The main reading movements consist of a series of small, 2-degree, rightward or forward moving, "progressive saccades" jumping from word to word. When the end of a line is reached, a larger leftward saccade (about 10 degrees in amplitude) jumps to the beginning of the next line. These "line return saccades" often have small corrective saccades to readjust eye position to the beginning of the next line. About 20 percent of the time, "regression saccades" are made. These are saccades moving leftward or backward. Regressions apparently serve a grammatical or syntactical function, whereby preceding key words such as verbs or important conjunctions in the sentence are rechecked; the French term for regressions is "verifications," emphasizing their linguistic function.

A normal reading rate for English is 250-300 words per minute. A nominal forward reading rate is calculated as the product of 1/fixation duration x saccadic span x 60 sec/min; with the common values of 250 msec/fixation and a span of 1.64 words, about 394 forward words per minute, wpm, are overviewed. If regressions are made 10% of the time and return-sweep and corrective saccades 15% of the time, the overall reading rate is 300 wpm.

Reading Chinese is almost equivalent to reading English. One and one-half Chinese characters is equivalent to one English word; the same packing occurs per page; and similar reading eye movement patterns are observed (Table 1) (Sun, Morita and Stark, 1985).

Skilled reading is a process requiring continued practice to maintain. Native Chinese scholars who have lived in Berkeley for over five years (mainly reading English for professional purposes) have decreased reading speed (in Chinese) compared to native Chinese who have just arrived in Berkeley. In 1926, native Chinese readers read vertically faster than horizontally. Since then, a reform in Chinese printing caused most material to be printed horizontally. Now, in 1985, native Chinese readers have slower reading speeds for vertical material than for horizontal material.

TABLE 1.   Reading Rate for English and Chinese.

	FIXATION DURATION (sec)	SPAN (words/min) or (char/fixation)	(words/min) or (char/min)
ENGLISH	0.27	1.8	380
CHINESE: HORIZONTAL (equivalent words)	0.26	1.7	390
UNSKILLED CHINESE (equivalent words)	0.29	1.1	240
CHINESE: VERTICAL (equivalent words)	0.29	0.8	170

Two components, fixation duration and saccadic span together
determine reading rate in wpm (words per minute). Note that normal
reading of English and Chinese are almost identical.   Lack of
continual practice yielded lower reading rates for unskilled
Chinese readers and for reading vertical Chinese (adapted from Sun,
Morita and Stark, 1985).

ZERO EYE MOVEMENT READING.

     Zero eye movement reading is accomplished by bringing up words
rapidly and successively in the center of a computer monitor screen
so that the subject can apprehend the stimulus without having to
move his eyes (Hannaford, Krischer and Stark, 1985). However, it
should be stated at the outset, that only the reading speed
normally attained with eye movements can be approached with zero
eye movement reading.

     Backward and forward masking restricts presentation to about
the same rate as reading eye movements attain (Table 1).   A
blanking period, possibly similar to saccadic suppression, helps in
maximizing this presentation rate (Figure 4).   There is perhaps a
positive effect with zero eye movement reading in that the return
sweep to the beginning of the line is eliminated; perhaps the
evolving printed page format toward a multi-column presentation is
an attempt to move in this direction in ordinary printing.   The
loss of control with respect to the general speed of word
presentation and to the absence of regressions/verifications more
than negatively compensates for the time saved due to the absence
of these regressions. Attempts to use a larger peceptual span than
the saccadic span were ineffective; increased errors negated the
advantage of presenting two words at a time. Interestingly enough,
micro-fixations, absent in ordinary reading, show up with zero eye
movement reading (Figure 5).

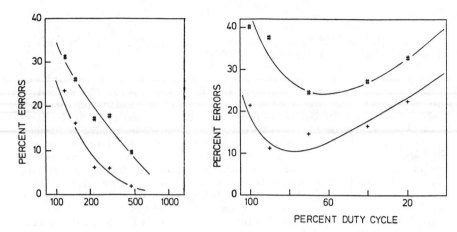

FIG 4   Attainable Rates for Zero Eye Movement Reading.
A. (left). Percent errors (ordinate) increases as repetition time decreases (abscissa) so that about 6% errors occur when 300 wpm, (words per minute), are presented. Error rates increase when two words are presented together, (double crosses) so that no increase in reading rate is obtained. Thus the 2.5 Hz sampled-data frequency for generating saccades is not rate-limiting.
B. (right diagram). An 80% duty cycle is optimum for one word presentations. Evidently a blanking (dark) period for 20% of the time is helpful in reducing backward and forward masking. Is this a role for saccadic suppression?

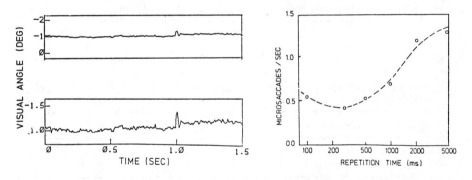

FIG 5   Microsaccades during Zero Eye Movement Reading.
A. (left diagram) Recordings of microsaccadic eye movements during zero eye movement reading. Upper trace, with moderate amplification (visual angle in degrees as ordinate) shows absence of usual eye movements over the few seconds (abscissa) of the recording. Lower trace, with expanded scale, shows one sizable (18 arcminutes) microsaccade and perhaps some smaller ones.
B. (right diagram) Microsaccade production rate (ordinate) shows increase with increase in repetition time over 500 ms (abscissa).

DYSLEXIA.

Reading Eye Movements in Dyslexia with Abnormalities Secondary to the Linguistic Problem. Dr. Deborah Adler did a careful study of eye movements in dyslexic children and concluded that "(1) normal and dyslexic children respond similarly to a meaningless target that is suddenly displaced in the visual field; (2) saccadic eye movements can be used, therefore, as an indicator of more complex behavior in both groups; (3) dyslexics have no difficulty with pictorial stimuli; (4) dyslexic children do not have a visual perception deficit, if we define visual-perception as appreciation of and task-solving competence in the visually presented environment; (5) the substitution of printed words for nonverbal stimuli causes a decrease in the visuomotor performance of only the dyslexic children; and (6) the information-processing obstacle appears to lie beyond visual perception, perhaps in the language area itself, and the dyslexic's characteristic deficit must, therefore, involve the integration of the visual input into the language-acquisition function" (Adler and Stark, 1981).

As can be seen (Table 2), the reading eye movements are significantly different in normal and dyslexic children. It appeared to be a reflection of the linguistic difficulty. Careful analysis of the literature and careful study of the normal eye movements of dyslexic children, lead us to conclude that there were no abnormalities in saccadic trajectories or latencies to meaningless targets, there were no differences in eye movements

TABLE 2. Reading Eye Movements in Dyslexic Children.

MEASURE	NORMAL		DYSLEXIC	
	$\overline{X}$	SD	$\overline{X}$	SD
Duration of forward fixations (msec)	280	33	340	45
Percentage regressions	22.0	6.6	22.9	5.3
Recognition span (words/fixation)	1.2	0.3	0.9	0.3
Reading rate (words/min)	164	57	105	33

Both major components that contribute to reading speed in wpm are altered in dyslexics. Duration of forward fixations is increased from 280 ms to 340 ms, and saccadic span in words between fixations decreased from 1.2 to 0.9. Percent regressions is the same, but of course, that still means more regressions per line (adapted from Adler and Stark, 1978).

during visual perception tasks involving linguistic symbols. A surprising finding was the increase in saccadic smooth pursuit movements. Saccadic smooth pursuit is not related to reading eye movement performance or consistently to specific neurological or motor deficits.

Possible Specific Eye Movement Abnormalities in Dyslexia. A possibility that has excited a number of researchers is that an eye movement abnormality will be discovered that is primary, associated with dyslexia, and not only secondary to the linguistic defect, such as the main eye movement findings of Adler, above. Candidate factors proposed have been met with scepticism by the dyslexia research community. Among these factors are difficulties in prediction of regular staircases (Pavlidis, 1981), cerebellar abnormalities (Frank and Levinson, 1973), mild smooth pursuit abnormalities (Adler and Stark, 1978) (although these authors did not make much of this non-specific and non-reading eye movement), Hering's Law violations (Ober: personal communication), vergence abnormalities (Stein, 1982), reaction time asymmetries (Hermann, Sonnabend and Zeevi, 1986), and backward staircases (many researchers including Jones and Stark, 1983) (Figure 6).

Speculations on the Motor Speech Code. Finally, we may speculate on how the visual interpretation of words impinges upon the phonolinguistic code. In this volume several chapters deal with the latest research on the epidemiological correlations between difficulties in phonological segmentation awareness in pre-readers and development of reading difficulties at a later date.

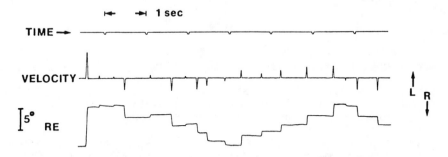

FIG 6   Backward Staircase in Reading Pattern of a Dyslexic. Right to left or backward staircase is seen in place of a single-saccade return-sweep in the reading eye movement pattern of a young person with specific dyslexia. Note 5 degree calibration (ordinate) for eye angle trace (lower) and directional arrows (left upward). Time in seconds shown in upper trace. This abnormal pattern of normal saccades should not be considered as secondary to the linguistic reading defect (from Jones and Stark, 1983).

Most likely, speech production in motor control is discrete in two dimensions. One dimension is time; a sampled-data control mechanism was proposed about 10 years ago at a "Conference on Speech Production in Santa Barbara, California", by Stark (unpublished). Another dimension would be the individual motor mechanisms for speech production, thorax and diaphragm, vocal cords, palate, tongue, jaw and lips, that reside in some region of the brain between Broca's area for motor speech and the individual mechanism representations in frontal cortex. Unlike the actual sound waves carrying speech, this discrete code would not be smeared by output filter characteristics in the co-articulation process, so phonological segments would be discretely available.

This motor code must be in a feedback loop so that hearing of one's own speech production can be continually compared with the desired output. Since we all have this loop for controlling speech output, we must all have the sensory-to-discrete-code mechanism for translating received speech. This does, of course, not answer the question posed --- How is the visual word decoded onto the phono-logical-segment code? However, these suggestions raise the question to a more concrete level of analysis and speculation. Again, the process developed later by skilled readers of directly decoding visual linguistic information, should be considered in terms of building upon and interfacing with the earlier decoding processes.

Acknowledgement: To NASA-Ames Research Center for partial support and to Drs. Fuchuan Sun, Ashby Jones, and Samuel Giveen for helpful discussions, and especially to the Rodin Remediation Academy and Drs. Per Udden and Curt von Euler for educating the senior author about dyslexia.

References

Adler-Grinberg, D. and Stark, L, (1978). Eye Movements, Scanpaths and Dyslexia. Amer. J. Optom. Physiol. Optics, 55, 557-570.

Bahill, T., Clark, M, and Stark, L. (1975). Glissades - Eye Movements Generated by Mismatched Components of the Saccadic Motoneuronal Control Signal. Math. Sci., 26, 303-318.

Clark, M. and Stark, L. (1975). Time Optimal Behavior of Human Saccadic Eye Movements. IEEE Trans. Autom. Control, 20, 345-348.

Cook, G. and Stark, L. (1968). The Human Eye Movement Mechanism: Experiments, Modeling and Testing. Arch. Ophthal., 79, 428-436.

Frank, J. and Levinson, H. (1973). Dysmetric Dyslexia and Dyspraxia. J. Amer. Acad. of Child Psychiatry, 12, 690-701.

Hannaford, B., Krischer, C. and Stark, L. (1985). A Device for Zero Eye Movement Reading. IEEE Trans. Biomed. Engr., 32, 86-89.

Hering, E. (1977). The Theory of Binocular Vision. (eds. B. Bridgeman and L. Stark). Plenum Press, New York, 1-210.

Hermann, H., Sonnabend, N. and Zeevi, Y. (1986). Interhemispheric Coordination is Compromised in Subjects with Developmental Dyslexia. Cortex, 22, 337-358.

Hsu, F., Krishnan, V. and Stark, L. (1976). Simulation of Ocular Dysmetria Using a Sampled Data Model of the Human Saccadic System. Annals of Biomed, Engr., 4, 321-329.

Jones, A. and Stark, L. (1983). Abnormal Patterns of Normal Eye Movements in Specific Dyslexia. In Eye Movements in Reading: Perceptual and Language Processes. (ed. K. Rayner). Academic Press, New York, 481-498.

Lehman, S. and Stark, L. (1979). Simulation of Linear and Nonlinear Eye Movement Models: Sensitivity Analyses and Enumeration Studies of Time Optimal Control. J. Cybernetics Inform. Sci., 2, 21-43.

Noton, D. and Stark, L. (1971). Eye Movements and Visual Perception. Sci. Amer., 224, 34-43.

Pavlidis, G. (1981). Sequencing, Eye Movements and the Early Objective Diagnosis of Dyslexia. In Dyslexia Research and its Applications to Education. (eds. G. Pavlidis and T. Miles). John Wiley and Sons, Chichester.

Stark, L. (1971). The Control System for Versional Eye Movements. In The Control of Eye Movements. (eds. Bach-y-Rita, Collins and Hyde). Academic Press, New York.

Stark, L. and Ellis, S. (1981). Scanpaths Revisited: Cognitive Models Direct Active Looking. In Eye Movements, Cognition and Visual Perception. (eds. Fischer, Monty and Senders). Erlbaum Press, New Jersey, 193-226.

Stein, J. and Fauler, S. (1982). Diagnosis of Dyslexia by Means of a New Indicator of Dominance. Brit. J. Ophthal., 66, 332-336.

Sun, F., Morita, M. and Stark, L. (1985). Comparative Patterns of Reading Eye Movement in Chinese and English. Perception and Psychophysics, 37, 502-506.

Yarbus, A. (1967). Eye Movements and Vision. Plenum Press, New York.

Young. L. and Stark, L. (1963). Variable Feedback Experiments Testing a Sampled Data Model for Eye Tracking Movements. IEEE Trans. Human Factors in Electr., 4, 38-51.

28
Eye Movements and the Perceptual Span in Beginning and Dyslexic Readers

Keith Rayner

INTRODUCTION

A great deal of recent research makes it clear that understanding the nature of eye movements is very important in understanding the reading process and quite a bit is known about the characteristics of skilled readers' eye movements (Rayner, 1978; Rayner & Pollatsek, 1987). The eye movements that occur during reading, called **saccades,** serve the function of placing a given region of text in foveal vision for detail processing. It is only when the eye is relatively still in a **fixation** that new information is extracted from the text. The average fixation duration for skilled readers is between 200-250 msec and the eyes typically move 7-9 character spaces with each saccade (Rayner, 1978). In addition, skilled readers **regress** (or move their eyes back) to material that they have already read about 10-15% of the time. It is important to realize that the values presented here are averages and that for any given reader there is a considerable amount of variability associated with each of the mean values. Much of the variability is related to the reader's cognitive processes involved in understanding the text; readers tend to look at difficult words longer than easier words and when text processing is difficult readers make shorter saccades and more regressions (Rayner & Pollatsek, 1987).

In comparison to skilled readers, the eye movement characteristics of both beginning and disabled readers are quite different. Beginning readers and disabled readers tend to make more and longer fixations, shorter saccades, and more regressions than skilled readers. These facts have been known for some time and have often been used to argue that (1) eye movements are a causative factor in poor reading and (2) since they make shorter saccades each time they move their eyes, beginning and disabled readers have smaller perceptual spans than skilled readers. In this chapter, these two topics will be discussed.

EYE MOVEMENTS OF BEGINNING AND DISABLED READERS

Children who have not yet successfully mastered the skill of reading, and hence can accurately be described as beginning readers, take considerably longer to read a simple sentence than do skilled readers. Their average fixation duration tends to be between 300-400 msec, they move their eyes about 4 character positions, they regress about 25% of the time, and they make roughly two fixations per word (Rayner, 1986a). While beginning readers have to learn to gain cognitive control over their eye movements during reading and to process parafoveal information effectively, it is clear that the eye movements per se are not the reason that beginning readers read slowly. The primary difficulties that beginning readers have are at the level of word decoding and integration. Hence, it seems that their problems are due to language processing difficulties and their eye movements simply reflect these difficulties. Thus, because they encounter many words that they are not familiar with, they fixate frequently and for long periods of time on these words. And, because they have problems in identifying words and integrating them together with other words, they make many regressions.

As indicated above, disabled readers' eye movement characteristics are also quite different from those of normal readers. This general statement is true of any type of disabled reader, whether they are categorized as backward readers (children whose poor reading can be accounted for by low intelligence), poor readers (children with normal intelligence who read below grade level), or developmental dyslexics (children with normal intelligence who read two or more grade levels below normal). In this chapter, the focus will be on a group of adult dyslexic readers, who read quite poorly in the absence of any type of known brain damage. When their eye movement characteristics are examined, we find that their average fixation duration is between 300-350 msec, they typically move their eyes about 5-6 character spaces, and about 25-35% of their fixations are regressions when reading age-appropriate text (Rayner, 1986b). However, there are some interesting differences between dyslexic readers that lends credence to the idea that there are different types of dyslexic readers (Rayner, 1986b). Table 1 shows a summary of some eye movement

Table 1.   Average eye movement measures for skilled readers (SR), beginning readers (BR), and dyslexia readers. DB is a language-deficit dyslexic, JB is a visual-spatial dyslexic, and SJ is an attentional-deficit dyslexic.

	SR	BR	DB	JB	SJ
Fixation duration (milliseconds)	225	315	310	335	240
Forward saccade length (letter spaces)	8	4	5	7	5
Regressive saccade length (letter spaces)	3	3	5	8	5
Frequency of regressions (percentage)	17	25	35	30	20

characteristics of skilled readers, beginning readers, and three types of adult dyslexic readers which shall be referred to as language-deficit dyslexics, visual-spatial dyslexics, and attentional- deficit dyslexics. Of the dyslexic readers observed in our laboratory, the vast majority are of the language-deficit type.

In essence, the eye movement characteristics of the majority of these dyslexic readers seem much more like those of beginning readers than those of skilled readers. Thus, it would seem most parsimonious to assume that, like beginning readers, the problem that these dyslexic readers have with text are due to language processing deficiencies and that their eye movements reflect these problems. This general conclusion has certainly been the most widely accepted view of the relationship between dyslexia and eye movements (Tinker, 1958; Rayner, 1985). However, the conventional wisdom had been challenged by some work by Pavlidis (1981). Pavlidis reported that a group of dyslexic readers he tested showed abnormal eye movement patterns not only in a reading situation, but also in a non-reading situation. Although he was not entirely clear in his original report if he thought the problem was due to eye movements per se or to some type of more central dysfunction, others have certainly interpreted his results as indicating that abnormal eye movements are a cause of dyslexia.

Pavlidis (1981) tested 12 dyslexic and 12 normal readers in a task, which he has referred to as the "lights test", in which subjects were asked to fixate continuously on a fixation target that jumped from left-to-right or right-to-left across a screen. When the target moved from left-to-right, the dyslexics showed significantly more right-to-left saccades (or regressions) than the normal readers. Pavlidis' results are consistent with a number of case studies (Ciuffreda, Bahill, Kenyon, & Stark, 1976; Pirozzolo

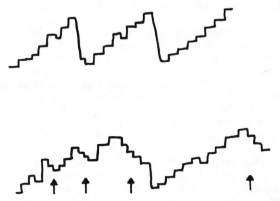

Figure 1.   Examples of staircase and reverse staircase patterns during reading. The upper part of the figure shows a typical staircase pattern in which saccades proceed primarily from left-to-right across the line followed by a return sweep to the beginning of the next line. The lower part of the figure shows examples of the reverse staircase pattern (marked by arrows) in which there are clusters of right-to-left saccades.

& Rayner, 1978; Zangwill & Blakemore, 1972) which have demonstrated erratic eye movements in dyslexic readers. In these case studies, dyslexic readers have been described who have a tendency to move their eyes from right to left during reading. Zangwill and Blakemore (1972) characterized their dyslexic reader as having an **irrepressible tendency** to move his eyes from right to left. Pirozzolo and Rayner (1978) reported the case study of a dyslexic reader who (like Zangwill and Blakemore's subject) would often end a line of text by dropping her eyes down to the next line and moving them from right to left. Pavlidis reported that his dyslexic subjects, when reading text, showed the characteristic **reverse staircase pattern** in which there are clusters of right to left saccades (see fig. 1). Hence, he concluded that erratic eye movements (moving from right to left when the task calls for movements from left to right) and the reverse staircase pattern are characteristic of dyslexic readers. In subsequent studies, Pavlidis (1983; 1985) has replicated his findings with dyslexic subjects and also reported that backward readers (whose poor reading can be accounted for by low intelligence) did not differ from normal readers.

On the basis of Pavlidis' (1981) original report, a number of attempts were undertaken to confirm his findings. However, all of these attempts to replicate his findings were unsuccessful (Black, Collins, De Roach, & Zubrick, 1984; Brown, Haegerstrom-Portnoy, Adams, Yingling, Galin, Herron, & Marcus, 1983; Olson, Kliegl, & Davidson, 1983; Stanley, Smith, & Howell, 1983). In fact, in all of the studies, there was no indication that dyslexic subjects differed from normal readers in the frequency of regressions during the lights test. Stanley et al. further pointed out that they found no difference between their dyslexic and normal readers' eye movement patterns on a visual search task. When asked to read text, the two groups of subjects differed markedly. Adler-Grinberg and Stark (1978) and Eskenazi and Diamond (1983) reported similar findings.

How can we account for the discrepancy between Pavlidis' results and these attempts to replicate his work? Elsewhere, I have suggested (Rayner, 1985) that Pavlidis may have a large portion of visual-spatial dyslexics in his sample of subjects. Thus, there may be a group of dyslexic readers who have unusual eye movement patterns and frequently show reverse staircase patterns when reading. Indeed, Pirozzolo and Rayner's subject (JB in Table 1), as indicated above, frequently dropped her eye from the end of one line to the end of the next and then started reading from right-to-left across the line. Interestingly, when the text was rotated 180 degrees (so that it was upside down), she read much more fluently and her pattern of eye movements looked much more like normal (except, of course, that her eye movements were from right-to-left). In addition, though JB's reading comprehension score was around 5th grade level when reading normal text, her comprehension score improved markedly when reading rotated text.

It is interesting to note that Inhoff, Pollatsek, Posner, and Rayner (1988) reported some experiments in which they asked normal readers to read distorted text (mirror image, upside down, rotated) and found, not surprisingly, that their subjects' eye movement characteristics changed dramatically. In terms of these subjects' reading rate and comprehension levels, it could be argued that their performance was much like dyslexic readers. But, the eye movements per se were not the cause of the problems that they had in reading the text. Text presented in distorted fashions that violated the normal visual-spatial array was very difficult for them to process. Likewise, JB's eye movements are not the cause of her reading problems. Rather, they reflect the visual-spatial deficit (amply documented by Pirozzolo & Rayner) that she has. For a visual-spatial dyslexic, like JB, the eye movement pattern is irregular quite independent of the difficulty of the text.

For the language-deficit dyslexics, it is also the case that their eye movements reflect their problem understanding written language; in their case the problem is one of comprehending the words printed on the page. While their eye movement characteristics are somewhat irregular when reading text above their reading level, when they read text consistent with their reading level their eye movement characteristics are very similar to those of children at that level. Thus, if they read at fourth grade level, their eye movement characteristics are much like those of children reading at fourth grade level. Analogously, in a recent experiment (Rayner, 1986a) it was demonstrated that when fourth grade children where given text above their grade level their eye movements looked much like those of language-deficit dyslexic readers; they made longer fixations, shorter saccades, and more regressions than they typically do.

It is probably also the case that among dyslexic readers with a language-deficit, differences in eye movement characteristics exist. For example, Olson, Kliegl, Davidson, and Foltz (1984) identified two reading styles among a sample of disabled readers that they referred to as **plodders** and **explorers.** The plodders displayed relatively few regressions between words and rarely skipped words on forward movements. They tended to move steadily forward, with more frequent forward saccades within words and to the immediately following word. Explorers, on the other hand, displayed relatively more regressions and word-skipping movements. The plodders and the explorers might finish reading a given text in the same amount of time, but the pattern of eye movements would be markedly different. In our laboratory, we have also observed such differences among language-deficit dyslexics.

In summary, the evidence that exists on the eye movement characteristics of dyslexic readers strongly indicates that eye movements per se are not a causative factor in reading disability. Rather, eye movements reflect the difficulties that dyslexic readers have in processing text. The evidence also suggests that there are different types of dyslexic readers.

THE PERCEPTUAL SPAN OF BEGINNING AND DYSLEXIC READERS

Beginning readers and dyslexic readers make more fixations per word than skilled readers. Hence, it has sometimes been suggested that they have smaller perceptual spans than skilled readers (see Pirozzolo, 1979 for a review of such suggestions). In fact, it has often been suggested that the size of the perceptual span in beginning and skilled readers is about half that of skilled readers. The perceptual span is the area around the fixation point

Table 2. Example of a moving window on three consecutive fixations. The dot marks the location of the fixation. The window size is 11 characters.

The clock in the kitchen was broken

Fixation n   The clock ixxxxxxxxxxxxxxxxxxxxxxx
                                       .

Fixation n+1   xxxxxlock in thexxxxxxxxxxxxxxxxx
                                          .

Fixation n+2   xxxxxxxxxxxxhe kitchen xxxxxxxx
                                             .

from which readers are able to obtain useful information. There have been many paradigms used to estimate the size of the perceptual span (see Rayner, 1978; 1986a), but the most informative technique is the moving window paradigm developed by McConkie and Rayner (1975). In this paradigm, subjects are asked to read text presented on a Cathode Ray Tube (CRT) controlled by a computer and their eye movements are monitored (by the same computer) as they do so. Then display changes contingent upon eye position are made as they read.

As can be seen in Table 2, the experimental situation creates a "moving window" of text in which the reader's eye movements determine the location of the window. Wherever the reader looks, text is exposed within the window region. The experimenter can vary the size of the text on each fixation, but the subject is always free to look anywhere in the text. A number of important conclusions have been reached about the characteristics of the perceptual span in skilled readers (Rayner, 1978; Rayner & Pollatsek, 1987). It has been found that the perceptual span extends from the beginning of the currently fixated word (but no more than 4 letters to the left of fixation) to about 15 characters to the right of fixation. Within the span region, different types of information are acquired.Information useful in identifying words and letters is acquired from

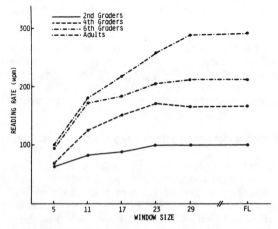

Figure 2. Reading rate in words per minute as a function of window size.

a region extending to about 7-8 characters to the right of fixation. Beyond that region, more gross types of information (such as word length) are acquired and used in guiding the eye movements.

The moving window paradigm has been used to determine the size of the perceptual span of beginning readers. Figure 2 shows the results of an experiment reported by Rayner (1986a). Here, it can be seen that the perceptual span for beginning readers is smaller than that of adults, but it is not half the size of skilled reader. It appears that the perceptual span extends about 11 characters to the right of fixation for beginning readers. Interestingly, Rayner (1986a) did find that the span was asymmetric for beginning readers. Apparently, the reason that the perceptual span is smaller in beginning readers than skilled readers is that beginning readers devote so much attention to processing the fixated word that reading is slowed down. Indeed, Rayner (1986a) showed that when fourth grade children read difficult text, the size of their perceptual span became comparable to that of beginning readers. Thus, difficulties in processing the foveal word lead to a smaller perceptual span.

Language-deficit dyslexic readers also appear to have a slightly smaller perceptual span than skiller readers. However, it is the case that it is not that much smaller than normal readers. Underwood and Zola (1986) found that the size of the span was fairly similar in good and poor fourth grade readers. In our laboratory, we have tested language-deficit readers and found that their span is a bit smaller than skilled readers (and very similar to that of beginning readers).

Recently, we (Rayner, Murphy, Henderson, & Pollatsek, 1988), observed an adult dyslexic reader with an attentional-deficit who actually reads better with a small window than when normal text is presented to him (without any restricting window). The dyslexic reader SJ (whose eye movement characteristics are included in Table 1) showed markedly better comprehension when listening to text than when reading. He reads quite slowly and laboriously and claims that he often looses his place in text. In the course of our testing, we asked him to read with a moving window. He found that when the window was relatively small (11-15 characters), reading was considerably easier than when it was large or when no window was present (that is, normal text). Figure 3 shows the results of one experiment. Here the window was defined in terms of words boundaries (rather than simply in terms of character spaces), but a window size of 2 words (2W) would be equal to a window size of about 11 characters and a window size of 3 words would be equal to a window size of about 15-16 characters. The figure shows the data from a group of control normal readers and from some language-deficit dyslexics, as well as SJ. The normal subjects showed the typical result wherein their reading performance reached asymptote when the window was 3 words. The language-deficit dyslexics reached asymptotic performance when the window was 2 words. However, SJ showed the interesting pattern that reading performance was better when the window was 2 words than when it was 3 words (or a full line). The data shown in Figure 3 are from conditions in which the letters outside of the window were replaced with Xs (as in Table 2). However, if the letters outside of the window were replaced with random letters, SJ showed a very different pattern; under this condition, his reading performance was constant across the different window sizes.

It would appear that SJ's problem in reading is related to an attentional deficit in which he is unable to selectively attend to the letters from the words or words near fixation and thus letters from parafoveal vision interfere with reading. It is difficult to specify exactly the nature of this interference. However, since reading was equally poor with normal text and with window conditions where the material outside of the window was random letters, it seems likely that the level of interference is below the level of word meaning. It appears that irrelevant parafoveal letters get in the way of the word identification process and/or the clearly demarcated window with **X̄**s allows his covert attention and eye movement system a better target for moving ahead in the text.

It is clearly the case that SJ's reading problem is not characteristic of most (or even many) dyslexic readers. However, there do seem to be other dyslexic readers who experience the kinds of problems that SJ exhibits. Geiger and Lettvin (1987) conducted some tests on dyslexic readers to examine how well they could identify letters in parafoveal vision*. They found that their dyslexic subjects could identify parafoveal letters better than normal readers. (We also found that SJ was superior to normal readers in this type of task.) Geiger and Lettvin concluded that dyslexic readers have better parafoveal and peripheral vision than normal readers and hence they suffer interference from parafoveal letters when they try and process foveally fixated text. In some remediation work, Geiger and Lettvin cut a small hole in the middle of an index card and printed a large cross just to the left of the hole. The dyslexic readers were instructed to fixate on the cross and to read the text through the small aperture. Thus, if the dyslexic continued to fixate on the cross while reading, the text would be read from parafoveal vision. They reported marked improvement in reading for the dyslexic readers who practiced this task for only a relatively short period of

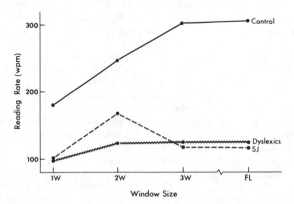

Figure 3. Reading Rate in words per minute as a function of widow size.

---

* see also Geiger and Lettvin in this Volume (Eds' comm.)

time (see Geiger and Lettvin, 1987).

Rayner et al. (1988) conducted a similar type of experiment with SJ in which there were no foveal words to process and any reading that could be done would have to be from parafoveal vision (see Rayner & Bertera, 1979). All of the letters in whichever word SJ fixated on were replaced by X̲s (as were all letters to the left of the fixated word) and the only words available were the two words to the right of the fixated word. In our situation, where we know exactly where the reader's eyes are (unlike Geiger and Lettvin), SJ found it virtually impossible to read under these circumstances. Indeed, though he was given a great deal of practice in the task, he found it very frustrating and his level of performance was very poor.

At first glance, it might seem a bit contradictory that SJ has such problems with reading under these conditions, when he is able to read parafoveal words better than normal readers. However, like normal readers, his performances dropped off markedly as the word was moved from the fovea and his recognition of words even at 1 degree eccentricity was far from perfect. Since a parafoveal window condition (in which there was not a foveal word) forced him to read words that were on average about 2 degrees from fixation, it is not surprising that his reading in this condition was labored.

It thus seems that there is good reason to question whether Geiger and Lettvin's subjects were doing what they were instructed to do when presented with their remediation procedure. One possibility is that rather than looking at the fixation cross on the index card and reading from parafoveal vision, they simply looked directly inside the aperture. Certainly, SJ found that reading with a small window was much more comfortable than when the entire line of text was present; in small window conditions he indicated that he experienced an ease of reading which he had never felt before. SJ also tried reading with an index card with a small aperture (of about 15 characters) and he found reading more comfortable than it normally is. Techniques such as this have often been used with dyslexic readers in attempts to improve their reading performance. The problem is that it is clear that such techniques will not work with all dyslexic readers because they do not all experience the same kind of selective attentional deficit that SJ (and at least some of Geiger and Lettvin's subjects) exhibited. His primary complaint with the index card procedure was that reading was very slow (in comparison to the speed with which a small window moved contingent upon his eyes movements). In any event, it does seem reasonable to conclude that at least a small segment of developmental dyslexics do have selective attentional deficits in which they are unable to focus attention exclusively on the word in the center of vision.

In summary, the evidence suggests that some language-deficit dyslexic readers may have a slightly smaller perceptual span than normal readers. However, as with beginning readers, the smaller span is not the reason for their reading problems, but rather reflects the difficulties they have in processing the fixated word. Interestingly, there also appear to be some dyslexic readers who read better when the window of visible text is quite small. Such dyslexics appear to have an attentional-deficit.

SUMMARY

Examination of some adult dyslexic readers reveals quite clearly that their eye movement characteristics and the size of the perceptual span are somewhat different than those of normal readers. However, I have argued that the eye movements per se are not the cause of the reading problems; the eye movement patterns simply reflect different problems that beginning and dyslexic readers have in processing text. Likewise, the size of the perceptual span is not a cause of reading problems. It is clearly the case that patients with lesions in various parts of the brain known to have some relationship to the oculomotor system often, though not always, have reading problems (Pirozzolo & Rayner, 1979). Likewise, patients with low vision due to macular degeneration, optic nerve atrophy, ocular histoplasmosis, etc. have difficulties in reading (Legge, Rubin, Pelli, & Schleske, 1985), but such patients would not be classified as developmental dyslexics. For most developmental dyslexics (the language-deficit type), eye movements reflect the difficulties the reader has in processing the fixated word. For the visual-spatial deficit dyslexics, eye movements reflect some underlying visual-spatial or perceptual problem. For attentional-deficit dyslexics, eye movements per se are not particularly diagnostic, but the nature of processing within the perceptual span region appears to account for their reading problems. Characteristics of dyslexic readers' eye movements and perceptual span may thus enable us to differentiate between different types of dyslexic readers, but it still seems safe to conclude, as Tinker did thirty years ago (Tinker, 1958), that eye movements are not a cause of dyslexia.

ACKNOWLEDGMENTS

This chapter was written while the author was a Fellow at the Netherlands Institute for Advanced Study. Support also came from grant BNS86-09336 from the National Science Foundation.

REFERENCES

Adler-Grinberg, D. and Stark, L. (1978). Eye movements, scan paths, and dyslexia. Amer. J. Opto. & Physio. Optics, 55, 557-570.

Black, J.L., Collins, D.W.K., DeRoach, J.N., and Zubrick, S. (1984). A detailed study of sequential saccadic eye movements for normal and poor reading children. Perc. & Motor Skills, 59, 423-434.

Brown, B., Haegerstrom-Portnoy, G., Adams, A.J., Yingling, C.D., Galen, D., Herron, J., and Marcus, M. (1983). Predective eye movements do not discriminate between dyslexic and control children. Neuropsych., 21, 121-128.

Ciuffreda, K.J., Bahill, A.T., Kenyon, R.V., and Stark, L. (1976). Eye movements during reading: Case studies. Amer. J. Opto. & Physio. Optics, 53, 521-530.

Eskenazi, B. and Diamond, S.P. (1983). Visual exploration of non-verbal material by dyslexic children. Cortex, 19, 353-370.

Geiger, G. and Lettvin, J.Y. (1987). Peripheral vision in persons with dyslexia. New Eng. J. of Med., 316, 1238-1243.

Inhoff, A.W., Pollatsek, A., Posner, M.I., and Rayner, K. (1988). Covert attention and eye movements during reading. Q.J. of Exp. Psych., in press.

Legge, G.E., Rubin, G.S., Pelli, D.G., and Schleske, M.M. (1985). Psychophysics of reading, 11: Low vision. Vis. Res., 25, 253-266.

Olson, R.K., Kliegl, R., and Davidson, B.J. (1983). Dyslexic and normal readers' eye movements. J. Exp. Psych.: HP & P, 9, 816-825.

Olson, R.K., Kliegl, R., and Davidson, B.J., and Foltz, G. (1984). Individual and developmental differences in reading. In Reading Research: Advances in Theory and Practice. (ed. T.G. Waller). Academic Press, New York.

Pavlidis, G.T. (1981). Do eye movements hold the key to dyslexia. Neuropsych., 19, 57-64.

Pavlidis, G.T. (1983). The 'dyslexia syndrome' and its objective diagnosis by erratic eye movements. In Eye Movements in Reading: Perceptual and Language Processes. (ed. K. Rayner). Academic Press, New York.

Pavlidis, G.T. (1985). Eye movement diferences between dyslexics, normal, and retarded readers while sequentially fixating digits. Amer. J. Opto & Physio. Optics, 62, 820-832.

Pirozzolo, F.J. (1979). The Neuropsychology of Developmental Reading Disorders. Praeger, New York.

Pirozzolo, F.J. and Rayner, K. (1978). Disorders of oculomotor scanning and graphic orientation in developmental Gerstman syndrome. Brain & Lang., 5, 119-126.

Pirozzolo, F.J. and Rayner, K. (1979). The neural control of eye movements in acquired and developmental reading disorders. In Studies in Neurolinguistics (eds. H.A. Whitaker and H.A. Whitaker). Academic Press, New York.

Rayner, K. (1978). Eye movements in reading and information processing. Psych. Bull., 85, 618-660.

Rayner, K. (1985). Do faulty eye movements cause dyslexia? Dev. Neuropsych., 1, 3-15.

Rayner, K. (1986a). Eye movements and the perceptual span in beginning and skilled readers. J. of Exp. Child Psych, 41, 211-236.

Rayner, K. (1986b). Eye movements and the perceptual span: Evidence for dyslexic topology. In Dyslexia: Its Neuropsychology and Treatment. (eds. G.T. Pavlidis and D.F. Fisher). Wiley, Chichester.

Rayner, K. and Bertera, J.H. (1979). Reading without a fovea. Science, 206, 468-469.

Rayner, K., Murphy, L., Henderson, J.M., and Pollatsek, A. (1988). Selective attentional dyslexia. Manuscript submitted for publication.

Rayner, K. and Pollatsek, A. (1987). Eye movements in reading: A tutorial review. In Attention and Performance 12: The Psychology of Reading. (ed. M. Coltheart). Erlbaum, London.

Stanley, G., Smith, G.A., and Howell, E.A. (1983). Eye-movements and sequential tracking in dyslexic and control children. Brit. J. of Psych., 74, 181-187.

Tinker, M.A. (1958). Recent studies of eye movements in reading. Psych. Bull., 55, 215-231.

Underwood, R. and Zola, D. (1986). The span of recognition of good and poor readers. Read. Res. Q., 21, 6-19.

Zangwill, O.L. and Blakemore, C. (1972). Dyslexia: Reversal of eye movements during reading. Neuropsych., 10, 371-373.

29
Some Characteristics of Readers' Eye Movements

George W. McConkie and David Zola

While reading, a person's eyes execute a series of rapid
movements, termed saccades. The pauses between saccades, called
fixations, are the periods during which the text is actually
perceived. The locations of these eye fixations play the role of
both cause and effect in reading. Eye position is an effect because
it results from stimulus, cognitive and physiological factors that
influence where the eyes go. At the same time, eye position is
causal in that it determines the nature of the stimulus information
available to the mind during the fixation, and influences where the
eyes will be sent next. This chapter will deal with eye behavior as
an effect, examining some of the factors that influence this
behavior.

A longstanding question in the study of dyslexia is whether
abnormalities in eye behavior can play a causal role in the
development of reading disability, that is, whether by responding in
an abnormal manner to normal controlling influences, inappropriate
eye positioning can change the nature of visual input enough to
increase the difficulty of reading or of learning to read.

The role of eye movements in dyslexia has not been a focus of
our research, and we are not prepared to take a strong position on
the issue. Rather, this chapter will describe some of the
currently-known characteristics of eye behavior during reading that
must be taken into account in attempting to deal with the role of
eye behavior in dyslexia. We first describe some characteristics of
the eye behavior of adults, then compare this with the eye behavior
of children learning to read, and finally consider possible
relations with dyslexia.

This paper reports research supported by the National Institute for
Child Health and Human Development, Grant No. HD18116, and by the
Office of Educational Research and Improvement, Grant No. 1-5-32308.

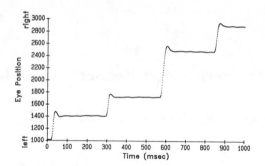

Figure 1. A graph of a college student's eye movements during one second of reading. Time is represented on the ordinate and eye position on the abscissa. Flat regions in the curve are eye fixations.

ADULT READER'S EYE MOVEMENTS

Figure 1 charts a college student's horizontal eye movements during one second of reading. Time is represented on the abscissa and eye position on the ordinate. Data are recorded from the reader's right eye, taking 1000 samples per second. Where the curve is flat, the eyes are in a fixation. Where the curve rises, the eyes are moving to the right along the line. This figure shows that the eye is stable during an eye fixation, then quickly accelerates as a saccade begins. Deceleration begins about halfway through the saccade and the eye finally reaches the extent of its forward motion. There is then a period, represented in the figure as leftward motion at the end of each saccade, during which the eyes are settling into position. Finally, the eye stabilizes once again, and another fixation is underway. This episode is repeated about four times per second during reading.

Figure 2 shows the locations of the eye fixations made by a college reader reading two lines of text. A letter is placed below each character in the text on which the eyes paused for a fixation, and the order of the letters indicates the sequence of the fixations. Below each fixation indicator is a number that shows how many milliseconds (1/1000's of a second) the eyes paused at that location. As can be seen in the figure, there is a considerable amount of variation in both the lengths of saccades and the durations of fixations as a person reads. In a set of 43,000 eye fixations recorded from 69 college students reading chapters from a contemporary novel, the median progressive (rightward) saccade length was 7.5 character positions (i.e., 1.88 degrees of visual angle), the median regressive (leftward) movement was 4.4 character positions (i.e., 1.1 deg), and the median fixation duration was 180 ms or 200 ms, depending on the algorithm used to define the beginning of a fixation. The frequency distribution for lengths of

```
the confluence of a large stream with a small river, a river
    a    b          c       d        e       f    g       h
   298  535        199     325      243     197  262      366

of the combined watercourse bubbled over rocks as it flowed into
    a    b    c       d          e           f          g    h
   160  185  141     314        274         297        303  334
```

Figure 2. Two lines of a passage read by a college student, with the
locations and durations (in ms) of his eye fixations indicated.

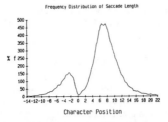

Figure 3. Frequency distribution of the lengths of saccades made by 69
college students reading chapters from a novel.

saccades is presented in Figure 3, illustrating the variability in
the data. Using this large data set, we have been studying the two
basic oculomotor decisions that are made during reading: where to
move the eyes and when to move them.

The Spatial Decision: Where are the Eyes Sent?

Saccades are launched with the goal of taking the eyes to a
specific word during reading. This is illustrated in Figure 4.
Here we have plotted two landing site distributions for 7-letter
words (McConkie, Kerr, Reddix & Zola, in press). Each landing site

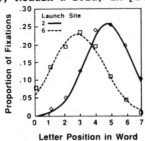

Figure 4. Landing site distributions on 7-letter words. These two
distributions show the proportion of fixations falling at each letter
position in the word when the prior fixation was either 2 or 6 letter
positions to the left of the word.

distribution shows the proportion of all fixations on the word that
were centered on each letter of the word, following saccades that
came from a specific location during reading. In Figure 4, the
left-most distribution shows where the eyes land when coming from 6
letter positions to the left of the word; the right-most
distribution shows where they land when coming from 2 letter
positions to the left of the word.

Landing site distributions show four properties of interest.
First, they are well fit by the normal curve, making it possible to
obtain estimates of the mean and standard deviation of these
distributions. The landing site distributions in Figure 4, for
example, have means of 2.8 and 4.8 character positions and standard
deviations of 1.8 and 1.5.

Second, the size of the standard deviation of the landing site
distribution is not affected by the length of the word to which the
eyes are sent. Thus, the shape of the distribution is the same for
saccades going to four-letter words as to eight-letter words. There
appears to be a functional target within the word to which the eyes
are being specifically sent when a saccade is made to it, with this
target determined by the region of space occupied by the word rather
than by individual characteristics of the word. It is as if some
higher mental function selects the word to be considered next, and
the perceptuo-oculomotor system then aims a saccade at a standard
target location within the space occupied by the word, apparently
close to its center.

Third, the mean of the landing site distribution in a word
varies with the distance of the prior fixation (i.e., the launch
site) from the center of the word. Saccades that come from locations
further to the left of the word produce mean landing sites that are
further to the left as seen in Figure 4. In our data, a launch site
that was 1 letter position further to the left of the word produced
a mean landing site 1/2 letter position further to the left within
the word. This data pattern is very similar to that described by
Poulton (1981) as a commonly-observed "range effect" in motor
control: a tendency for the mean landing site to be beyond the
target when the launch site is close to it, and to fall short of the
target when the launch site is farther from it. "Close" and "far"
here are judged relative to the range of motor movements being made
in the situation. Cöeffé and O'Reagan (1987) have attributed this
error to systematic error in spatially locating objects in
peripheral areas of vision.

Fourth, between the systematic error in mean landing sites,
just described, and the nonsystematic error represented by the
standard deviation of the landing site distributions, it appears
that some proportion of the time the eyes actually land on the wrong
word. That is, though the eyes were targeted for one word, they
fall on another. This is most likely to occur with shorter words

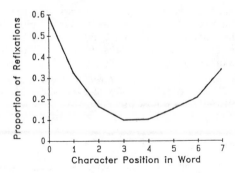

Figure 5.   Refixation frequency curve for 7-letter words, showing the percentage of initial fixations on different letter positions in the word that were followed by a second fixation on the word.

and with longer saccades. Of course, the targeted word may still be read even though the eyes are not centered directly on it.

These landing site distributions take on greater significance when it is recognized that where the eyes land in a word has a substantial effect on whether or not the word is identified on that fixation (O'Reagan, 1984). Figure 5 shows that the location of the reader's initial fixation on a 7-letter word greatly influences the frequency with which the next fixation is also on that word. When the initial fixation is at the center of the word, the word is refixated only about 10% of the time. When the eyes are centered just two letters away from the center of the word, refixations rise to 23%, and at three letters away, 38%. Thus, characteristics of oculomotor control that result in misplacing the eyes by just a letter or two can have sizeable effects on the word identification processes during reading. We assume that this is due to the rapid drop in visual acuity, even within the fovea, with distance from the center of vision.

It is not necessary to directly fixate a word in order to identify it. A 4- to 5-letter word that begins three letter positions to the right of the fixation location is skipped over about 38% of the time. This figure drops to 18% at five letters to the right and to 8% at seven letters. These figures also drop for longer words. For example, 6- to 7-letter words beginning three letter positions to the right of a fixation are skipped only 10% of the time. Fisher & Shebilske (1985) present evidence that words not directly fixated are sometimes identified. Characteristics of the words, such as their frequency in print, and of their context, such as the degree to which it constrains the words, can influence the likelihood that words will not be directly fixated (Rayner & Ehrlich, 1981) or refixated (Zola, 1984) during reading.

For adult readers, we presume that most eye movements are made
in response to the need for additional visual input for the purpose
of identifying the words of the text. Most words receive no more
than a single eye fixation. Many are identified without direct
fixation. The likelihood of identifying a given word during a
fixation appears to be determined by the location of the eyes with
respect to that word, the acuity characteristics of the retina, and
characteristics of the word and its context.

The Temporal Decision: When are the Eyes Moved?

The reaction time of the eyes, when asked to move to a target
when it appears, differs depending on the uncertainty of the target
location. With a perfectly predictable stimulus, the reaction time
can be as low as 185 ms, but with some uncertainty in the target
location, values around 210 msec are more commonly observed (Rayner,
Slowiaczek, Clifton & Bertera, 1983). The fact that there is so
little difference between the eyes' reaction time and the median
fixation duration has led to speculation that decisions of where to
send the eyes cannot be made on the basis of information acquired
during the fixation preceding a saccade (Shebilske, 1975). However,
demonstrations of immediate effects (e.g., cases where aspects of
the stimulus present during a fixation are shown to affect the onset
time, length or direction of the immediately following saccade)
indicate that this is not the case (McConkie, 1983).

Recent research has found a much shorter response time of the
eyes. When a change in the stimulus occurs, such as moving a target
location (Becker & Jurgens, 1979) or masking the stimulus (McConkie,
Underwood, Zola & Wolverton, 1985), changes in saccade onset time
and/or length can be observed within about 90 ms. Furthermore, there
are conditions under which saccades can be initiated to a target
within about that same period of time (Fischer & Ramsperger, 1984).
Thus, it appears that the basic response time of the eyes (e.g., the
time for information to be transmitted from retina to brain, there
to affect the ongoing activity in such a way as to change the
programming of the following saccade) is about 90 ms. In skilled
readers, the effects of processing at the orthographic and lexical
levels can be observed in fixations lasting only 150 ms and effects
of processing at the syntactic and semantic levels can be observed
in fixations lasting about 210 ms (McConkie, et al, 1985; McConkie,
Reddix, & Zola, 1985).

With these considerations in mind, it is instructive to examine
the frequency distribution of fixation durations following rightward
saccades, as shown in Figure 6. It shows the typical rightward
skewed distribution, with a mode at about 160-180 ms. It can be seen
that some saccades are launched in less than the basic response time
of the eyes. These must necessarily have been ordered by the brain
prior to the onset of the fixation. Other saccades, while occurring
after the eyes' response time, were launched before word-level or

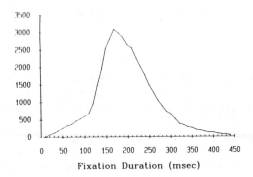

Figure 6. Frequency distribution of the durations of eye fixations made
by 69 college students reading chapters from a novel.

language-level information from this fixation can begin influencing
saccade decisions. These saccades were probably initiated on the
basis of processing from an earlier fixation. Perhaps a saccade
request was issued to take the eyes to a particular word, but before
visual information arrived from the new fixation, that word was
identified. Orders for a saccade to the next word may then be sent,
even before the first saccade was completed. Whether there are
instances in which multiple saccades are programmed simultaneously
(Morrison, 1984), as well, is an issue requiring further study.

     The information just presented about fixation durations, or the
time at which saccades are launched during fixations in reading,
leaves a somewhat confusing picture. Sometimes saccades are ordered
even before information from a fixation becomes available, sometimes
after visual information has become available but before higher-
level language processes are initiated, and sometimes only later.
While different characteristics of the language can influence the
durations of fixations on which they are encountered, at other times
the effects only show up on the following fixation (McConkie,
Underwood, Wolverton & Zola, 1988). In many tasks in which eye
behavior is studied, the signal for a saccade is the onset of a
target in the stimulus array. In reading, since the page of text
does not change, the decision that it is time to move the eyes is
made on some basis internal to the reader. At the present time, we
do not know the cognitive event or events that serve to signal that
it is time to move the eyes.

CHILDREN'S EYE MOVEMENTS DURING READING

     Figure 7 presents an example of the eye fixation pattern made by
two different first grade children in reading a line of text. Both
children are near average in reading ability. As is typical for

```
    across a large meadow.   They walked in the woods.
 c bd  a gh ijl   nmp    q     r st     u vx  y z
    e   f   k      o                    w


    across a large meadow.   They walked in the woods.
    b a   e d    c          g f         h    i
```

Figure 7. Fixations made by two first grade readers as they read a line
of text. Letters are placed under the text positions where fixations
were made. The order of the letters indicates the fixation sequence.

children this age, there is a large number of fixations, often with
multiple fixations on a single word. Furthermore, in the data
presented here, the two children show rather different eye movement
patterns. The first child exhibits a sequential, left-to-right
progression, that Olson, Kliegl and Davidson (1984) have labelled
the "Plodder" pattern, whereas the second child exhibits a pattern
containing more long progressive and regressive movements, labelled
the "Explorer." Olson et al. provide evidence that among poor
readers, children showing the explorer pattern tend to show higher
reading levels.

Children's Saccades During Reading

    Figure 8 presents frequency distributions of the lengths of
saccades for three first grade children all of about the same
reading ability as they read from a child's novel. The distributions
contain between 1000 and 4000 saccades. Two characteristics of the
data are striking. First, there are many very short saccades, as
Kowler & Martins (1982) have observed in preschool children.

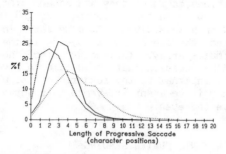

Figure 8. Frequency distributions of the lengths of saccades for three
first grade children of similar reading ability.

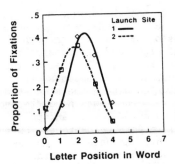

Figure 9. Landing site distributions on 4-letter words for a group of 6 first grade children showing similar saccade length distributions.

Among a group of first grade children we have studied, 14% of all progressive saccades were less than 2.0 letter positions (.5 deg) in length. Second, children at the same reading level show very different saccade length distributions. Reports of average lengths of saccades seems to capture relatively little of the actual variability among children. We suspect that these differences reflect differences in the approaches the children are taking to their reading.

First grade children show landing site distributions that are much like those of adults, as seen in Figure 9. These data are from a group of 6 children whose saccade length distributions are similar in shape. As with adults, the landing site distributions are normal in shape, shift as launch site changes, and show no effect of word length. Apparently these children are directing their eyes to word-units, much as adults do. In this and other tests of children's eye movements during reading, we have found no evidence for oculomotor development as children learn to read.

In her doctoral dissertation, Nancy Bryant (1988) examined the eye movements of children on selected words as they read sentences containing those words. She first identified words that individual 2nd and 3rd grade children could read without difficulty and others they could not. These words were then embedded in sentences that the children read silently as their eyes were monitored.

On the average, the children made 3.0 eye fixations on the words that they could read without difficulty, with 301 ms per fixation. On unfamiliar words, they made an average of 4.6 eye fixations, averaging 322 ms. Children with lower reading skills made more and longer fixations than children of higher skill on both familiar and unfamiliar words.

Why do young children need to make so many eye fixation on words as they read? One obvious possibility is that, even

when not overtly decoding, the children are "sounding out" the words
to themselves as they read. If this were so, we would expect to see
a left-to-right progression of the eyes through the words. We might
also expect this regular rightward progression to be more pronounced
in the data of the better readers. Neither of these expectations
was confirmed. Of all within-word saccades (e.g., saccades that
were initiated and terminated within the same word) made on familiar
words, 41% were regressive. There was no difference between better
readers (3.3 - 3.9 reading grade level) and poorer readers (2.2 -
2.6 reading grade level) in this percentage. Furthermore, on the
less familiar words the children made 40% regressions, almost
identical to the percentage for familiar words. It should be noted
that in an absolute sense there were more regressions with lower
ability children and less familiar words, but only because there
were more total fixations on the words; the percent of within-word
saccades that were regressive was similar in all cases. The number
of fixations made on a word is a primary difference between the eye
behavior of adults and children, but the role of children's multiple
fixations is not currently known.

     Twenty percent of all between-word saccades were regressive,
which is quite similar to the frequency of regressions in adult
readers. Reading skill did have an effect: contrary to
expectations, better readers produced a higher percentage of
regressions (24% vs. 17%). Thus, the number of between word
regressions does not appear to vary much with reading skill.

EYE MOVEMENTS AND DYSLEXIA

     In considering the relationship between eye movements and
dyslexia, we can quickly discard two extreme possibilities, viz., that
oculomotor control factors are the basic cause of all reading
difficulties, and that oculomotor factors have no relation to
reading difficulty. Many children with reading disabilities are
greatly helped using techniques that would seem to have little or
no effect on oculomotor control. On the other hand,
ophthalmologists deal with people having oculomotor disorders that
clearly make reading difficult. However, people with obvious visual
or oculomotor disorders are typically excluded from studies of
dyslexia (Vellutino, 1979).

     A basic question is whether or not there are cases in
which subtle and undiagnosed oculomotor difficulties make
learning to read difficult and result in severe reading
disabilities. Second, if there are such oculomotor difficulties,
what is their nature? Third, in what proportion of reading
disabilities do such oculomotor difficulties play a role? The fact
that these questions have had such an important place in the
dyslexia literature over several decades, yet still remain without
convincing answers, indicates that they cannot be answered simply.

We wish to make four comments about research in this area. First, there has been speculation that difficulties in the binocular coordination of the eyes may lie at the basis of some reading problems (Bedwell, Grant & McKeown, 1980). It is important to realize that this is an extremely difficult question to investigate. It is not possible to obtain an exact record of the eyes' behavior; it is only possible to obtain a record of the response of an eyetracking instrument to the eyes' behavior. The significance of this statement is that, in order to study questions of binocular coordination, it is necessary to have devices that track the two eyes in exactly the same way. No two eyetracking devices are identical; the question is whether they are similar enough that their differences are well below the level of differences exhibited in the behavior of the two eyes. Furthermore, even if the eyetracking devices are identical themselves, there may be differences between the two eyes that lead to the appearance of differences of behavior of the eyes that in fact do not exist. Differences in the shapes or reflective properties of the two eyes, or in the shapes of their lenses or other internal structures, could cause differences in the signals coming from two eyetrackers even when the two eyes are moving in perfect synchrony. Therefore, the onus is on the researchers who address this issue to convince their audience that differences observed in the data coming from the two eyes is truly indicating differences in the eyes' behavior. If no differences between the eyes are observed, then it is necessary to demonstrate that the equipment used has the capability of detecting differences if they exist. Otherwise, true problems in binocular coordination may be going undetected.

Second, in our own research, we have been surprised that where the eyes fixate in a word is so important. The fixation location greatly influences the likelihood of refixating, presumably reflecting the clarity of information about letters in the word. Thus, the potential effects of oculomotor error and perhaps of slight differences in visual acuity appear to be more severe than we had previously imagined. Studies are needed to examine individual differences in perceptuo-oculomotor accuracy of children and to determine whether this has any relation to progress in learning to read.

Third, we have suggested that eye movements are executed in response to needs of the higher cognitive processes for visual information. This implies a careful coordination between the different systems, one that is partially represented by the concept of visual attention. Each saccade takes the eyes to a new location, and in turn requires that the system then identify the spatial location, in the new stimulus array, of the word or words from which information is being sought. This dynamic coordination between saccade control, visual attention and the processes seeking visual information for word identification during reading is another area in which some children could experience difficulty, and in which further research is needed.

Fourth, we are concerned that global eye behavior indicators, including mean fixation duration and mean saccade length, frequently fail to reveal eye movement differences that actually exist between individuals or conditions. Fine-grained analyses reveal patterns and regularities in the data that lead to more sensitive and interpretable indicators of the processes taking place. We suspect that these will be more useful in coming to understand dyslexia.

While we ourselves are skeptical that oculomotor factors play a significant role in the reading problems of very many children, there is certainly a need for good research on this issue. However, we suspect that eye movement research is most likely to play quite a different role in the study of dyslexia, viz., providing a source of information about the ongoing perceptual and language processing taking place as people with reading disabilities attempt to read. Even if oculomotor factors are found to play no causative role in the development of dyslexia, eye movement research will still prove very useful in investigating the specific perceptual and language processing difficulties faced by dyslexic children and adults, and how dyslexics attempt to deal with these problems in learning to read.

It seems clear that whether causes of severe reading disorders sometimes lie within the oculomotor realm, or whether the causes lie elsewhere, eye movement research will continue to play an important role in the study of dyslexia. Basic research on eye movement control during reading and on the relation between eye movements and higher cognitive functioning are important in laying the foundation for this work.

REFERENCES

Balota, D.A., Pollatsek, A., & Rayner, K. (1985). The interaction of contextual constraints and parafoveal visual information in reading. Cognitive Psychology, 17, 364-390.

Becker, W., & Jurgens, R. (1979). An analysis of the saccadic system by means of double step stimuli. Vision Research, 19, 967-983.

Bedwell, C.H., Grant, R., & McKeown, L.R. (1980). Visual and ocular control anomalies in relation to reading difficulty. The British Journal of Psychology, 50, 61-70.

Bryant, N.R. (1988). Children's eye movements and the learning of words. Doctoral Dissertation, University of Illinois, Urbana, Illinois.

Cöeffé, C. & O'Regan, J.K. (1987). Reducing the influence of nontarget stimuli on saccade accuracy: Predictability and latency effects. Vision Research, 27, 227-240.

Ehrlich, S.F. & Rayner, K. (1981). Contextual effects on word perception and eye movements during reading. Journal of Verbal Learning and Verbal Behavior, 20, 641-655.

Fischer, R., & Ramsperger, E. (1984). Human express-saccades: Extremely short reaction times of goal directed eye movements.

Experimental Brain Research, 57, 191-195.

Fisher, D.F. & Shebilske, W.L. (1985). There is more that meets the eye than the eyemind assumption. In Eye Movements and Human Information processing. (eds. R. Groner, G.W. McConkie & C. Menz). Amsterdam: North-Holland.

Kowler, E. & Martins, A.J. (1982). Eye movements of preschool children. Science, 215, 997-999.

McConkie, G.W. (1983). Eye movements and perception during reading. In Eye movements in reading: Perceptual and language processes. (ed. K. Rayner). New York: Academic Press.

McConkie, G.W., Kerr, P.W., Reddix, M.D., & Zola, D. (In press). Eye movement control during reading: I. The location of initial eye fixations on words. Vision Research, in press.

McConkie, G.W., Reddix, M., & Zola, D. (1985). Chronometric analysis of language processing during eye fixations in reading. Paper presented at the Annual Meeting of the Psychonomic Society, Boston, MA.

McConkie, G.W., Underwood, N.R., Zola, D., & Wolverton, G.S. (1985). Some temporal characteristics of processing during reading. Journal of Experimental Psychology: Human Perception and Performance, 11, 168-186.

McConkie, G.W., Underwood, N.R., Wolverton, G.S. & Zola, D. (1988). Some properties of eye movement control during reading. In Eye movements research: Physiological and Psychological Aspects. (eds. G. Lüer, U. Lass, & J. Shallo-Hoffmann). Göttingen, Germany: Hogrefe.

Morrison, R.E. (1984). Manipulation of stimulus onset delay in reading: Evidence for parallel programming of saccades. Journal of Experimental Psychology: Human Perception and Performance, 10, 667-682.

Olson, R.K., Kliegl, R., & Davidson, B.J. (1984). Individual and developmental differences in reading disability. In Reading research: Advances in theory and practice, Vol. 4. (ed. T.G. Waller). New York: Academic Press.

O'Regan, J.K. (1984). How the eye scans isolated words. In Theoretical and applied aspects of eye movement research. (eds. A.G. Gale & F. Johnson). Amsterdam: North-Holland.

Poulton, E.C. (1981). Human manual control. In Handbook of Physiology, Sect. 1, Vol. II, Part 2. (ed. V.B. Brooks). Bethesda, MD: American Physiology Society.

Rayner, K., Slowiaczek, M.L., Clifton, C., & Bertera, J.H. (1983). Latency of sequential eye movements: Implications for reading. Journal of Experimental Psychology: Human Perception and Performance, 9, 912-922.

Shebilske, W. (1975). Reading eye movements from an information-point of view. In Understanding Language. (ed. D.W. Massaro). New York: Academic Press.

Vellutino, F. R. (1979). Dyslexia: Theory and research. Cambridge, MA: MIT Press.

Zola, D. (1984). Redundancy and word perception during reading. Perception & Psychophysics, 36, 277-284.

Index